Integrated Cancer Care
Holistic, complementary
and creative approaches

Integrated Cancer Care

Holistic, complementary and creative approaches

Edited by

Jennifer Barraclough

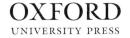
OXFORD
UNIVERSITY PRESS

OXFORD
UNIVERSITY PRESS

Great Clarendon Street, Oxford OX2 6DP

Oxford University Press is a department of the University of Oxford. It
furthers the University's objective of excellence in research, scholarship,
and education by publishing worldwide in

Oxford New York

Athens Auckland Bangkok Bogotá Buenos Aires Calcutta Cape Town
Chennai Dar es Salaam Delhi Florence Hong Kong Istanbul Karachi
Kuala Lumpur Madrid Melbourne Mexico City Mumbai Nairobi
Paris São Paulo Singapore Taipei Tokyo Toronto Warsaw

with associated companies in
Berlin Ibadan

Oxford is a registered trade mark of Oxford University Press in the UK
and in certain other countries

Published in the United States by Oxford University Press Inc., New York

British Library Cataloguing in Publication Data available

Library of Congress Cataloguing in Publication Data
Integrated cancer care: holisic, complementary, and creative
approaches/edited by Jennifer Barraclough
    p. cm
    Includes bibliographical references and index.
    1. Cancer—Alternative treatment. 2. Holistic medicine.
    I. Barraclough, Jennifer.
    [DNLM: 1. Neoplasms—therapy. 2. Alternative Medicine. 3. Holistic
Health. 4. Mental Healing. 5. Palliative Care. QZ 266 1557 2000]
    RC271.A62 155 2000   616.99'406—dc21   00-047889

1 3 5 7 9 10 8 6 4 2

ISBN 0 19 263095 4

Typeset in Minion by EXPO Holdings, Malaysia
Printed in Great Britain on acid-free paper
by Biddles Ltd, Guildford & King's Lynn

Preface

Jennifer Barraclough qualified in medicine from Somerville College, Oxford in 1970 and has been involved for many years with clinical, teaching and research aspects of psycho-oncology. The present book was inspired by her work as consultant in psychological medicine with the cancer clinical centre of the Oxford Radcliffe Hospital NHS Trust during the 1990s. She now lives mainly in New Zealand (e mail: starflower@paradise.net.nz) and has a life coaching practice.

Choosing the title for a book is seldom easy; this one posed a particular challenge.

'Complementary' 'holistic' 'integrated' — which was the key term and should the others be included too? I proposed various combinations, but none of them satisfied all of the relevant people. For example, some colleagues objected to the word 'holistic' which I had wanted to put first. This lack of consensus reflects a subject in which terminology, definitions and boundaries may be rather vague, but strong feelings and contrasting opinions abound.

Contrasting approaches to healthcare

Orthodox Western medicine: 'Yang'	Holistic healing model: 'Yin'
Logical, analytic, objective, evidence-based	Intuitive, subjective
Focus on pathology	Focus on wellbeing, self-development potential
Narrower focus: disease-specific pathogens & treatments, linear cause & effect models	Broader focus: whole person (body, emotions, mind & spirit) in context of environment; interweaving processes
Works with measurable material phenomena	Concepts of subtle energies, pyschospiritual meanings
Doctor–patient relationship detached, prescriptive, 'doing-to'	Healer–client relationship involved, collaborative, 'being-with'
Powerful, invasive, synthetic treatments working against disease (allopathic)	Gentle, natural complementary therapies encouraging self-healing capacity
Aims towards cure, death regarded as failure	Aims towards healing, acceptance of death as part of renewal/continuity of life force
Best results with acute illness	Best results with chronic illness

Background

Like many doctors, I was educated in an approach which I have since heard called 'the Western medical model'. It was not quite what I had expected when my teenage ideals had led me to enter the profession, but it seemed to prevail within all the National Health Service specialties — oncology, general practice, even psychiatry — in which I practised as a young doctor, and I adopted it without much question. I had reached my mid-forties before a series of new encounters, including work with the hospice movement and then a course at the College of Healing in West Malvern, made me aware of a different approach which I shall call the 'holistic healing model' flourishing in other settings. Although in one sense the two approaches represented opposite extremes (see Table), both seemed to contain much of value and I saw little reason why they should not run in parallel or be combined, rather than conflict. I studied some of the specific 'complementary' therapies which are grounded in the holistic healing model, and experienced some first-hand. I tried to develop an integrated approach in my own psycho-oncology practice (Barraclough 1999).

These stages in my personal career development have mirrored a more general trend within Western healthcare. Many therapies once dismissed as 'alternative' are now styled 'complementary,' and receive serious consideration by orthodox healthcare professionals (see for example Lewith *et al.* 1996; Zollman and Vickers 2000; Vincent and Furnham 1997). The concept of 'integrated medicine' (Coates *et al.* 1998) implies an even wider acceptance.

Turning specifically to the cancer field, surveys indicate that many cancer patients in Europe and the USA are now using one or more types of complementary therapy. Though much of this activity takes place in the private sector, often informed by self-help books (for example Lerner 1994; Simon 1999), provision within the orthodox healthcare system has also increased, both in palliative care (hospice) services and in oncology overall.

Within orthodox cancer care settings, complementary approaches are usually provided with the aims of relieving physical symptoms, and easing emotional reactions to illness. These benefits — now supported by a considerable body of evidence — may be due partly to a specific effect of a particular therapy, and partly to general features: providing extra time and attention, offering more opportunity for active participation and choice, bringing positive meaning to the illness experience. The comparatively low costs of the therapies, and their relative freedom from toxic effects if correctly applied, would further support their use for improving 'quality of life'.

Much more controversial are the claims that complementary therapies and the holistic approach offer prolonged survival or improved prospects of cure. Modern scientific work in psychoneuroimmunology (Lewis *et al.* 2000) and related disciplines does provide some theoretical rationale for these claims, but the published clinical evidence is rather slender, and like many clinicians I have always felt wary about the potential risks: fostering unrealistic hopes, rejecting orthodox treatments which could have had clear benefit, guilt about becoming ill or failing to recover. Such professional caution stands in distinct contrast to many patients' own robustly positive attitudes, as displayed in the personal contributions to this book.

Evaluation is complicated. Patients often choose to try more than one kind of complementary therapy, at different times in the course of their illness; therapists often tailor the content of their intervention to the particular case. When standardized regimes are delivered within randomized controlled trials, these untidy variations of 'real life' are eliminated, but at the risk of discounting the individuality and choice which may be crucial ingredients of success. What study designs and outcome measures are most appropriate to determine the benefits and costs, clinical and economic?

This book

Despite the recent moves towards integration, it is still commonplace to hear orthodox healthcare professionals — usually doctors — dismissing complementary therapy as 'magic' or 'mumbo-jumbo,' and complementary therapists expressing open antagonism towards orthodox medicine. Such polarization may be perpetuated by the system of competitive bids for health service funding which can force a choice between, for example, prescribing a new chemotherapy agent or staffing a cancer information and support centre. I hope this book will contribute to greater understanding between two cultures.

Part I presents the background: clinical principles of the holistic approach, and discussion of general issues about evaluating complementary therapies, and providing them within state-funded systems of healthcare.

Part II describes some specific therapies (listed alphabetically) to illustrate the great diversity of approaches included under the umbrella term 'complementary'. Written by experienced practitioners, these are designed to give a clear account of what the interventions comprise; the benefits of, and barriers to, combining them with more mainstream approaches; and the current state of evidence about their effects. Some of the therapies involve primarily practical interventions, others work on the emotional or spiritual planes or through expression of creativity. However, several contributors refer to simultaneous action at several 'levels' (body, emotions, mind, and spirit), and suggest that a combined package of several therapies may be more powerful than one alone. Some of these therapies truly merit the term 'complementary' in that they are already widely used for the supportive care of patients within cancer hospitals; others are still seen as 'alternative' and less compatible with mainstream treatments. Some of the contributors are practising within orthodox hospitals or hospices, others independently. It would have been impossible to include all available therapies but I hope this selection is reasonably representative.

Part III includes chapters about delivering, and receiving, therapies within a variety of healthcare disciplines and settings.

Different contributors have adopted different styles, ranging from academic review to personal testimony, and although most of them are supporters of an integrated approach, others are more sceptical. This variety is in keeping with the current state of the field, and I hope will add to the interest and value of the book for the widest possible readership. I, as editor, do not necessarily agree with all that is written here. In my view, however, one clear unifying theme does emerge from the case histories, and this is summed up in the adage 'all true healing is self-healing'. Patients who benefit most from these approaches are not passive recipients, but people who take the initiative and responsibility to seek out a programme of therapies to support changes in their own behaviour, attitudes, and beliefs. Whether the example of these remarkable individuals can be adapted to the needs of the majority, within the framework of evidence-based standardized packages demanded by modern healthcare systems, is a challenge for the future.

The book is primarily for doctors, nurses, and other healthcare professionals in oncology units. Nowadays, such clinicians are often called upon for advice about the role of complementary therapies, but many lack the knowledge or experience to give an informed response. Other readers may include clinicians in other hospital settings and in primary care; health service planners, purchasers, and managers; complementary practitioners seeking to integrate their work within orthodox settings; and patients wishing to make informed choices from the many options available today.

References

Barraclough, J. (1999). *Cancer and emotion* 3rd edn. (especially Chapter 10). Wiley, Chichester.

Coates, J., Jobst, K., Fielding, S., *et al.* (1998). Integrated healthcare: a way forward for the next five years? A discussion document from the Prince of Wales Initiative on Integrated Medicine. *Journal of Alternative and Complementary Medicine.* 4, 209–47.

Lerner, M. (1994). Choices in healing. MIT Press, Cambridge, Mass.

Lewis, C., O'Brien, R., and Barraclough, J. (in press). *Psychoimmunology of cancer* (2nd edn) Oxford University Press, Oxford.

Lewith, G., Kenyon, J., and Lewis, P. (1996). *Complementary medicine: an integrated approach.* Oxford University Press, Oxford.

Simon, D. (1999). *Return to wholeness.* Wiley, Chichester.

Vincent C., and Furnham A. (1997). *Complementary medicine: a research perspective.* Wiley, Chichester.

Zollman, C. and Vickers, A. (2000). *ABC of complementary medicine.* BMJ Books.

Acknowledgements

I would like to thank Lesley Atkinson and Meg Roberts at Sobell House, Churchill Hospital, Oxford for their help in preparing the manuscript.

Contents

List of contributors

Sally and Edward Baldwin freelance
contributors, Oxford

Mandy Barnett
Centre for Primary Health Care Studies
University of Warwick
Conventry CV4 7AL

Michael Baum
Department of Oncology
University College London Medical School
3rd Floor Bland Sutton Institute
48 Riding House St
London W1P 7PL

Beata Bishop, freelance contributor, London
Beatabishop@clara.co.uk

Thurstan Brewin
82 Pegasus Grange
Oxford OX1 4QQ

Camilla Connell
Wrexham Lodge
Ealing Green
London W5 5EN

Alastair Cunningham
Ontario Cancer Institute/Princess Margaret
  Hospital
Division of Epidemiology and Statistics
610 University Avenue
Toronto
Ontario M5G 2M9
Canada

Rosy Daniel
Bristol Cancer Help Centre
Cornwallis Grove
Clifton
Bristol BS8 4PG

Claire Edmonds
Ontario Cancer Institute/Princess Margaret
  Hospital
Division of Epidemiology and Statistics
610 University Avenue
Ontario M5G 2M9
Canada

Jacqueline Filshie
Royal Marsden Hospital
Downs Rd
Sutton
Surrey

Heather Goodare
1 Heron Way
Horsham
West Sussex
RH13 6DF

Sandra Goodman
Positive Health
51 Queen Square
Bristol BS1 4LH

Sheila Hallissey
Medical Oncology
The London Clinic
20 Devonshire Place
London W1N 2DH

Nest Howells, freelance contributor, Wales

Julian Kenyon
The Dove Centre for Integrated Medicine
Hockley Mill
Church Lane
Twyford
Winchester
Hamsphire SO21 7NT

Colin Lee
Head of Music Therapy
Wilfrid Laurier University
Ontario
Canada
NZL 3C5

George Lewith
University Medicine
Southampton General Hospital
Tremona Rd
Southampton SO16 6YD

Tony and Ann Neate
10 Hatley Court
81 Albert Rd South
Malvern WR14 3DX

Catherine Philips
Ontario Cancer Institute/Princess Margaret
  Hospital
Division of Epidemiology and Statistics
610 University Avenue
Toronto
Ontario M5G 2M9
Canada

Rebecca Rees
EPPI Centre
Social Science Research Unit
Institute of Education
University of London
18 Woburn Square
London WC1H 0NS
0171612 6854/6397/6400

Robert Ross
32 William St
Marston
Oxford OX3 OER

Joanne Stephen
Ontario Cancer Institute/Princess Margaret
  Hospital
Division of Epidemiology and Statistics
610 University Avenue
Toronto
Ontario M5G 2M9
Canada

Caroline Stevensen
The London Haven
Breast Cancer Resource Centre
Effie Road
Fulham
London SW6 1TB

Hilary Thomas
St Luke's Cancer Centre
Royal Surrey County Hospital
Egerton Rd
Guildford
GU2 5XX

Kimberley Watson
Ontario Cancer Institute/Princess Margaret
  Hospital
Division of Epidemiology and Statistics
610 University Avenue
Toronto
Ontario M5G 2M9
Canada

Sheila Weitzman
Dept of Oncology
Hospital for Sick Children
555 University Avenue
Toronto
Ontario
Canada

Adrian White
Department of Complementary Medicine
School of Postgraduate Medicine and Health
  Sciences
University of Exeter
25 Victoria Park Rd
Exeter EX2 4NT

Chris Worth
Janssen-Cilag Ltd
P.O. Box 79
Saunderton
High Wycombe
Buckinghamshire
HP14 4HJ

Judy Young
The Lynda Jackson Macmillan Centre
Mount Vernon Hospital
Northwood
Middlesex
HA6 2RN

Catherine Zollman
Division of Primary Health Care
University of Bristol
Canynge Hall
Whiteladies Road
Bristol
BS8 2PR

Part 1

The background

Chapter 1

Overview of complementary therapies in cancer care

Mandy Barnett

Mandy Barnett is Consultant in Palliative Medicine at Walsgrave Hospital, Coventry and Myton Hamlet Hospice, Warwick, and Honorary Senior Lecturer at the University of Warwick. Mandy obtained a degree in psychology prior to qualifying in medicine in London in 1982. Her postgraduate training included general medicine, clinical oncology, and general practice in addition to clinical and research work in palliative medicine. She has undertaken introductory studies in aromatherapy, reflexology, shiatsu, homoeopathy and massage applied to palliative care, and courses at the Bristol Cancer Help Centre. She is a long-term member of the British Psycho-Oncology Society. In her work she actively supports the development and evaluation of complementary therapies.

In this chapter I shall consider a number of issues which affect the integration of complementary therapies into cancer care: these include a historical perspective of developments within medicine as well as in complementary therapies and changing expectations of patients themselves. I have also placed some emphasis on the question of accountability and measuring benefits of complementary therapies as a further step on the road to integration. However, before considering these wider issues, the first knotty problem is to decide what is meant by the term complementary therapies.

What makes a therapy complementary?

In considering the application of complementary therapies in cancer there are a number of terms such as 'complementary therapies', 'alternative medicine', or 'holistic approaches' which are sometimes used interchangeably but can lead to confusion (Zollman and Thompson 1998).

The World Health Organization (WHO) defines alternative medicine as all forms of healthcare provision which 'usually lie outside the official health sector'. A more explanatory definition of complementary medicine arising from the Cochrane Collaboration (1996) reflects both a medical and sociological perspective: 'Complementary medicine (CM) is a broad domain of healing resources that encompasses all health systems, modalities and practices and their accompanying theories and beliefs, other than those intrinsic to the politically dominant health system of a particular society or culture in a given historical period. CM includes all such practices and ideas self-defined by their users as preventing or treating illness or promoting health and well-being. Boundaries within CM and between the CM domain and that of the dominant system are not always sharp or fixed.'

Although these definitions are broad based, they do not particularly clarify the practices concerned; in addition they have become slightly confounded by the incorporation of some complementary therapies into the mainstream health service. If the term 'complementary therapy' or 'holistic approach' is employed the definition becomes broader still and the number of potential therapies included increases.

This chapter focuses on the 'alternative' end of the 'complementary' spectrum, using the glossary listed by the British Medical Association (BMA) (1993), acknowledging that this may be considered an arbitrary selection. It excludes art and music therapy and the various psychotherapies (including counselling); although these are often included under the 'complementary' or 'holistic' umbrella, they have a long-term history of use within a variety of healthcare settings and are not considered 'alternative'.

Historical perspective of the role of doctors

Historically, the practice of medicine has many of its foundations in religious healing. With a paucity of effective treatments to offer, the doctor in centuries past concentrated on the relief of suffering, both physical and spiritual, which may sometimes have contributed to patient survival (Suchman and Matthews 1988; Maclean 1994). Although the concept of medicine as a science was established during the Renaissance, the 'bedside manner' of the doctor continued to be his most important skill well into the twentieth century.

Before the Great War of 1914, there were no antibiotics, few safe surgical procedures and environmental health and preventive medicine were almost unknown. The average life expectancy in England was less than 50 years (Fry 1993), with high infant mortality, endemic TB, and frequent epidemics of infection. Death was a fact of life for both young and old.

In the last half-century however, enormous technical advances have changed our expectations of life dramatically. In particular, we anticipate good health and longevity as the normal course of events, with death no longer commonplace in our experience as individuals. Medical training and practice have become geared towards diagnosis, treatment, and cure, or at the very least effective maintenance. However, this fails to recognize the fact that death is universal, and that chronic illness and disability still affect many people's lives.

Doctors face the same limitations in their powers to cure conditions such as acquired immune deficiency syndrome, motor neurone disease, and many forms of cancer as did their predecessors with tuberculosis, but medical training does not prepare them to face this. As the new millennium approaches we have come full circle and begun to realize the danger of sacrificing valuable human skills at the altar of medical technology (Colditz 1983). The call for medical practitioners to adopt a 'patient-centred' rather than 'doctor-centred' approach was originally expounded by Balint (1957) over forty years ago and has received considerable attention in the primary care setting (Pendleton 1984). However, it

Non-conventional therapies (BMA 1993)

Acupuncture

Alexander technique

Aromatherapy

Bach flower remedies

Chiropractic

Crystal therapy

Healing

Herbalism

Homoeopathy

Hypnotherapy

Iridology

Kinesiology

Massage

Osteopathy

Radionics

Reflexology

Shiatsu

has only recently impinged on undergraduate medical training, with the implementation of the General Medical Council's 1993 recommendations which place a new emphasis on enabling medical students to develop a more holistic view of their patients and a more problem-solving approach to the conditions with which they present.

Power to the people — the demand for patient information and autonomy

Changes to medical training and practice are not before time, as over the last three decades, there have been significant shifts in public health awareness and expectations of healthcare systems. While the public still applauds technical advances, they are no longer overawed by them. They also recognize a number of areas in medicine where science appears to hold few answers; cancer being one such area. Patients are today a vocal consumer group with more access to medical information through the media and the internet than ever before. This has led to a more critical appraisal of medical care and practitioners themselves, and increasing demands for improvements in provision of medical information for the individual. A number of studies have monitored this trend (Cassileth *et al.* 1980; Degner and Russell 1988; Sutherland *et al.* 1989). Most have supported the view that patients are both more satisfied with their doctors' care and also cope better when provided with information, even when the news is bad, suggesting that it is hardest to live with uncertainty and fear of the unknown (Dunn *et al.* 1993).

This has necessitated a change in perspective for the medical profession, from the viewpoint that patients were better off not knowing about a poor prognosis (Ward 1974; Knight and Field 1981) to an acknowledgement of patients as individuals with a right both to diagnostic information and to participate in decisions about treatment options that may radically affect their future. Even if cure is not possible, for many patients cancer is a chronic disease, which they may live with for a number of years, thus an all-round approach to their management is crucial (Broadwell 1987). Much of their dissatisfaction and distress relates not so much to the failure to achieve a cure, as to the interpersonal aspects of the care they receive (Pruyn *et al.* 1985). Conversely, if medical carers adopt an open and honest approach, it is easier to develop a mutual bond of trust which will facilitate dealing with problems in the terminal phase of illness (Steinmetz and Gabel 1992).

At its extreme, this has led some doctors (particularly in the US) to devolve all decision-making to patients, irrespective of their professional opinion (Quill and Brody 1996). In the UK, although the trend is to offer more discussion and negotiation, decisions tend to be shared or handed back to the doctor (Degner and Russell 1988), especially as the patient's condition deteriorates (Degner and Sloan 1992).

The rise of complementary medicine

In parallel with the demand for more autonomy has come a rise in interest in self-help in various forms and and in complementary therapies in particular. This applies both in the primary care setting and perhaps especially in cancer care.

During the 1980s, many studies focused on patient motivation for seeking complementary therapies as much as on the therapies themselves, perhaps reflecting a growing concern in the medical and research establishment that patients might be rejecting conventional treatment in favour of complementary approaches. Some studies did indeed demonstrate a certain level of disillusionment and dissatisfaction with what was perceived to be available in 'orthodox' medical practice (Furnham and Smith 1988; Pruyn *et al.* 1985). However, many patients felt it was appropriate to use both orthodox and complementary treatments (Donnelly *et al.* 1985), a trend which has continued (Thomas *et al.* 1991).

Current use of complementary therapies

Prevalence studies in the US show that 30–50% of the general population use complementary therapies in some form or other either in health maintenance or for illness or symptom conditions (Astin *et al.* 1998). In the UK, surveys have been fraught with methodological inconsistencies (Zollman and Vickers 1999), but have produced similar results of 33% 'ever used'. Most patients who turn to complementary therapies do so either alongside or after consulting their medical practitioners, most frequently for chronic conditions which have not responded to conventional treatment.

Prevalence amongst cancer patients

Although many people are aware of complementary therapies, recent surveys among cancer patients have come up with widely differing estimates of use. Ernst and Cassileth (1998) attempted to determine the prevalence of complementary therapies usage among cancer patients by a systematic literature review: they retrieved a total of 26 surveys from 13 countries, including 4 among paediatric patients. The average prevalence among adults was 31%, but with a wide range (6–64%) which the authors concluded could reflect differences in terms of reference as much as usage. They also suggested that most of this use reflected an adjunctive approach, rather than a turning away from orthodox medicine.

Certainly surveys among attenders at cancer centres in various countries have still found only relatively small numbers in this patient population were actively using complementary therapies: they tended to be younger, of higher socio-economic groups and more frequently female than the overall cancer patient population. They were also likely to have used complementary therapies prior to their cancer diagnosis (Coss et al. 1998; Downer et al. 1994; Crocetti et al. 1998). Notwithstanding their familiarity with complementary therapies however, 75% would prefer that the referral came from a doctor, and 85% wanted complementary therapies to be offered as part of the service of the cancer centre itself (Coss et al. 1998).

Consistent with the findings among other patient populations, the motivation for cancer patients to use complementary therapies arose from dissatisfaction with conventional treatment either because of lack of curative effect or experience of distressing side-effects, rather than as a primary choice of active cancer treatment. Although they cited anticancer hopes as their main motivation, the overall benefits obtained were more often psychological, and high levels of satisfaction were reported irrespective of the disease outcome (Downer et al. 1994).

Attitudes of healthcare professionals towards complementary therapies — historical obstacles to integration

If complementary therapies are to be integrated into mainstream cancer care, the attitudes of doctors are an important factor, particularly given the finding that patients would prefer their clinicians to be involved in the referral process.

Traditionally, clinicians in orthodox medicine have been mistrustful of complementary therapies that they regarded as unscientific and unproven, and this has tended to be perpetuated by lack of exposure and training. However, this view has gradually softened over the last two decades, reflecting either a similar disillusionment with conventional treatment or increased openness.

As far as conventional treatment for cancer is concerned, doctors working within cancer treatment centres have generally been more positive than those in other fields (Cohen et al. 1982), but a more recent study found that they were less inclined to advise their patients, or to accept for themselves, toxic regimes with minimal chance of benefit (Slevin et al. 1990). Interestingly, this contrasted with the attitudes of patients in the study, who favoured the aggressive approach.

A study of primary care physicians in the United States demonstrated varying degrees of acceptance of complementary therapies according to age, exposure in training, and the therapy concerned, but were generally positive (Berman *et al.* 1998). Perhaps more significant for future reference is the recent survey finding that a significant proportion of North American medical schools are now offering courses in complementary therapies within the medical curriculum (Wetzel *et al.* 1998).

So what is the UK experience? Surveys of general practitioners since the early 1980s (Reilly 1983) have shown both increasing awareness of the potential benefits of a variety of complementary therapies and increasing willingness to refer patients, at least to the more recognized therapists such as osteopaths, acupuncturists, and aromatherapists. While they remain sceptical of the more extravagant claims for cure, GPs accept that such treatments enhance psychological well-being, and possibly confer physiological benefits, especially in chronic conditions. There has also been steadily increasing interest especially among younger practitioners who are obtaining training in fields such as acupuncture and homoeopathy (Reilly 1983; Wharton and Lewith 1986).

However a complicating factor is the medico-legal responsibility of doctors to ensure not only their own adequacy to practise whatever therapy they offer, but to satisfy themselves of the competence of another therapist, before either referring or delegating care, as defined by the General Medical Council in its guidance document for doctors: *Professional conduct and discipline: fitness to practise*[1]. The regulation of medicine as a profession[2] was introduced to protect both patients and doctors from the potential damage (in the former case, to their health and wallet; in the latter, to their professional reputation) which could be caused by untrained 'quacks' purporting to offer cure-all remedies.

In the modern context, although the public may not always consider the regulatory process adequate, it is clearly described and legally enforcible. Many complementary therapies have no such regulatory processes in place; practitioners may work with patients with no professional insurance after extremely variable levels of training. In the worst case, this may put patients at risk, but on a practical day-to-day level it poses problems for a doctor wishing to refer a patient to an external complementary therapist, as it is difficult to determine the competence of such a therapist, particularly if the doctor has little knowledge of the therapy concerned.

Equally, it may not be easy for medical practitioners to assess the quality of courses offered when they are considering training for themselves; one mid-80s survey of 200 GPs in Avon in south-west England found that 38% of respondents (75% response rate) claimed

---

[1] In the first instance, the doctor hands the decision-making process over to the therapist for diagnosis or treatment where this falls outside of the scope of care normally provided by the doctor, whereas in the latter the doctor requests another professional to perform a specific task or function which might otherwise be carried out by him/herself, retaining clinical responsibility and accountability for the patient's treatment. Within orthodox medical practice, referral normally occurs between different medical practitioners (e.g. from a general practitioner to a specialist consultant) or from a medical practitioner to a non-medical practitioner within another recognised professional field e.g. dentist, whereas delegation is likely to occur within various forms of team working.

[2] Introduced in the Medical Act of 1858.

to have received some training in complementary therapies, albeit mostly limited to short courses (Wharton and Lewith 1986).

Moving towards integration — the impact of NHS reorganization and regulation of complementary therapies on availability

Although regional variations occur, prior to 1990 few complementary therapies could be accessed through NHS practitioners, directly or indirectly. Thus patients had to be responsible for seeking information and choosing both therapy and therapist, which was likely to deter all but the most motivated and autonomous individuals. A study of home-based patients with advanced cancer (Barnett 1995) found only a very small minority (6/106) were using complementary therapies, all of whom were self-referrals.

However, a variety of therapies have begun to be provided either within or alongside NHS departments, reflecting several sea changes in the Health Service. In primary care, the introduction of fund-holding enabled general practitioners to be more experimental in their budgeting priorities at practice level: since 1991 they have been able to claim reimbursement for employing complementary therapists. Patient views are also being sought more actively and used in service development, although it remains to be seen how much impact this will have on primary care groups and their choices of service commissioning.

There have also been moves within a number of complementary therapies to regulate and standardize their training and practice[3]. This has both clarified the medico-legal position for individual clinicians, and has also facilitated more formal contractual arrangements between NHS units and complementary practitioners.

Contrary to the reservations sometimes expressed by clinicians, complementary practitioners tend to be cautious both in their use of therapeutic approaches and their claims of success. This was demonstrated by a UK survey of 250 aromatherapists and reflexologists carried out within the region served by a North London Cancer Centre (Howells and Maher 1998): 104 responders described their qualifications, cancer-related experience, work patterns, contribution of therapies to cancer care, and interest in cancer-related training. Therapists felt they needed more information on cancer, and were working sensitively or even overcautiously. Subsequent training workshops were organized which improved therapists' understanding and improved liaison between themselves and the cancer centre. This in turn led to an improved referral network for patients.

Another factor has been the increasing availability of training in these areas for medically qualified practitioners. In general practice, a recent UK survey (Wearn and Greenfield 1998) of complementary therapy provision by practices within a single health authority area found that half the responding practices (response rate 68.9%) offered an in-house service. This was likely to have been developed after 1990 and was mostly provided by the doctors themselves. The most common therapies offered were acupuncture, osteopathy, chiro-

---

[3] Osteopathy was the first therapy to put forward a system of statutory regulation — following on from a King's Fund working party report in 1991, formal legislation was introduced through Parliament in 1993.

practic, hypnotherapy, and homoeopathy. In the south-west of England, a survey across a wide range of practices found that over two thirds of GPs used complementary therapies, although here a smaller number (16%) practised them themselves (White and Ernst 1997).

Increasing recognition of therapies has also led to improved access within secondary care. Homoeopathy has been provided at specialist NHS hospitals for a considerable time, and other therapies such as acupuncture, osteopathy, aromatherapy, and massage are now being offered in a number of hospital settings (Burke and Sikora 1993[4]). This provision is determined by individual trusts rather than any coherent national policy.

The model for integrated care varies according to the needs and preferences of individual services: in some instances practitioners are salaried directly by a trust or primary care centre, elsewhere patients are referred to an established complementary therapy centre whose practitioners remain independently employed (Paterson 1997). Commonly a therapist is employed on a sessional basis but retains an external private practice.

Many nursing staff have undertaken training in complementary therapies (frequently massage) which they integrate into their general nursing care (Malkin 1994). Indeed, the nursing profession as a whole has taken a generally positive view towards complementary therapies, particularly those involving hands-on techniques, and this may also have influenced health trust policies.

The BMA (1993) recommended that doctors should be enabled to become both better informed about non-conventional therapies and offered training opportunities by approved bodies. It concurred with the US view that the undergraduate medical curriculum should offer basic courses to familiarize students. However, a recent survey of British medical schools has indicated that although this is an area of curriculum development no formalized teaching has yet been established (Rampes *et al.* 1997).

Evaluation

Both practitioners and patients are beginning to agree that complementary therapies have a place in the conventional medical setting; however, their effectiveness needs to be evaluated.

Much of the existing research on complementary therapies has arisen from the historical context of needing to 'prove' valid treatment outcomes in comparison with orthodox approaches. Where this is relevant to modifying or discontinuing either therapeutic approach this is clearly important, particularly if it leads to symptom or health benefits to the patient in the long term.

However, in life-threatening conditions such as cancer such therapeutic comparisons may be erroneous. The ill-fated study at Bristol Cancer Help Centre (Bagenal *et al.* 1990) which considered survival benefits to cancer patients treated by orthodox vs. complementary approaches illustrates this problem well (in hindsight). On closer examination, the study suffered from a number of significant methodological flaws, particularly with regard to the comparability of the patient populations. Nevertheless, the results and initially published conclusions (that Bristol patients demonstrated a higher mortality rate than those treated in orthodox settings alone) led to a public furore which proved highly damaging both to the

---

[4] Burke and Sikora describe an especially innovative programme developed at Hammersmith Hospital in consultation with the Bristol Cancer Help Centre, one of the first true attempts at integration.

parties involved and the reputation of complementary therapies in general. This led to a loss of confidence amongst a vulnerable patient group and considerable reluctance on the part of therapists to expose their practice to further scrutiny.

Ironically, although there has in the past been mutual antagonism between those with extremely 'orthodox' views and the more radical complementary practitioners, the potential for common ground has always existed.

Despite dramatic improvements in long-term survival in some diagnostic groups and the participation of thousands of patients in clinical trials, the prognosis for many solid tumours remains poor. Even where survival is enhanced, differences between treatments may disappear if the time in which the patient benefits from the positive effects of treatment is set against the time during which toxicity is experienced (Priestman 1986). Whereas clinical trials prior to 1980 used only tumour response and disease free survival as outcome measures[5], there has been steadily increasing emphasis on quality of life over the last two decades.

In those cancers where long-term survival or cure remains unlikely, or even in good prognosis groups where different treatments may be equally effective but of varying toxicity, the inclusion of a quality of life outcome measure provides a more balanced viewpoint of the overall cost:benefit ratio of a particular treatment option[6]. Funding bodies such as the Medical Research Council now require their inclusion in all relevant trial protocols.

Similarly, the evaluation of benefit of complementary therapies in cancer care has moved away from the curative to the quality of life dimension.

Potential benefits of evaluation of complementary therapies and improved integration

There are two approaches to considering quality of life benefits associated with the use of complementary therapies:

1) the effect of an individual therapy;

2) the indirect effect of active participation in disease management.

In the first case there are potential psychological benefits which may be held in common by a number of therapies, and in addition physiological effects specific to a particular therapy which may guide choice of treatment. These are considered further in later chapters.

In the second case, people who take a 'fighting' approach to their cancer diagnosis fare better in terms of psychological adjustment, including those who are helped to do so through psychological intervention (Watson *et al.* 1991). Thus patients who seek out or take up opportunities to use complementary therapies may benefit psychologically from the very action of taking a positive role in their management, quite apart from the effects of treatment itself.

---

[5] In Bardelli and Saracci's review of clinical trials between 1956–76, only 5% referred to the impact of treatment toxicity on quality of life (Bardelli and Saracci, 1978).

[6] The importance of this is demonstrated by the sometimes counter-intuitive results obtained, as in Sugarbaker's seminal study on osteo-sarcoma (1981), in which the treatment options of amputation and chemotherapy were compared with limb-sparing surgery combined with radiotherapy and chemotherapy in terms of resulting quality of life. Contrary to expectation, amputation resulted in a better long-term outcome from the patient's point of view.

There is also some evidence that survival outcome may be influenced (Spiegel *et al.* 1989), although this is more contentious. Certainly there is interest in areas such as immunological marker responses indicating neurophysiological effects of psychological responses (Walker and Eremin 1995). This might not only be useful in itself, but could point out routes for combining complementary therapies with conventional cancer treatment.

For example, in HIV-related illness, complementary therapies may affect a variety of immune factors which in turn affect survival. Calabrese *et al.* (1998) reported on a survey of 117 practitioners in the US, offering a total of 115 different therapies: 90% of providers claimed benefits at all disease stages, particularly for symptom management and quality of life, but also for specific disease outcome measures such as raising or maintaining CD4+ lymphocyte levels, slowing progression to full-blown AIDS, and extending survival.

Methodological issues in evaluation: qualitative vs. quantitative approaches

This is a long-running debate that extends to areas of research far broader than the complementary therapies, but it impinges on any attempts to clarify either the benefits or drawbacks of their usage. To some extent the argument represents a cultural divide between researchers with nursing and/or social science backgrounds and those with medical backgrounds (Roter and Frankel 1992). Social scientists value qualitative methods such as the analysis of interview transcriptions using small numbers of patients. Medical researchers tend to regard this as less scientifically sound, preferring to use standardized instruments and larger samples, to obtain numerical data which lends itself to statistical analysis and facilitates cross-study results comparisons. Which is the best method to apply when investigating subtle psychological issues? Both methods are valid, but they provide different types of data.

Our aim should be to start by defining outcomes and then look for the best methods. This was supported by a consensus meeting in the US examining the application of research methodologies to complementary therapies. It concluded that despite reservations held by complementary practitioners, existing methods of research analysis can be applied both to biological and clinical efficacy outcome measures. The authors cite observational epidemiology and social survey techniques as well as conventional experimental trials as appropriate methodologies (Levin *et al.* 1997), a view echoed by researchers in the UK (Vickers 1996).

However, there are inherent limitations when applying scientific criteria,: for example, where the therapeutic approach involves different manipulative techniques, as in the comparative study of orthodox versus chiropractic treatment of low back pain (Meade *et al.* 1990) double blind principles cannot be applied. Equally one should not dismiss the therapeutic relationship purely in terms of 'placebo effect' as many complementary therapists view this as an integral part of their treatment and question the validity of outcomes measured independently from the patient's experience and understanding (Anthony 1987).

This is exemplified by a recent case-controlled study (Rao *et al.* 1998) which attempted to assess the impact of a complementary therapy programme on quality of life among palliative care patients, using a combination of standardized questionnaires and qualitative self-reports. The results from the standardized questionnaires showed no significant benefit, whereas the self-reports indicated highly positive effects. Although there is the risk of a placebo effect, patient views in this area are as valid as in symptom assessment; the problem lies with finding the right measurement tool rather than a lack of significance in the effects of the therapy being assessed.

Even in the context of a randomized trial (Wilkinson 1995), the therapist was considered part of the therapeutic process, supporting the view that this needs to be taken into account in trial design, rather than viewed simply as a confounding variable.

Another lesson comes from the use of focus groups among cancer patients to consider the research questions which patients themselves deem important, rather than the traditional outcomes determined by scientific or clinical opinion (Bradburn *et al.* 1995). This led into a call for more patient involvement in the design of clinical trials, and would provide a useful model for an evaluation process in complementary therapies.

To summarize, as a clinician and researcher who has struggled to apply scientific principles to evaluating concepts of quality in human relationships (Barnett 1995), I do not underestimate either the value of the therapeutic relationship, or the difficulty entailed in attempting to measure the effectiveness of complementary approaches in isolation from the effect of the individual therapist. However, if complementary therapies are to be fully integrated into cancer care directly or indirectly accessed through the NHS, they must be judged by the same yardsticks as other treatments.

Potential advantages of integrating complementary therapies into cancer care — future areas for research

1) Improving access for patients. Many people use complementary therapies. They are not equally distributed, with women, younger age groups, and those of higher socio-economic status disproportionately represented. It is probably overly simplistic to assume that a free and direct referral system would correct this imbalance completely, as patients' awareness and health beliefs are a significant factor, but it would at least ensure that those who wished to use complementary therapies could do so.

2) Improving symptom control for patients. Whether undergoing curative or palliative treatment, living with its long-term effects, or dealing with progressive disease, many patients experience a wide variety of unpleasant and sometimes intolerable symptoms. Increasingly, palliative care clinicians are involved at all stages of cancer to provide an all-round approach to these problems; whereas the conventional armamentarium relies heavily on pharmacological or procedural interventions, these are neither the only nor sometimes the most appropriate solutions. Just as the value of palliative radiotherapy is better appreciated by those who have had some direct experience of working in departments of clinical oncology[7], better understanding of individual complementary therapies by 'orthodox' clinicians will lead to more referrals and better symptom control.

3) Improving patient well-being. This is perhaps the most commonly reported benefit, both anecdotally and in some instances using standardized measurements (Wilkinson 1995). In the palliative care setting, it is often the main aim of treatment (see Chapter 20) but patients with good prognoses have long been recognized to experience psychological

---

[7] The conclusion of a survey of training experience conducted among palliative care physicians by the Association for Palliative Medicine

distress, particularly in the initial period following diagnosis and during treatment (Maguire *et al.* 1980), and would benefit from therapies which enhance overall well-being.

4) Enhancing patient satisfaction. Although not easy to define or measure, it is an important issue both for patients and indirectly for NHS trusts. It is all too easy for patients to feel that they are just another number being processed through a treatment centre. Where support teams or clinical nurse specialists become involved with patients and their families, it is often the time spent listening and the perception of individual worth that is valued as much if not more than any specific advice (personal communication). Similarly, the benefit of touch therapy may relate as much to the affirmation of the patient as a touchable person as for example the direct effect on a swollen limb. In cancer treatment centres which currently offer complementary therapies, anecdotal reports suggest that patients perceive the overall service as more holistic and satisfactory. It would be interesting to measure this formally, particularly if wishing to address the concerns of health trust management over increasing litigation.

5) Cost effectiveness. This is also a difficult area to measure, especially if the quality rather than quantity of the service needs to be part of the equation. However, some aspects could be evaluated relatively simply, such as the effect on conventional drug prescribing (Cannard 1996).

Potential disadvantages

1) Devaluation of therapeutic relationship. This is a purely speculative argument, but if complementary therapists work within the NHS, it may become increasingly difficult for them to protect the amount of time spent with individual patients as their caseload increases. While time itself is not the most important factor, an overstretched and stressed complementary therapist risks burnout as much as any other healthcare professional (Ullrich and Fitzgerald 1990; Ramirez *et al.* 1995), which may in turn affect the quality of care offered. It is also possible that providing a service which is free at the point of delivery may itself lead to devaluation of its benefit by patients.

2) Loss of perception of self-help. Apart from any financial element, the necessity of taking responsibility for seeking out a practitioner confers a sense of positive self-help. Whether or not this aspect is lost when a therapy is provided within a conventional treatment centre has not been measured.

Conclusion

In the last decade, there has been a greater focus on developing an integrated approach to cancer care, with complementary therapies increasingly recognized as having a part to play. The potential uses of individual therapies need to be considered and evaluated, and some of these points will be addressed in the rest of this book. Although financial limitations cannot be ignored, the future for complementary therapies within the health service looks positive.

References

Anthony, H. M. (1987). Some methodological problems in the assessment of complementary therapy. *Statistics in Medicine*, 6, 761–71.

Astin, J. A. Marie, A., Pelletier, K. R., *et al.* (1998). A review of the incorporation of complementary and alternative medicine by mainstream physicians. *Archives of Internal Medicine*, 158, 2303–10.

Bagenal, F. S., Easton, D. S., Harris, E., *et al.* (1990). Survival of patients with breast cancer attending Bristol Cancer Help Centre. *Lancet,* **336,** 1186–8.

Balint, M. (1957). *The doctor, his patient and the illness.* Pitman, London.

Bardelli, D. and Saracci, R. (1978). Measuring quality of life in cancer trials: a sample survey of published trials. *UICC Technical Report,* **36,** 75–94.

Barnett, M. (1995). *The doctor–patient relationship in advanced cancer.* MD Thesis, University of Bristol.

Berman, B. M., Singh, B. B., Hartnoll, S.M., *et al.* (1998). Primary care physicians and complementary-alternative medicine: training, attitudes, and practice patterns. *Journal of the American Board of Family Practitioners,* (127) **11,** 272–81.

Bradburn, J., Maher, E. J., Adewuyi-Dalton, R., *et al.* (1995). Developing clinical trial protocols: the use of patient focus groups. *Psycho-Oncology,* **4,** 107–12.

British Medical Association (1993). *Complementary medicine: new approaches to good practice.* Oxford University Press.

Broadwell, D. C. (1987). Rehabilitation needs of the patient with cancer. *Cancer,* **60** (Suppl), 563–8.

Burke, C. and Sikora, K. (1993). Complementary and conventional cancer care: the integration of two cultures. *Clinical Oncology,* **5,** 220–7.

Calabrese, C., Wenner, C.A., Reeves, C., *et al.* (1998). Treatment of human immunodeficiency virus-positive patients with complementary and alternative medicine: a survey of practitioners. *Journal of Alternative and Complementary Medicine,* **4,** 281–7.

Cannard, G. (1996). The effect of aromatherapy in promoting relaxation and stress reduction in a general hospital. *Complementary Therapies in Nursing and Midwifery,* **2,** 38–40.

Cassileth, B. R., Zupkis, R. V., Sutton-Smith K., and March, V. (1980). Information and participation preferences among cancer patients. *Annals of Internal Medicine,* **92,** 832–6.

Cochrane Collaboration Complementary Medicine Field (1996). The Cochrane Library, Update Software Ltd, Oxford.

Cohen, R. E., Ruckdeschel, J. C., Blanchard, C. G., *et al.* (1982). Attitudes toward cancer. II: A comparative analysis of cancer patients, medical students, medical residents, physicians and cancer educators. *Cancer,* **50,** 1218–23.

Colditz, G. A. (1983). Medical education meeting community needs. *Medical Education,* **17,** 291–5.

Coss, R. A., McGrath, P., and Caggiano, V. (1998). Alternative care. Patient choices for adjunct therapies within a cancer center. *Cancer Practice,* **6,** 176–81.

Crocetti, E., Crotti, N., Feltrin, A., *et al.* (1998). The use of complementary therapies by breast cancer patients attending conventional treatment. *European Journal of Cancer,* **34,** 324–8.

Degner, L. F. and Russell, C. A. (1988). Preferences for treatment control among adults with cancer. *Research in Nursing and Health,* **11,** 367–74.

Degner, L. F. and Sloan, J.A. (1992). Decision making during serious illness: what role do patients really want to play? *Journal of Clinical Epidemiology,* **45,** 941–50.

Donnelly, W. J., Spykerboer, J. E., and Thong, Y. H. (1985). Are patients who use alternative medicine dissatisfied with orthodox medicine? *Medical Journal of Australia,* **142,** 539–41.

Downer, S. M., Cody, M. M., McCluskey, P., *et al.* (1994). Pursuit and practice of complementary therapies by cancer patients receiving conventional treatment. *British Medical Journal,* **309,** 86–9.

Dunn, S. M., Patterson, P. U., Butow, P. N., *et al.* (1993). Cancer by another name, a randomized trial of the effects of euphemism and uncertainty in communication with cancer patients. *Journal of Clinical Oncology,* **11,** 989–96.

Ernst, E. and Cassileth, B. R. (1998). The prevalence of complementary/alternative medicine in cancer: a systematic review. *Cancer,* **83,** 777–82.

Fry, J. (1993). *General practice — the facts,* p9. Radcliffe Medical Press, Oxford.

Furnham, A. and Smith, C. (1988). Choosing alternative medicine: a comparison of the beliefs of patients visiting a general practitioner and a homeopath. *Social Science and Medicine*, 26, 685–9.

General Medical Council (1993). *Tomorrow's doctors*. GMC, London.

Howells, N. and Maher, E. J. (1998). Complementary therapists and cancer patient care: developing a regional network to promote co-operation, collaboration, education and patient choice *European Journal of Cancer Care*, 7, 129–34.

Knight, M. and Field, D. (1981). A silent conspiracy: coping with dying cancer patients on an acute surgical ward. *Journal of Advanced Nursing*, 6, 221–9.

Levin, J. S., Glass, T. A., Kushi, L. H., *et al.* (1997). Quantitative methods in research on complementary and alternative medicine. A methodological manifesto. NIH Office of Alternative Medicine. *Medical Care*, 35, 1079–94.

Maclean, I. (1994). Dr Rabelais's 500 year old prescription. *British Medical Journal*, 308, 803–4.

Maguire, G. P., Tait, A., Brooke, M., *et al.* (1980). Psychiatric morbidity and physical toxicity associated with adjuvant therapy after mastectomy. *British Medical Journal*, 281, 1179–80.

Malkin, K. (1994). Use of massage in clinical practice. *British Journal of Nursing*, 3, 292–4.

Meade, T. W., Dyer S., Browne W., *et al.* (1990). Low back pain of mechanical origin: randomized comparison of chiropractic and hospital outpatient treatment *British Medical Journal*, 300, 1431–37.

Paterson, C. (1997). Complementary practitioners as part of the primary health care team: consulting patterns, patient characteristics and patient outcomes. *Family Practice*, 14, 347–54.

Pendleton, D., Schofield, T., Tate, P., and Havelock, P. (1984). *The consultation: an approach to learning and teaching*. Oxford Medical Publications, Oxford University Press.

Priestman, T. J. (1986). Measuring the quality of life during cancer therapy. *Update*, June, 987–96.

Pruyn, J. F. A., Rijckman, R. M., van Brunschot, C. J., and van den Borne, H. W. (1985). Cancer patients' personality and characteristics, physician–patient communication and adoption of the Moerman diet. *Social Science and Medicine*, 20, 831–47.

Quill, T. E. and Brody, H. (1996). Physician recommendations and patient autonomy. *Annals of Internal Medicine*, 125, 763–69.

Ramirez, A. J., Graham, J., Richards, M. A., *et al.* (1995). Burnout and psychiatric disorder among cancer clinicians. *British Journal of Cancer*, 71, 1263–9.

Rampes, H., Sharples, F., Maragh, S., and Fisher, P. (1997). Introducing complementary medicine into the medical curriculum. *Journal of the Royal Society of Medicine*, 90, 19–22.

Rao, A. S., Chronicle, E. P., and McIllmurray, M. B. (1998). Investigating the impact of an innovative cancer care programme on the quality of life of cancer patients. *Psycho-Oncology*, 7, 64.

Reilly, D. T. (1983). Young doctors' views on alternative medicine. *British Medical Journal*, 287, 337–9.

Roter, D. and Frankel, R. (1992). Quantitative and qualitative approaches to the evaluation of the medical dialogue. *Social Science and Medicine*, 34, 1097–103.

Slevin, M. L., Stubbs, L., Plant, H. J., *et al.* (1990). Attitudes to chemotherapy: comparing views of patients with cancer with those of doctors, nurses and the general public. *British Medical Journal*, 300, 1458–60.

Spiegel, D., Bloom, J. K., Kraemer, H. C., and Gottheil, E. (1989). Effects of psychosocial treatment on survival of patients with metastatic breast cancer. *Lancet*, ii, 888–91.

Steinmetz, D. and Gabel, L. L. (1992). The family physician's role in caring for the dying patient and family: a comprehensive theoretical model. *Family Practice*, 9, 433–6.

Suchman, A. L., Matthews, D. A. (1988). What makes the patient-doctor relationship therapeutic. Exploring the connexional dimension of medical care. *Annals of Internal Medicine*, 108, 125–30.

Sugarbaker, P. H., Barofsky, I., Rosenberg, S. A. and Gianola, F. J. (1981). Quality of life assessment of patients in extremity sarcoma clinical trials. *Surgery*, 91, 17–23.

Sutherland, H. J., Llewellyn-Thomas, H. A., Lockwood, G. A., and Tritchler, D. L. (1989). Cancer patients: their desire for information and participation in treatment decisions. *Journal of the Royal Society of Medicine*, 82, 260–3.

Thomas, K. J., Carr, J. Westlake, L., and Williams, B. T. (1991). Use of non-orthodox and conventional health care in Great Britain. *British Medical Journal*, 302, 207–10.

Ullrich, A. and FitzGerald, P. (1990). Stress experienced by physicians and nurses in the cancer ward. *Social Science and Medicine*, 31,1013–22

Vickers, A. (1996). Methodological issues in complementary and alternative medicine research: a personal reflection on 10 years of debate in the United Kingdom. *Journal of Alternative and Complementary Medicine*, 2, 515–24.

Walker, L. G. and Eremin, O. (1995). Psychoneuroimmunology: a new fad or the fifth cancer treatment modality? (Editorial). *American Journal of Surgery*, 170, 2–4.

Ward, A. W. M. (1974). Telling the patient. *Journal of the Royal College of General Practitioners*, 24, 465–8.

Watson, M., Greer, S., Rowden, L., *et al.* (1991). Relationships between emotional control, adjustment to cancer and depression and anxiety in breast cancer patients. *Psychological Medicine*, 21, 51–7.

Wearn, A.M. and Greenfield, S. M. (1998). Access to complementary medicine in general practice: survey in one UK health authority.*Journal of the Royal Society of Medicine*, 91, 465–70.

Wetzel, M. S., Eisenberg, D. M., and Kaptchuk, T. J. (1998). Courses involving complementary and alternative medicine at US medical schools. *Journal of the American Medical Association*, 280, 784–7.

Wharton, R. and Lewith, G. (1986). Complementary medicine and the general practitioner. *British Medical Journal*, 292, 498–500.

White, A. R., Resch, K. L., and Ernst, E. (1997). Complementary medicine: use and attitudes among GPs. *Family Practice*, 14, 302–6.

Wilkinson, S. (1995). Aromatherapy and massage in palliative care. *International Journal of Palliative Nursing*, 1, 21–30.

Zollman, C. and Thompson, E. (1998). Complementary approaches to palliative care. In *Handbook of Palliative Care* (ed. C. Faull, Y. Carter, and R. Woof), pp. 333–55. Blackwell Scientific Publications.

Zollman, C. and Vickers, A. (1999). ABC of complementary medicine — users and practitioners of complementary medicine. *British Medical Journal*, 319, 836–8.

Chapter 2

Holistic approaches to cancer: general principles and the assessment of the patient

Rosy Daniel

Rosy Daniel has specialized in holistic medicine since completing her GP vocational training in 1989. She worked for ten years at the Bristol Cancer Help Centre (1989–99), becoming Medical Director in 1995. Since leaving this post she has been working to help develop Integrated Healthcare Systems in Britain as well as Health Creation initiatives for the promotion of health and well-being among the general public. Day to day she works as a holistic doctor in Bristol and London as well as teaching, writing, and broadcasting on the subject of the Holistic Approach to Health.

General principles

The holistic approach involves viewing our state of health or illness as the result of the inter-acting influences of mind, body, and spirit, and the environment in which we live. This gives many perspectives on how illness may have developed, and provides the vital clues needed to create an individually tailored programme of psychological therapy, complementary medicine, support, healing, and orthodox medicine to promote recovery. The holistic approach is entirely complementary to medical treatment, and can enhance its effectiveness by helping individuals cope with diagnosis, symptoms, and treatment whilst helping them to work to recover their health. Through therapeutic, self-help programmes, lifestyle review, and re-orientation of life around (new) core values the quality of living and dying can be improved greatly. In cancer medicine aspects of this approach are implemented in three settings:

- *Psychosocial care* given within hospitals, hospices, voluntary sector support groups, or within the community via health visitors, social workers, or the Church to ease psychological distress and the existential angst caused by the diagnosis, and to give spiritual comfort and guidance;

◆ *The supportive care setting*, used in hospitals, hospices, and the community where there is increasing use of complementary therapies, particularly by nurses for symptom control, comfort, and palliative care; and

◆ *The patient self-help movement*, where a mixture of self-help approaches, complementary and alternative therapies, nutrition, and psychological approaches are used with the aim of improving health, well-being, and prognosis.

The holistic model

The holistic model is a health-based model in which individuals and therapists work in partnership to achieve the best levels of health, energy, emotional and spiritual well-being, whether as a preventive measure, to promote health in the presence of illness, or to facilitate spiritual growth through times of adversity. The word 'holistic' comes from the Greek word *holos* which means 'the whole which is greater than the sum of the parts'. This gives a sense of not only the interconnecting levels of mind, body, and spirit but also the profound way in which we are interconnected, to each other and all that is around us. This fits with the Buddhist belief that all of 'reality' is in fact one and that the root of all suffering is the 'illusion' that we are separate.

In the West we have a model of medicine which is reductionistic, or mechanistic. The body is viewed like a machine and the focus is on the disease and not the person. In modern medicine we look at tissues, cells, DNA, and biochemistry, with many brilliant outcomes and technical solutions becoming possible. However, many patients feel that they become lost in the process. People often say that the doctor no longer seems to be thinking about them and that they find this a frightening and alienating process; they feel bereft and abandoned with their emotions and fear, and that their own involvement and insight into their illness or problem is being over-looked. In the holistic approach each person is seen as being the greatest expert on themselves and many important factors and behaviours which affect health are felt to be within the indi-vidual's control — hence the need for partnership with healthcare professionals. Herein lies another essential element of the approach — the importance placed on the caring connection made between the patient and the professional helper or the great value of the 'therapeutic rela-tionship'. In the reductionistic model the professionals' value is a function of their knowledge and technical skills and modern scientific research controls out the effect of the practitioner in order to measure the 'real' therapeutic benefit of any given intervention.

Within the holistic model the factors primarily affecting an individual's state and health are seen as:

◆ the state of the individual's 'spirit', purpose in living, and will to live;

◆ the emotional/mental state both current and chronic, and the underlying beliefs and past experiences which determine behaviour and the relationship to oneself;

◆ the physical state — nutrition, fitness, posture, and breathing;

◆ the environment — socially and physically;

◆ the lifestyle — particularly the balance of work with recreation and pleasure, and busyness with stillness and regenerative time.

State of the spirit

If an individual has lost their will to live, then no medicine, orthodox or complementary, will help them. Similarly, if individuals have become dispirited or had their spirit crushed by hurt, loss, disappointment, abuse, social disadvantage, grief, or continual stress, the body's ability to heal is severely compromised. The accent within the holistic approach is therefore placed strongly on helping to revive the individual's spirit through holistic therapies and individual and group psychotherapeutic processes. These aim to help the individual to discover a sense of purpose and meaning in life; identify their core values and current choices; and find sources of uplift for their spirit. These may range from the beauty of nature, art, music, and children, to spiritual practices, following a religion, or helping others. Sometimes individuals have become dispirited by following the wrong life-path and ending up in occupations or 'ways of being' which do not fully express them. Here the emphasis is placed on helping individuals to make new choices and to find activities and occupations which excite and stretch them, helping them to reach their potential and achieve fulfilment. This is particularly important for individuals who have been repressed chronically, through abuse, abandonment, or social disadvantage.

Another common reason for depression of the spirit is loneliness, and here the need is to connect individuals to others either socially, in learning situations, or in community initiatives or support groups. Individuals must learn how to make good relationships and how to communicate their needs clearly. This may require assertiveness training. The overall aim is to enable individuals to rediscover their joy in living, a sense of purpose and belonging, and an outlet for authentic self-expression, and caring connections to other people and the community.

Spiritual enquiry often becomes activated if there is serious life-threatening illness. The kind of questions which come to the surface are: 'What is life all about? Is there a purpose to life or is this all there is? If there is a purpose, what is it, and how does it affect me? If it is a journey, where am I going? Is there any sense in it all and what will happen to me when I die?' Often through the very process of asking and thinking about these questions and working on the areas of faith, belief, and understanding, the inner spiritual essence within awakens and with this awakening a huge amount of energy for living life in the present can be released. Commonly times of extreme adversity are the times when individuals discover their spiritual nature and develop their own spirituality in very personal ways. This profoundly enriching process can be so important that there is sometimes a feeling that the illness has served to awaken the person to the real essence of life, 'transforming' them and enabling them to live a far happier life based on spiritual rather than material or fear based values.

The emotional and mental state

In the holistic model great attention is paid to the emotional state, both current (particularly relating to the diagnosis of cancer) and chronic, and to the way the individual handles their emotions. Because of the deleterious effects of fear and repressed emotion on the body, patients learn how to relax and to feel safe to express their emotions, helping them to identify and meet their emotional need. At a deeper level efforts are made to help individuals identify the beliefs and attitudes they hold, which dictate the relationship they have with themselves and others. Often those who have not been well cared for as children, and who do not have strong, positive self-images, will base a great deal of their behaviour on the desire to win approval and affection, stressing and exhausting themselves in the process. Simultaneously, they may be alienating those whose affections they are trying to win! Individuals are asked: 'What is their relationship to themselves; how are they looking after themselves; do they nourish, care for, and protect themselves from destructive influences, or do they chronically abandon, neglect, or even abuse themselves?' The establishment of a new, loving and nurturing relationship to one's self is one of the most important themes within the holistic model, and individuals are enabled, first through the therapies and then through self-help approaches, to learn to identify their needs and care for themselves properly. They can then model their new relationship to themselves on the therapeutic relationships they have developed.

The physical state

In the West most of us eat a very processed diet which is high in fat, sugar, and protein, with too few fruits, vegetables, vitamins, and minerals. This results in us becoming overfed and undernourished, and having too little fibre in our digestive tracts. Within the holistic model people are encouraged to have a whole-food, high vegetable/fruit diet, which is organic where possible, with vitamin and mineral supplements as required. In cancer the anti-oxidant vitamins and minerals beta-carotene, C, E, selenium, and zinc are most commonly recommended. Individuals are also encouraged to exercise and stretch daily, even if they have to do this on a chair or in bed. It is necessary to identify food allergies which may be seriously compromising to the health of some people.

Avoiding 'stagnation' of the body energies is seen as an important part of many holistic therapies, and a good posture is also encouraged. This is becoming increasingly relevant with the very sedentary office and computer-based Western lifestyle. Attention is also directed to breathing patterns. Often the combination of sedentary lifestyle, poor posture, and emotional tension or depression leads to very shallow breathing. This in turn affects the mental state, leaving the individual feeling sluggish, depressed, or anxious. Through yogic breathing, relaxation, and exercise in general it is possible to deepen the breathing, which in turn helps to oxygenate the body more fully and create a state of well-being and vitality.

Environment

Socially one's environment may be dominated by difficult, demanding relationships, or by inter-personal pressures in the workplace or home. Many have discovered, through their holistic explorations, that they had never before had the chance to find out 'who they are', or what their own needs are, because of having lived around extremely dominant family members, partners, or colleagues whose needs were always given priority. Re-establishing health and well-being may depend upon renegotiating boundaries and commitments; identifying and meeting personal needs and goals.

At the physical level our environments may be overtly toxic — smoky, airless, or very electro-magnetic. At subtler levels our environments may be subject to geopathic stress or radiation hazards. Certainly many individuals report never having felt well since moving into particular houses or offices, or find it difficult to maintain their health within the more polluted town environment. Developing the awareness of the toxicity of one's environment on all levels begins to give individuals choice about making the necessary changes to promote their health and well-being.

Lifestyle

An individual's lifestyle is usually a clear reflection of the nature of their relationship to themselves, and it may be necessary for the relationship to the self to change before changes in lifestyle become possible and sustainable. The overall aim is to bring the lifestyle into balance, helping those who have become workaholic to relearn how to play and relax; enabling people who have become addicted to being busy and constantly stimulated to learn how to become still. This process can be helped by spiritual healing and learning the self-help techniques of relaxation and meditation, which also enable the development of a rewarding inner life. This in turn can help to break the cycle of individuals requiring more and more stimulation and higher and higher achievement and excitement in order to have any sense of satisfaction. In relaxing and becoming more open, individuals regain their sensitivity and have an enhanced ability to experience pleasure and the subtler dimensions of life.

The energy model

Another key concept within the holistic approach is to think in terms of the effect of an individual's behaviour, lifestyle, and mental state on their energy levels or vitality. In all the old traditional holistic systems there is a concept for this energy. It is called the vital force in homoeopathy, chi in acupuncture, prana in yoga, and ki in shiatsu. During illness or debilitating treatment it is considered important in the first instance to have therapeutic help which will raise the energy level through passive input of energy. When clients are in a low energy state, self-help will be impossible and the first key to recovery is for them to be able to 'let go' and allow themselves to receive help and energy input. Individuals often need permission from therapists to do this. The energy levels can be lifted by spiritual healing, and the energy medicines of acupuncture, shiatsu, and homoeopathy. Touch therapies like massage, reflexology, and aromatherapy will also help to reduce fear levels and facilitate the letting go process.

Once the energy has returned, the second key is for people to learn the importance of putting themselves first; reorganizing their priorities and values in life, hanging on to this precious new energy and continuing to build it through self-help practices such as healthy diet, relaxation, meditation, visualization, exercise, and by becoming involved with that which is really exciting and inspiring. We can look at this energy equation in budgetary terms, getting clients to ask themselves 'How am I spending my energy, where is it all going, and is this right?' And the second, more important question 'How do I build my energy and am I spending more than I am generating?'

Illness and therapy

Within the holistic model, illness is seen to arise when the system's ability to resist disease has broken down due to a state of disharmony or imbalance in mind, body, spirit, or the individual's environment. All holistic therapies and self-help techniques are therefore designed to strengthen and rebalance the body, increasing the individual's ability to stabilize the disease process and recover from illness. The therapies aimed at any of the levels of mind, body, and spirit are seen as being able to affect all other levels because of the integrated nature of the system. After an initial exploratory assessment with the holistic doctor, nurse, or practitioner a therapeutic and then a self-help plan is negotiated which feels most appropriate to the individual.

Evaluation of the patient

To evaluate a person with cancer in relation to diagnosis and treatment it is necessary to assess:

+ The reaction of the individual to the diagnosis — What is the current emotional state? What are the current emotional needs? What support system does the individual have?

+ The person's state in relation to their treatment plan — Is the person emotionally ready for treatment? Have they recovered sufficiently from the shock of diagnosis to make informed decisions about treatment? Do they require psychological, nutritional, or complementary help to prepare for treatment?

+ The person's symptoms, either of cancer or side-effects from treatments — What symptoms do they have? What complementary help may be available to help control symptoms?

+ The individual's health beliefs and needs — Does the individual wish to become involved in the holistic approach? Does the individual wish to seek alternative cancer treatment?

In relation to holistic health promotion it is necessary to assess:

+ The state of the spirit — Does the individual have the will to live? Do they have meaning and purpose in their life, or something to live for? Do they have sources of uplift and nourishment for their spirit? Do they feel connected to life and society?

+ Emotional/mental state — What are the current mental and emotional states and needs? How does the individual deal with their emotions? Are they able to express emotion? Does the client have any long-term or recent triggers or stresses? Does the individual self-stress? What is their relationship to themselves? What are the underlying emotional beliefs and attitudes which determine their behaviour?

+ Physical state — What is their current nutritional state, the state of fitness and posture? What is the client's current breathing pattern?

+ Environmental state — Is the person experiencing health problems due to dominant social or physical environmental stressors? Are there subtle environmental factors affecting health?

+ Lifestyle — Is the client's lifestyle in balance? Are they in stress? Are they balancing work and leisure activities? Are they achieving stillness and reflective times to balance periods of high activity?

+ Energy levels — Is the client currently depleted energetically, requiring input of energy prior to the commencement of self-help (or even medical treatment in some cases)? Is the patient strong enough to embark upon treatment? Is the client ready to go from the therapeutic to the self-help phase of the holistic programme?

A holistic therapeutic programme for cancer is divided into therapeutic and self-help phases.

Therapeutic phase

The therapeutic phase ideally includes the assessment by a multidisciplinary holistic team including:

+ *Holistic doctors and nurses* for medical counselling needs, and lifestyle and stress assessment, symptom control, natural remedies (herbal and homeopathic), and specific nutritional advice.

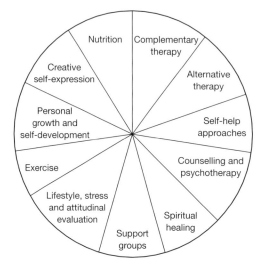

Fig. 2.1 The holistic approach

- *Counselling, psychotherapy, group work, and creative therapies* (art, music, drama,) aimed at:
  - promoting emotional expression;
  - examination of lifestyle, stress, and self-stressing attitudes;
  - re-orientation and rehabilitation of individuals towards more authentic and meaningful personal values and goals.
  - (Transpersonal and psychosynthesis counselling models are commonly used as part of the holistic approach.)
- *Nutritional approaches* based on replacing high fat, high protein, high salt, high sugar, highly processed Western diets with a wholefood, vegan, preferably organic diet, supplemented with anti-oxidant vitamins and minerals (A as beta-carotene; C and E; plus the minerals selenium and zinc). Nutritional changes should be introduced and supervised by qualified nutritional therapists and/or doctors to avoid stress, weight loss, and inappropriate dietary recommendations.
- *Complementary therapies*: at this stage should be the 'energy medicines' of acupuncture, shiatsu, and homoeopathy, which are helpful in lifting the patient's underlying energy and improving well-being and symptom control; or bodywork, such as massage and aromatherapy, which helps to reduce fear, tension, isolation, and the alienation felt by cancer patients towards their diseased or sometimes disfigured bodies.
- *Spiritual healing*: which lifts underlying energy, improves coping, is calming and has emotional and spiritual benefits.
- *Support groups*: aimed at giving encouragement, social contact, and support.
- *Alternative cancer therapies*: which are thought to be actively anticancer and in this sense are more like allopathic anticancer medicines than holistic health-based therapies *per se*. These therapies tend to fall into the categories of:
  - *Herbal remedies*: e.g. Rene Caisse herbs (Essiac), Iscador (mistletoe therapy), or Carnivora (Venus flytrap);

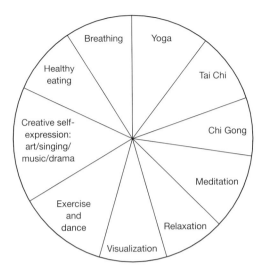

Fig. 2.2 The self-help phase.

- Metabolic approaches: which are thought to be immunostimulant e.g. MGN3, an extract from maitake mushrooms and 1P6 (Inositol Phosphate) an extract from Vitamin B;
- Dietary approaches e.g. the Gerson diet: which are based on fasting to 'detoxify' the body, followed by 'super nutrition' with very pure plant-based juice, raw food, or other 'spring cleaning' diets;
- Alternative remedies: which have a specific anticancer mechanism, e.g. shark's cartilage which has been shown to have angiogenesis inhibiting factor activity.

The self-help phase

A point will come when, through the application of holistic therapies, the patient feels sufficiently strong to embark upon self-help approaches at home. It is important not to encourage patients to take up self-help approaches before they are strong enough to do so, because if they are unable to implement this advice they will blame themselves and feel they have failed. The key self-help approaches are:

Mind/body approaches: These are aimed at calming the mind, inducing states of well-being and happiness (e.g. regular practice of relaxation and meditation). Another key practice is visualization where positive mental focus is achieved with pictures or words (affirmation) in an attempt to affect disease outcome and morale. Visualization is divided into guided imagery, where therapists guide individuals or groups with sequential use of pleasant visual images into happier states of mind, or personal imaging where a cancer patient creates images of their cancer being destroyed, or images of themselves completely recovered.

Exercise: Cancer patients are encouraged to take up holistic forms of exercise such as yoga, t'ai chi, or chi gong to the extent of their ability, which again promote emotional, physical, and spiritual well-being.

Healthy eating: Once the patient has been taught and guided through dietary changes, healthy eating can become incorporated into their lifestyle.

Creative self-expression: Patients are encouraged to live more balanced, expressive lifestyles where far more accent is placed on recreation, self-expression, and the fulfilment of personal goals and ambitions.

The scientific evidence underpinning the holistic approach

There is a growing body of scientific evidence for the holistic approach to health which has been developed intuitively over many centuries.

1. Important evidence comes from the study of the effects of stress on the body. The body's reaction to stress or fear is to direct resources to the brain and muscles, so that we can think, run or fight. This happens at the expense of the housekeeping functions of the body, such as digestion, absorption, growth, healing, immunity and repair, all of which are compromised greatly when we are frightened or stressed in sympathetic nervous system arousal. Many of the holistic therapies and self-help approaches work by reducing fear and anxiety, helping to establish predominantly parasympathetic 'self-healing' states within the body in which immune and repair functions are optimized.

2. Since the early 1980s a far more subtle level of connection between the mind and the body has been identified. The study of psychoneuroimmunology (PNI) has revealed mechanisms for the interconnections of the brain, neuroendocrine, immune, and repair tissues of the body. It started with the discovery of a receptor in the brain for an opiate-like substance, and shortly afterwards the substance itself was discovered which was called 'enkephalin' or 'endorphin'. The discovery that the brain made its own morphine-like compound initiated a search for other similar messenger substances, and over 200 messenger chemicals which are secreted by the brain and the tissues of the body have now been found. These are called 'neuropeptides' or 'informational substances'. There are receptors for these substances in all the tissues of the body, and when these molecules interact with the receptors they affect the cells' functioning either by activating the cells or by slowing down or deactivating them. The neuropeptides which are secreted in persistent states of depression or stress depress the tissue functioning. This may provide an explanation for the connection between the mind and the body which has been witnessed for centuries.

   This is crucially important in cancer and many other illness processes because healthy, active immune cells can recognize abnormal, infected, or cancerous cells and destroy them. However, in stressed, depressed, or unhappy people the immune blood cells multiply less fast and the activities of existing cells can be depressed by up to 50%. Even red blood cells have been shown to carry less oxygen in depressed people.

   PNI has shown that the reverse is also true: that when we are excited and happy and feeling loved or loving, our tissue and immune function increases greatly. There is therefore a physiological as well as emotional need to free cancer patients from chronically depressed states of mind and unexpressed emotion, by the use of counselling and group therapy, by encouraging involvement in that which excites and inspires (Coleman and Gurin 1998; Pert 1997).

3. Scientific work has also pointed to the crucial relationship between the dominant 'coping style' of patients and survival rates with cancer. Greer and Pettingale, working at the Marsden Hospital in the 1970s, realized that they were observing very different survival patterns in people with cancer depending on their reaction to the diagnosis. They

described the different coping styles as 'fighting spirit', 'denial', 'stoic acceptance, or fatalism' 'helplessness and hopelessness', or 'anxious preoccupation', and demonstrated a 60% survival advantage at thirteen years for those with fighting spirit compared with those who became helpless and hopeless (Greer *et al.* 1990). Subsequent work in this area has confirmed this, particularly linking the state of helplessness and hopelessness to significantly poorer prognosis. Greer has subsequently shown that people can be helped to develop a fighting spirit given sufficient psychological support (Greer *et al.* 1997). It is therefore crucial for those who are ill to become involved in the fighting of their illness and to be encouraged by both healthcare professionals and supporters who are looking after them.

4. Further evidence that support and emotional expression influence the body's response to disease has come from the support group studies of Spiegel *et al.* (1989) and Fawzy *et al.* (1993) in America. Spiegel has shown that expressive psychotherapeutic support given to women with breast cancer for one hour once a week for one year, doubled their mean survival time compared with women who did not receive this support. Fawzy showed that giving support to melanoma patients decreased the death rate from 10% in the control group who received no support, to 1% in the group who received support.

5. Seminal studies performed by Walker in Scotland have shown that the use of mind/body techniques such as visualization and relaxation are associated with strengthening of the immune response in patients with breast cancer (Walker *et al.* 1999) and extension of survival in patients with lymphoma (Walker 1998). There are many other studies which show the qualitative benefits of relaxation, aromatherapy, meditation, and visualization (Bristol Cancer Help Centre 1997).

6. Good nutrition is known to be important both in preventing cancer and promoting recovery. In 1994 Key and Thorogood, who had followed 11 000 vegetarians for seventeen years, showed that as a group they had between 40–50% lower death rate from cancer than the general population, after correcting for smoking (Thorogood *et al.* 1994). There are now several good treatment studies which show that the lives of those with cancer can be extended with healthy diet (Lechner and Kronberger 1990; Holm *et al.* 1993).

7. Several studies have shown that people with cancer who take high quality antioxidant vitamins and minerals can improve their survival rates (Li 1993). A study in China showed that taking antioxidant vitamins and minerals A, C, E, and selenium reduced the death rate from cancer by 13% overall and 20% in their two most common cancers.

8. There is also randomized control trial evidence for the power of prayer and spiritual healing. It was demonstrated that people in intensive care units who were prayed for, even without them knowing it, did significantly better than those who were not (Dossey 1993).

9. Placebo studies have shown that strong relationships between patient and doctor/ therapist, and belief in the therapy, can convey up to a 90% clinical effect. Because of the emphasis on the therapeutic relationship in complementary medicine and the conviction of the therapists it is likely that these therapists engender a powerful placebo effect (Mitchell and Cormacks 1998).

Patients' attitudes towards the holistic approach

A focus group study performed in 1998 entitled 'Meeting the needs of cancer patients for support and self-management' (The Bristol Study; Tritter *et al.* 1998) identified the fact that individuals' self-management strategies were aimed at three different levels:

- Attempts to mitigate the psychological and spiritual impact of the cancer diagnosis;
- Help to achieve symptom control from the cancer and side-effects of treatment;
- Actively fighting the disease through self-help, holistic, complementary and alternative health-promoting methods.

Although all participants had very marked emotional needs, a smaller number were using complementary therapies for symptom control, and a smaller group still were actively using the holistic approach to promote their health. Currently within mainstream hospital and hospice practice, both psychological and complementary therapies are offered within a supportive care paradigm, whereas clients wishing to embark upon either an holistic approach to health promotion in the presence of illness, or alternative cancer therapy must do so within the voluntary or private sectors. Interestingly in the Bristol Study, patients commented that their reasons for seeking the help of complementary therapists were that:

- They provided high quality loving supportive care by virtue of the therapists' skills and the emphasis placed on the empathic therapeutic relationship, the time given, and the engendering of feelings of security;
- They provided help in facing orthodox treatment due to relief of side-effects, symptom control, improved state of mind, and increased energy levels;
- They enabled people to feel that they were being treated as individuals; helping them to focus on themselves and their needs;
- They empowered people to take an active role, thereby bringing about a sense of control and involvement;
- They gave tangible and practical ways of improving health, e.g. healthy diet;
- They gave messages that individuals can play a role in restoring their health and well-being, however ill they are;
- They focused on 'natural' rather than 'chemical' or 'high-tech' medicine;
- They included the patient's own insights and self-healing abilities;
- They encouraged hope and positivity.

Certainly the benefits reported by individuals for use of the holistic approach include:

- Reduction in fear, anxiety, isolation;
- Achieving a sense of control, involvement, and partnership with healthcare professionals;
- Improvement in physical state, energy levels, and sleep;
- Improved symptom control and tolerance of treatments;
- Greatly improved quality of life, enabling the crisis of cancer, in many cases, to be turned into an opportunity for learning, increased self-understanding, and greater personal fulfilment, happiness and the establishment of spiritual values;
- Stabilization or reversal of disease process in some individuals;
- The rekindling of hope.

The issues

Despite the recommendations by Calman and Hine (1995) which have suggested that 'psychosocial care is provided at all stages of the cancer journey', and 'there should be access to information and complementary therapies', as well as 'a seamless provision of care', provision of and access to support, complementary and self-help resources is extremely random and haphazard throughout the UK. Most support initiatives are patient led and run within the voluntary sector. Although there is increasing provision of complementary therapies for supportive care, patients wishing to get involved in the promotion of their own health and their fight against cancer, may face the disapproval or even dismissal of their attempts by healthcare professionals. The current challenge in oncology is whether:

- Psychosocial screening and support can be made available routinely to all who receive a cancer diagnosis;
- Supportive complementary care can be offered routinely within hospitals;
- The model of holistic health promotion can be incorporated into the spectrum of options available within conventional healthcare settings, or whether at the very least information about, and access to, such resources can be made available routinely to patients from the point of diagnosis.

Current medical attitudes tend to inhibit patients' holistic therapeutic and self-help activities rather than encourage them, and often ignore or bypass the intense emotional problems of patients. In the light of the evidence for the protective role of 'fighting spirit', psychosocial support, mind/body techniques, nutritional approaches, and the placebo effect, these attitudes should be urgently reconsidered by all those involved in the provision of care and service for cancer patients. New policies should be made on both compassionate and ethical grounds which reflect these scientific developments and make provision of, and/or access to, these approaches routine.

References

Bristol Cancer Help Centre (1997). *Mind/Body database.*

Calman, K., Hine, D. (1995). A policy framework for commissioning cancer services: a report by the Expert Advisory Group on Cancer to the Chief Medical Officers of England and Wales. Department of Health, London.

Cohen, L. A., Rose, D. P., Winder, E. L. (1993). A rationale for dietary intervention in post-menopausal breast cancer patients; an update. *Nutrition & Cancer,* 19, 1–10.

Coleman, D., Gurin, J. (1998). *Mind/Body Medicine.* Consumer Reports Books.

Dossey, L. (1993). *Healing Words: The Power of Prayer and the Practice of Medicine.* Harper Collins, USA.

Fawzy, F. I., Fawzey, N. W., Hyun, C. S., *et al.* (1993). Malignant melanoma, effects of an early structured psychiatric intervention, coping and affective state on recurrence and survival six years later. *Archives of General Psychiatry,* 50(a), 681–9.

Greer, S., Moorey, S. (1997). Adjuvant psychological therapy for cancer patients. *Palliative Medicine,* 11, 240–4.

Greer, S., Morris, T., Pettingale, K. W., Haybittle, J. L. (1990). Psychological response to breast cancer and 15 year outcome. *Lancet,* 1, 49–50.

Holm, L. E., Nordevang, E., Hjalmar, M. L., *et al.* (1993). Treatment failure and dietary habits in women with breast cancer. *Journal of the National Cancer Institute,* 85, 32–36.

Lechner, E., Kronberger, L. (1990). Experiences with the use of dietary therapy in surgical oncology. *J. Akt. Ernahr.-med*, 15, 72–8.

Li, J. Y., Taylor, P. R., Li, B. (1993). Nutrition trials in Linxian. *Journal of the National Cancer Institute*, 85.18, 1492–98.

Mitchell, A., Cormacks, M. (1998). *The Therapeutic Relationship in Complementary Health Care*. Churchill Livingstone.

Pert, C. (1997). *Molecules of Emotion*. Simon & Schuster, USA.

Spiegel, D, Bloom, J. R., Kraemer, H. C., Gottheil, E. (1989). Effect of psychosocial treatment on survival of patients with metastatic breast cancer. *Lancet*, 2, 888–91.

Thorogood, M., Mann, J., Appleby, P., McPherson, K. (1994). Risk of death from cancer and ischaemic heart disease in meat and non-meat eaters. *British Medical Journal*, 308, 1667–70.

Tritter, J. A., Daniel, R., Cooke, H, Baldwin, S. (1998). *Meeting the needs of people with cancer for support and self-management*. Bristol Cancer Help Centre publication.

Walker, L. G., (1998). Hypnosis and cancer: host defences, quality of life and survival. *Contemporary Hypnosis*, 15, 34–38.

Walker, L. G., Walker, M. B., Ogston, K. *et al*. (1999). Psychological, clinical and pathological effects of relaxation training and guided imagery during primary chemotherapy. *British Journal of Cancer*, 80, 262–8.

Chapter 3

Casting off the spell

Robert Ross

55-year-old Robert Ross has had four careers — as a town planner, lecturer, student counsellor, and careers advisor. On being diagnosed with terminal cancer of liver and lungs, he consulted the Bristol Cancer Help Centre, took early retirement from Oxford Brookes University and reinvented himself as an author and playwright. One book and five stage plays later he is in remission, living positively and creatively, one day at a time.

'There is nothing alternative or scientifically dubious about the fact that what goes on inside someone's brain influences their physical health.' (Paul Martin 1997)

The bad news

'Pain and suffering are inevitable: misery is optional.' (Anon)

My first hint of trouble was a tingling sensation on the left side of my face which was diagnosed as atypical facial pain in the spring of 1990. This gradually worsened, became focused on the left side of my mouth, and proved difficult to alleviate by orthodox or complementary therapies. This chronic pain was largely to blame for a gradual descent into clinical depression, for which I was briefly hospitalized in April 1993. However, I made a surprisingly quick recovery before medication could have much effect, decided to take early semi-retirement and settled into a more relaxed and balanced lifestyle. What appeared to be toothache in March 1996, again on the left side, prompted a visit to the dentist who immediately referred me to hospital. I had adenoid cystic cancer of the mouth.

I remember reeling from the shock, but reassured by the positive attitude of the oral surgeon — the prognosis was good, I should regain the power of speech and be able to return to my part-time job as a careers counsellor. I had a rare form of cancer which was apparently slow growing (the good news) and could pop up anywhere (the bad news), but I was preoccupied with the scary prospect of surgery in one week's time to remove half my tongue and part of my jaw. I found it hard to believe that surgery, my only treatment option, was unlikely to affect the atypical facial pain.

When I awoke from an eleven hour operation to rebuild my face and neck I thought I was in heaven, being pain free for the first time in six years, but it was the ITU nurse reassuring me that everything had gone well. A series of complications resulting in a grand total of five operations kept me in hospital for seven weeks, but eventually I appeared to make a full recovery, and there was the unexpected bonus of being completely pain free. As a squeamish man who had spent a lifetime avoiding all forms of human confrontation, I was pleasantly surprised at my attitude to all this trauma and found the overall experience of hospital positive. I may have been unlucky in having to endure five operations in a sensitive area but I could not fault the quality of care. To keep myself amused as I recuperated, I finished off my first full-length play, a comedy aptly entitled *Climb Every Mountain.*

No doctor, nurse, or nutritionist discussed the need for me to change any aspect of diet, attitude, or lifestyle even though they might have contained potential seeds of destruction. On the contrary, I was actively encouraged to pick up the threads of my life and work as if I had never had the disease, an institutionalized form of 'denial' you might say. Hopefully in the new millennium health professionals will routinely invite cancer patients to review their lifestyles and actively participate in their own recovery/survival strategy.

> 'The art of medicine consists of amusing the patient while nature cures the disease.' (Voltaire)

The really bad news

> 'If negative thoughts, feelings and emotions can hold up health, what then can positive thoughts, feelings and emotions achieve?' (Robert Holden 1993)

I don't remember but my wife says she was told that my 'pop-up' cancer might possibly recur within 10 or 15 years; in fact it popped up inside six months, and a scan in December revealed metastases on liver and right lung, which my oral surgeon assumed should be operable. The liver specialist, who I met just once, was not so optimistic, described my condition as borderline for surgery and recommended another scan after Christmas. He politely suggested that I 'put my affairs in order', a classic example of oblique understatement.

Question: 'What's the worst scenario?'

Answer: 'You never leave hospital.'

Merry Christmas! A scan in January 1997 showed the liver was unchanged but there were now metastases in both lungs. 'There is nothing more we can do', said the liver expert, after consulting a chest expert who I had never even met.

Question: 'If I do everything in my power to look after myself, roughly how long have I got?'

Answer: 'Twelve months.'

I had been sentenced to death. My wife was shattered but I remember feeling strangely calm and relieved that I was not faced with any more invasive treatment. As I had feared a worse forecast, twelve months seemed quite a long time, enough to see my first book published. As apparently neither chemo nor radiotherapy were recommended I was at the end of the orthodox road, but my cancer journey had only just begun.

Fortunately I was not aware that the liver is a rather bad place to have cancer, so I clutched at three straws — firstly a dimly recollected TV programme on the Bristol Cancer Help Centre, secondly the fact that laughter stimulates the immune system, and thirdly that God moves in mysterious ways. I had a well developed, satirical sense of humour and was about to attend the opening night of *Climb Every Mountain*, so I recklessly contacted the local press and media and cheerfully explained, for the benefit of my fellow cancer patients, that I was going to try and beat cancer by the application of humour. With hindsight, I am struck by my balance of realism and optimism at the time — 'Perhaps I can slow it down,' I said. My wife badgered me into contacting Bristol, so I paid my first of four visits in February 1997 and this proved to be the turning point.

> 'Had she been light, like you, of such a merry, nimble, stirring spirit, she might have been a grandam ere she died; and so may you, for a light heart lives long.' (William Shakespeare *Love's Labours Lost* 1595)

The Bristol Cancer Help Centre

> 'Don't stop thinking about tomorrow, don't stop, it'll soon be here. It'll be here, better than before, yesterday's gone' (Fleetwood Mac 1988)

Following his own cancer scare in 1998, John Cleese quipped that he'd 'never met anyone who wished they had spent more time in the office'. As I now had more important things to do than my likeable, part-time job, I immediately retired, visited Bristol with an open mind, liked very much what I heard and reinvented myself. A typical day's holistic treatment (mind, body, and spirit) included individual sessions with doctor, counsellor, nutritionist, art therapist, and healer, and group sessions on guided meditation and relaxation. There was also empowering, informal interaction with other patients who, like me, were all fighters. I took up two new sports, was delighted to receive an honorary MA from Oxford Brookes University, joined the Methodist Church, and otherwise devoted myself to writing. I decided to risk self-publishing my book *Counselling as a Career* (originally commissioned by Sage) and wrote play number two, *The Awkward Squad* — a celebration of four early retirees who belatedly form a hugely successful rock band. I confronted my illness with humour, my fondness for satire taking on a new significance as I set out to prove that if you can laugh at something, you take away its power.

In October 1997 I crashed my motorcycle, landed in A & E and my regular oral surgeon patched up my shattered right cheekbone with a metal plate, by which time I really felt like 'bionic man'. A few days later, as he took out the stitches, my surgeon calmly announced that there was 'no change' in the lung tumours — scientific proof that I was in remission! It's a sobering thought that if my lung condition had *not* worsened over Christmas 1996, I would have opted for drastic surgery with doubtful quality of outcome. Two years later, almost to the day, I am writing this chapter and still feeling fine, although some facial pain has returned. It is not sinister and is almost certainly caused by the severed nerves attempting to grow, which I interpret as a healthy sign. Having no qualms about resorting to orthodox medicine when appropriate, I have it reasonably well controlled with amitryptiline and meditation.

In my experience the Bristol Cancer Help Centre holistic approach revolves around three central features:

- **Special projects in life:** I write, especially satirical comedy about my real and imaginary enemies. My goals are to see the millennium, hear one of my plays on radio, experience grandparenthood, and die at home of old age, in bed, with Dire Straights on the hi-fi.

- **Healing:** I go for Reiki every month, a very gentle, hands-on form of treatment.

- **Diet:** I eat mainly organic fruit and vegetables, organic corn fed chicken, and deep sea fish, plus a daily cocktail of vitamins, minerals, and liver herbs. However, I am no zealot and consume more caffeine and chocolate than I should.

The other important elements are:

- **Visualization:** In this technique my imagination runs riot with a rich mixture of themes including peace (e.g. a team of healers touring my tumours preaching early retirement), war (e.g. an army of killer cells attacking the aliens), and humour (e.g. a troupe of Tommy Coopers encouraging my cancer cells to die laughing). The regular hero is my immune system, known affectionately as 'Baldrick' because of his indefatigable optimism and cunning plans.
- **Relaxation/meditation:** I try to spend a few minutes every day, believing that it will boost my natural killer cell production.
- **Exercise:** I play badminton and bowls all the year round, and have even won three trophies in my first two seasons.
- **Counselling:** I go once a month for transpersonal counselling, which emphasizes the spiritual element. A standing joke is the notable absence of plans for 'termination'.

Formal religion does not feature in the Bristol approach but my Church is important to me and so, after 35 years lapsed, I finally joined the Methodist Church at Easter 1997. A doubting Thomas, I pray not for a cure, but for courage and enlightenment. 'May your God go with you,' quipped my oral surgeon after my last regular check-up.

'Sweet are the uses of adversity' (William Shakespeare *Love's Labours Lost* 1595).

Primitive and advanced labels

'Faith and hope are necessary to survive. Fatalism can be fatal.' (Bernie Siegel)

Tell bright six year olds that they are dim and they will behave according to dismal stereotype. When his teacher told me that my son would never, ever, pass O level German I discretely arranged a few extra, private lessons and he obtained a grade B pass. Studies have shown that some cancer patients are helpless and hopeless and the vast majority are at best stoical in the face of this awesome disease. It is a media cliché that many people 'lose their battle' with cancer but, sadly, most do not actually fight at all, being resigned to their fate. They say that 'information is power' but most patients are unaware that they might have an influence over the course of their own cancer largely because, in our culture, they are taught to be wholly reliant on having things done to them — namely high tech drugs, radiation, or surgery. There is an excellent local Cancer Information Centre, with masses of helpful literature, tapes (including an introduction to Bristol) and now even some holistic/complementary therapy, but I was not even made aware of its existence when I was, allegedly, dying of cancer less than one mile away.

In primitive cultures voodoo death will occur when a patient is:

- highly susceptible
- believing in the power of the doctor who 'curses'
- helpless
- surrounded by those who are of similar mind.

Had I passively accepted my doctor's death sentence I would have died years ago, another victim of sophisticated Western style voodoo. After I was in remission, my good friend the oral surgeon told me of another very strange case. Sadly, a young African student had arrived at the end of orthodox cancer treatment and, as there was nothing more advanced medicine could do for him (and my city is one of the better places to be seriously ill) he was sent home to die in his tribal home. Many years later, and now a robust, qualified lawyer, he visited my surgeon and described the treatment from his local traditional healer. Mind over matter? Act of God? Chance? Misdiagnosis? A fascinating example of the outer limits of the placebo effect? Take your pick, but I note Joan Borysenko's claim that most so called 'spontaneous remissions', including my own, actually come about from hard work, sometimes accompanied by significant ritual. I identify with Martin's assertions that to ignore the mind is an irresponsible waste, and that there is compelling evidence that psychological factors affect the chances of patients' survival/recovery.

What else do Western doctors habitually *not* tell you that might affect your chances, hopes, and fears? That cancer is a convenient subtitle for over two hundred diseases? That it is subject to wide individual variation? That they still don't understand it very well and sometimes get it wrong? That our brains are like pharmacies, compounding a wide range of drugs that affect both our moods and all of our biological systems, including the immune system? I agree with Bernie Siegal that doctors have no right to play God by extinguishing hope, just because they have run out of orthodox ideas. It may be too difficult or unethical to prove the efficacy of holistic/complementary medicine by the gold standard of double blind clinical trial, but why ignore something that works for some, just because we don't fully understand it? The intransigence and pessimism of many health professionals remind me of the occasion when a Scottish preacher was haranguing his flock:

Preacher: 'At the day of judgement there will be weeping, wailing, and gnashing of teeth!'

Voice from the congregation: 'What about people who've lost their teeth?'

Preacher (grimly): 'Teeth will be provided!'

Bristol does not come cheap but there is a bursary scheme and, anyway, what price improved quality or length of life? I estimate that my survival strategy has already cost me over £40 000 in lost salary alone, which does not bother me in the slightest. A lasting source of amusement for my wife and me is the fact that the Department of Social Security are effectively paying for my complementary therapies because, having been so labelled, I qualify for a modest Disability Living Allowance under special rules for the 'terminally ill'. They even rang me up to reassure me that this was not subject to income tax or periodic review, and politely inquired whether I had any mobility problems, for which there would be extra payments. 'Not for the time being' I heard myself saying in a quavery voice.

'Do not go gentle into that good night, Old age should burn and rage at close of day, Rage, rage against the dying of the light' (Dylan Thomas 1952)

Integration

'I am too much of a sceptic to deny the possibility of anything.' (T. H. Huxley 1886)

I was very sceptical about 'healing', coming as I do from a rational/scientific background and out of tune with new age gurus and charismatic faith pedlars. To this day I am unconcerned about whether or not my healer has special powers, or how she works with mysterious body energies and 'chakras' undetectable by Newtonian physics. What I do know is that I experience a profound sense of peace during healing sessions, sometimes spontaneous prayer and/or vivid healing visualizations. In my home city I have been able to integrate all elements of the Bristol approach into a coherent, creative, and idiosyncratic strategy for survival. I have regular sessions with both healer and counsellor and, between them, my support group and local cancer information centre offer discussion, guided meditation, and art therapy. I appreciate Bernie Siegal's view that 'to be 'healed' represents a condition of one's life, 'cured' relates strictly to one's physical condition'.

I don't believe I could achieve very much on my own: I thrive on the love and cheerful support from my wife, and I continue to dote on my two grown up, independent children. After my second day at Bristol I remember saying to my wife that I would always appreciate their complementary therapy for helping me to cope with cancer, even if I lived no longer than forecast. It was another two years before I came across research into therapy which, intended merely to help patients and their families cope with the disease and augment their quality of life for whatever time they had left, surprised the researchers by helping people to live longer. Common sense suggests that one would lead naturally to the other.

My principle motivation in writing this chapter is to convince health professionals of the wisdom of inviting many more patients to be what Bernie Siegal calls 'exceptional' — to join in the fight to heal themselves. Naturally I am reluctant to alter in any way my successful Bristol holistic formula, but I do not reject outright orthodox medicine — a consultant oncologist surprised me by suggesting that I might one day qualify for some new drug trial, so maybe complementary therapy will keep me in remission for long enough to seek an orthodox cure?

'Keep an open mind but don't let your brain fall out.' (Joan Borysenko 1995)

A patient-centred approach

'Tell me, I forget. Show me, I remember. Involve me, and I understand.' (Chinese proverb)

For twenty five years I worked in higher education and witnessed a quiet but significant revolution called 'student-centred learning'. The influx of bright, mature students made it increasingly obvious that it was wrong to regard lecturers as gurus and students as empty vessels. When I taught the final year part-timers the group included students who actually had more years of practical experience than myself, so it was self evident that I should treat their knowledge and experience with respect, and also learn from them. Substitute 'doctor' for lecturer and 'patient' for student and you have 'patient-centred medicine'.

I make a polite nuisance of myself at the occasional cancer conference and I was pleasantly surprised to hear recently of national moves towards a more patient-centred approach in the UK. At the time of writing the newly appointed Secretary of State for Health (Alan Milburn) is announcing new initiatives for the two main killers — heart disease and cancer, and a new cancer 'czar' has been appointed (Professor Mike Richards). But the focus, as ever, is on early detection, better and more uniform access to new and improved drugs — worthy but limited. A holistic approach seems hard for many doctors to embrace: they seem to me, at worst, to be obsessed with cancer by body part, mesmerized by global statistics, and enslaved by a reductionist view of biology. I get blank stares when I speculate that I may have blocked the blood supply to my tumours without the aid of drugs. Even the advocates of reform seem to see patient centredness as primarily about more skilful communication with better informed patients, and few acknowledge openly that patients themselves might have an active role to play in their own healing. Patient centredness involves a creative partnership, with health professionals really listening to individuals and seeking the best ways to mobilize their patients' psychological and other resources. Surely such an approach would produce more fighters than the dismal, estimated 15–20%?

More recently I have been curious to find out more about how, according to science, I am keeping myself alive, and I have been very impressed with Paul Martin's *The Sickening Mind*, intrigued by Joan Borysenko's *The Power of the Mind to Heal* and James LeFanu's *The Rise and Fall of Modern Medicine*, uplifted by Bernie Siegal's *Love, Medicine and Miracles* and amused by Robert Holden's *Laughter, The Best Medicine*. I find Martin especially convincing, considering that the book is primarily about how the mind can make us ill rather than well. He concludes that although it is a trickier proposition to condition an increase in the immune sytem, rather than suppressing it with drugs, it can be done such as in the enhancement of antibody production and natural killer cell activity. Borysenko claims it is easy to condition the immune system, for example by practising forgiveness and feelings of joy, but try explaining that to a reductionist! Siegal is appalled at the negative attitude of many doctors when they run out of orthodox treatment options, and LeFanu regards the 'obsession with the new' (fostered by the drug companies) as ignoring the wisdom of the past. Much of what I have read appeals to common sense — that hope, a humorous attitude, a fighting spirit and strong, supportive relationships are good for both mental and physical health. I now have scientific reasons for compelling my wife to continuing our cuddles after it is time for her to go to work.

Mary: 'I shall be late'

Robert: 'Ah, but you are boosting my antibody production!'

As I should know from my counselling background, it is not so much the actual control individuals have over stressors, but the degree of control they believe they have. Perceptions are all important and Paul Martin shrewdly observes that complementary medicine typically offers patients a greater sense of personal control over their problems, which helps to explain its broad and growing appeal. In the USA, complementary medicine consultations have long since outstripped orthodox ones. LeFanu links the popularity to the undivided attention (and sometimes the physical manipulation) offered by its practitioners, in contrast to expensive overinvestigation and overtreatment in a hospital bed.

Some of my visualizations of late have been X certificate as I attempt to go one stage further — to regress my tumours. Woody Allen's film *Antz* provided the inspiration for my most violent psychodrama, in which wave upon wave of ants (my killer cells) do battle with the predatory termites (cancer cells), eventually overwhelming them by sheer force of numbers. According to Siegal visualization takes advantage of a 'weakness' of the body, in that it cannot distinguish between vivid mental and actual physical experiences.

'Belief shapes the power of the treatment.' (Bernie Siegal)

Personality and change

'Presume not that I am the thing I was; for God doth know, so shall the world perceive, that I have turned away my former self'. (Hal, in *Henry IV Part 2*, William Shakespeare 1598)

I have long been fascinated by the concept of determinism and, in my early days as a lecturer I used to tantalize planning students with questions like — 'Can design breed crime?' Later I would discuss environmental determinism within the wider nature/nurture debate and, three careers later, I have addressed the question of the likely links between my personality, behaviour, and cancer. I am close to the 'type C' personality and I have had clinical depression which are, allegedly, predisposing factors for cancer. However, I refuse to blame myself entirely for getting cancer in the first place, or to believe my personality was 'hard wired' by the age of six. Being married to an uncomplicated optimist helps me to believe in change.

At first I struggled to embrace the idea of lasting change, so on a bad day I was a 'retired careers counsellor' and on a good day a 'writer'. My counsellor is particularly good at reminding me of the intrinsic and therapeutic value of my writing: it does not require a breakthrough with the BBC Drama Department to justify my efforts. I took enormous satisfaction from not only completing my first book *Counselling as a Career*, but marketing and selling it too (copies for readers available direct from Baldrick Press, at 32 William Street, Oxford, OX3 0ER, at a bargain price of £4.95!). There was a predictably mixed reception to my politically incorrect cartoons, Basil Fawlty on the front cover, and the outrageous (spoof) chapter on 'Counselling in sport and entertainment', but customer satisfaction was high and the excellent reviews were terrific for morale. Audience laughter at my 1997 autumn production of *The Awkward Squad* was music to my ears, never mind the fact that it was only an amateur production, running for three nights in a village hall.

I listened recently to a fascinating lecture on 'Solution focused counselling' in which clients are encouraged to focus on what was going well, rather than badly in their lives. This reminded me of Bernie Siegal's passionate plea to remember the, say, two out of ten who survive a cancer rather than highlighting the eight out of ten who do not. In *The Choice* (BBC Radio 4, October 1999) a young mother of four described her harrowing decision to have a double mastectomy because she had a genetically determined 85% chance of later getting breast cancer. What saddened me was the absence of discussion on why 15% did not get the disease. By chance? I doubt it.

I determined to change in healthy ways such as avoiding stress but taking calculated risks with my writing, not bottling up emotions such as anger, and trusting my intuition. A lifetime devotee of writing and performing satirical comedy, I have applied this to my new status as a terminally ill cancer patient. For example, on those rare occasions when anybody asked me about my cancer I might answer in the manner of Hyacinth Bucket (TV sitcom: *Keeping Up Appearances*) — 'Well of course mine is very rare you know, not one of these more common cancers, such as the bowel'. More seriously, I choose to interpret the rarity of my cancer as an advantage — because they knew relatively little about it, maybe its progress would be less predictable and subject to much individual variation. Uncertainty nurtures hope.

'To live is to suffer: to survive is to find meaning in the suffering.' (Victor Frankl)

Conclusions

'The secret of reaping the greatest enjoyment from life is to live dangerously.' (Nietzsche)

I would not wish my cancer onto anybody, neither would I dream of calling it a 'gift', or 'God's will' as some do, and yet it is true to say that the three and a half years since diagnosis have been amongst the best of my life. This is partly explained by the fact that I have lived life positively and creatively one day at a time, a philosophy I generally recommend. Cancer gave me an excuse to take risks, to plunge myself into creative writing and it has given me, paradoxically, a new lease of life. Of course I am biased about complementary medicine and, if my head is in the clouds, then my feet are on the ground, my heart is roughly in the right place and rules my head.

There is compelling evidence that we patients can play an active, creative part in palliative care, or prevention, or remission, or cure of our cancers. We can exert some positive influence over our own immune systems. We are more than bundles of cells and symptoms, all with the same average forecast five year survival rate, to be drugged, irradiated, or operated upon by body-part mechanics. I am flattered to be regarded by some kind people as exceptional, courageous, and so on, but the fact is I have no desire to be a maverick patient — the exception that proves the rule. I want others to have the chance to work in genuine, creative partnership with health professionals in order to, if not ultimately defeat cancer, then at least take away some of its awesome power. To exercise some control, to feel better, to live better, and probably longer.

'Who wants to be 98 anyway? Someone who is 97.' (George Melly)

References

Borysenko, J. and Miroslav, (1995). *The power of the mind to heal.* Eden Grove Editions, Enfield, Middlesex.

Fleetwood Mac (1988). *Don't Stop,* Warner Bros.

Holden, R. (1993). *Laughter, the best medicine.* Thorsons, London.

LeFanu, J. (1999). *The rise and fall of modern medicine.* Little Brown and Co, London.

Martin, P. (1997). *The sickening mind.* Flamingo, London.

Ross, R. (1997). *Counselling as a career.* Baldrick Press, Oxford.

Siegal, B. (1988). *Love, medicine and miracles.* Arrow.

Chapter 4

Researching complementary therapies in cancer care

Rebecca Rees

Rebecca Rees worked for five years promoting research and audit with the independent charity, the Research Council for Complementary Medicine. She is now working on synthesizing research findings in the fields of health promotion and education at the Institute of Education's Evidence-informed Policy and Practice Information and Co-ordinating Centre.

This chapter provides a brief overview of research issues in complementary medicine and describes further sources of information and support. Since people who have had a diagnosis of cancer use complementary therapies to a significant degree, healthcare professionals need to provide advice and make clinical and management decisions about these therapies. This work should be informed by research evidence wherever possible.

Unfortunately, the research base in complementary medicine is extremely patchy. Some therapies are far more researched than others but high quality research into their use for cancer is scarce. An assessment of the past climate for complementary medicine research provides insights into how research needs to be driven in future. There is a burning need in cancer care, as in other areas of healthcare, for a systematic appraisal of research already done. The priorities set for future work should take into account a wide range of perspectives so that we start to have research studies centred on patients' and carers' needs.

Why do research into complementary therapies in cancer care?

Complementary therapies appear to be a relatively permanent feature of cancer care. One recent population study (Rees *et al.* 2000) found that over a third of women diagnosed with breast cancer in the South Thames NHS region had visited a complementary therapist since their diagnosis. A further 15% had not visited a complementary therapist but had bought an over-the-counter product. An earlier survey of people attending two London oncology departments (Downer *et al.* 1994) found that 16% had used a complementary approach. Use in cancer care settings is common. One early national survey (Wilkes 1992) found that approximately 70% of UK hospices were offering massage and aromatherapy services. A more recent, unpublished, nationwide hospice study by the Sara Lee Trust (Whitehead, personal communication) appears to have found similar levels. Over half of the hospices responding to this survey claimed to provide at least three therapies.

This level of interest means that, increasingly, people working in cancer care will have to make decisions about complementary therapies that will affect the care of patients. Clinicians will be asked for advice as to which therapy their patients should try; managers and clinicians will be asked to work together to produce guidelines for therapy use. Some centres are employing independent complementary therapists on a pilot basis and are having to decide which therapies to provide. Many health professionals have now received some complementary medicine training and, to varying degrees, will be applying this in day-to-day practice.

There is growing agreement that clinical decisions such as these must be informed by reliable information from well designed research studies (Higginson 1999; Sackett *et al.* 1996): individual or even group beliefs are not enough. We all have perceptions about what is going on around us but these can be misleading. Our memories deceive us, tending to hold examples of the extreme, rather than a balanced overview of all that we have experienced.

Practitioners may tend, for example, to remember patients whose care went particularly well or particularly badly, rather than the far larger number whose care was more routine. We all also tend to have pet subjects or interests that stay at the front of our minds, influencing the things we remember and the way we see things.

A variety of research methods have been developed in an attempt to overcome some of these biases. These methods allow us to answer questions in a systematic and transparent way that itself is also open to scrutiny and criticism. The results of research, along with personal and group experience, can make up a kind of evidence jigsaw. As we get more and more pieces we slowly start to describe the complex picture of care.

Research has been carried out in complementary medicine but it can be hard to find. Anyone turning unprepared to the complementary medicine literature will find themselves faced with a large number of descriptive pieces that introduce therapies and present competing claims for effectiveness. Research papers are scattered throughout a large number of journals, often ones that are not indexed by *Medline* or other well known bibliographic databases. Luckily there are a growing number of initiatives working to make complementary medicine research findings more accessible and usable (Box 1).

Box 1. Sources of information and support for complementary medicine research

Research Council for Complementary Medicine (RCCM). The RCCM is an independent research charity founded in 1983. It carries out, promotes, and facilitates rigorous research in complementary medicine to encourage safe and effective practice and improved patient care. The organization runs an information service based on CISCOM, an in-house database of over 60 000 published papers. CISCOM is regularly updated with specialized searches of bibliographic databases such as *Medline, Embase,* and the British Library's *AMED,* along with citation tracking. It covers both clinical and

Box 1. Sources of information and support for complementary medicine research (continued)

social aspects of complementary medicine. Searches can distinguish between research studies and opinion pieces. A subset of the CISCOM database forms part of the trials register for the Cochrane Collaboration's complementary medicine field (see below). The RCCM provides a selection of references and advice for researchers on-line via its internet web page. Contact: Research Council for Complementary Medicine, 10 Church St, Steeple Bumpstead, Haverhill, Suffolk CB9 7DG. Tel: +44(O) 1440 730901. Fax: +44 (O) 1440 730088. Email: info@rccm.org.uk. Internet: www.rccm.org.uk.

The Cochrane Collaboration complementary medicine field. Cochrane fields work with Cochrane Collaboration review groups (see below). The fields focus on dimensions of healthcare other than health problems, such as the setting of care (e.g. primary care), the type of consumer (e.g. older people), the type of provider (e.g. nurses), or the type of intervention (e.g. physical therapies). Field activities include the hand-searching of specialist journals, commenting on reviews related to the field's specialist area and the compilation of specialist databases of reviews. At the start of 1998, 11 systematic reviews had investigated complementary therapy approaches and a further 12 reviews were at the protocol development stage. Topics include: St John's Wort for depression, music therapy for dementia, therapeutic touch for wound healing, acupuncture for lower back pain, headache and arthritis. Contact: Cochrane Collaboration complementary medicine field, Dr Brian Berman, Convenor, University of Maryland School of Medicine, Kernan Hospital Mansion, 3rd Floor, 2200 N Forest, Park Avenue, Baltimore MD 21207–6697, USA. Telephone: +1 410 448 6871. Fax: +1 410 448 6875. Email: bberman@compmed.ummc.ab.umd.edu.

The Cochrane Collaboration. This prepares, maintains, and promotes the accessibility of systematic reviews of the effects of healthcare. It is an international initiative, founded in 1993 by 77 people from 11 countries. The Collaboration has over 40 review groups covering different health problems. Review group members include researchers, healthcare professionals, consumers, and others. The groups produce systematic reviews which are published electronically in successive issues of *The Cochrane Database of Systematic Reviews*. The Cochrane Database is available in bigger healthcare libraries. It is accessible via the internet, where abstracts of reviews can be browsed without a subscription. Contact: UK Cochrane Centre, Dr Iain Chalmers, Director, UK Cochrane Centre, Summertown Pavilion, Middle Way, Oxford OX2 7LG, UK. Telephone: +44 (0)1865 516300. Fax: +44 (0)1865 516311. Email: general@cochrane.co.uk. Internet: http:// hiru.mcmaster.ca/cochrane/default.html.

The National Center for Complementary and Alternative Medicine (NCCAM). This centre was established by the US government in 1998, as a part of the US National Institutes of Health (NIH). The Centre has a $50 million budget for 1999. It funds 11 specialty CAM research centres, with average budgets over three years of $850 000. Specialties include pain, ageing, immunology, cancer, and HIV/AIDS. The Centre runs a public information clearinghouse. Contact: NCCAM Clearinghouse, Box 8218, Silver Spring, Maryland 20907–8218, USA. Telephone: + 1 888 644 6226. Fax: +1 301 495 495. Internet: http://nccam.nih.gov/.

What kinds of research have been carried out?

A review of research into complementary medicine needs to be systematic if it is to produce meaningful and valid results. Systematic reviews involve an extensive search for both published and unpublished studies and a thorough appraisal of the study methods and results of each relevant paper. There have only been a small number of systematic reviews of complementary therapy approaches. Good sources for these are CISCOM, the Research Council for Complementary Medicine's in-house register of research, and the Cochrane Library (see Box 1). However, few of these systematic reviews cover questions relevant to cancer care.

Several authors have presented preliminary, non-systematic overviews of complementary medicine research (e.g. Cassileth 1999; Vickers 1996). A recent, more general introduction to complementary medicine has assessed the research base on a therapy by therapy basis (Zollman and Vickers 1999). These studies help put some of the recent research into a clinical context. This section aims to outline the extent of research in various areas, highlighting the gaps and opportunities for further research, rather than identifying therapies or conditions that have been well covered.

Research into the effectiveness of different complementary approaches to cancer has been carried out. Careful searches in bibliographic databases for complementary medicine research can find several hundred studies of different degrees of relevance to cancer care. For example, a broad search of CISCOM for randomized controlled trials (RCTs) involving people diagnosed with cancers will find over 150 studies. At the time of writing, CISCOM held sixteen or so RCTs that involved patients in receipt of palliative care. We find slightly more RCTs if we broaden our search to include trials that look at well-being and at symptoms related to cancer and cancer treatments. Over five hundred RCTs have looked at complementary approaches to pain, for example. A further 100 or so RCTs have looked at the effects of various therapies on nausea.

A wide range of research methods have been applied to the study of complementary therapies. The randomized controlled trial research design aims to answer the question, 'Which approach appears to be the most effective?' By randomly allocating patients to two or more treatment groups. the groups should differ only in terms of the treatment they receive. Thus the differences seen between groups after treatment are likely to be due to the treatments alone.

An important, if far smaller, body of research has asked different kinds of questions about complementary cancer care. Surveys, as illustrated earlier, can provide essential information about the level of use and attitudes towards complementary therapy use. In addition, a small number of studies have evaluated the processes of complementary cancer care, asking, for example, 'What do patients say they want from their treatment and what are we providing?' (e.g. Kite et al. 1998). In-depth qualitative studies have also provided valuable information (e.g. Montbriand 1997).

The remainder of this chapter focuses on controlled trials, mainly because this is the study type most investigated. The value of different research methods to complementary medicine research is covered in a number of introductory texts (e.g. Vickers 1995).

The complementary therapy research literature is dominated by a small number of therapies. The RCTs found on CISCOM give an idea of where most cancer care research interest has centred. Of the palliative care studies, six look at the potential impact of relaxation techniques, three at herbal treatments, three at acupuncture, and the remainder at healing, hypnosis, and aromatherapy massage. Of the RCTs of cancer treatments, almost half look at the effects of herbal treatments. The majority of the remainder are either studies of so-called 'talk therapies', such as counselling, or of a variety of meditation or relaxation approaches. Most of the studies of treatments for pain investigate acupuncture or relaxation techniques. Over three-quarters of the studies that compare nausea treatments look at acupuncture.

Some approaches are seriously lacking in a research base. Research has only just started in some of the therapies that appear to be most used within cancer care. Reflexology, where points on the feet are used to identify and treat problem areas elsewhere in the body, is a case in point: this therapy has been the subject of fewer than ten published controlled trials, none of which involve cancer patients. Several studies have looked at the effects of essential oils in a laboratory environment, on micro-organisms, for example, or on experimental animals. However databases such as CISCOM currently identify fewer than twenty published studies involving patients where aromatherapy massage using essential oils has been compared with other treatments. Only a fraction of these trials involve cancer patients.

The quality and findings of this research base

Unfortunately, much of the complementary medicine research published to date has serious methodological shortcomings. As an indication of this, most systematic reviews of research in complementary medicine note that the poor quality of studies makes it very difficult to reach firm conclusions (Hammerschlag and Morris 1997; Kleijnen *et al.* 1991; Seers and Carroll 1998 are examples of potential relevance to cancer care). Authors frequently provide insufficient details of their methods or results, leaving readers unable to give a study the critical appraisal that it needs. In further cases, study methods are quite seriously flawed. Another problem is the small size of many studies. Very few published complementary medicine trials have involved the numbers of patients routinely expected of conventional treatments.

Perhaps the most important problem with complementary medicine research is that the vast majority of studies have been designed to answer questions that are of little relevance to people having to make clinical decisions. Acupuncture, one of the most researched areas of complementary medicine, can be used to illustrate this point. A palliative care specialist might want to know, for example, whether acupuncture is at least as effective for chronic pain as available medication options. The research base for acupuncture initially looks promising: there is a considerable body of high quality preclinical research that helps explain how stimulation of acupuncture points might have physiological effects on the body; 40 or so systematic reviews of controlled trials of acupuncture have been published; there are over 500 randomized controlled trials involving some form of acupuncture. However, a large proportion of these studies have: a) attempted to establish whether acupuncture is a placebo or not; or b) investigated the effect of acupuncture on experimentally induced or acute pain, often postoperative; or c) measured the outcomes of treatment over extremely short periods of time. The specialist's question remains unanswered.

Why is the complementary medicine research base in this state?

Box 2 outlines some of the problems that have faced those wanting to research complementary approaches to date. Most of these can be seen to be practical, rather than theoretical in nature. One assumption that is sometimes made by people relatively new to the complementary medicine field is particularly important to deal with: the idea that complementary therapies need a completely different set of research methodologies and that conventional approaches to research should be discarded. Complementary practitioners have historically been concerned that research would fail to measure the essence of their therapies. Common themes are the need to account for the therapist's individualized approach to patients and the subtleties of clinical improvement in complementary therapy patients.

Box 2. Factors influencing complementary medicine research

The environment for therapist training and practice

Historically, most therapists were trained at private colleges and practised privately. A recognition of the value of research and what it requires has only recently begun to emerge among training centres. For the more established therapies, courses are becoming available within university settings. Training in research methods and in critical appraisal of published research are being introduced. An academic infrastructure is starting to develop, providing access, for example, to computer and library facilities, university research grants, and supervisory and methodological support. Therapists are also being introduced to research through increased levels of complementary therapy provision on the NHS.

Lack of funding

The pharmaceutical industry has been most interested in funding complementary medicine research when this has the potential to lead to a patentable, over the counter product. Herbal preparations are therefore relatively well represented in the research literature. Conventional funding bodies have been hesitant to award funds to previously unresearched areas. In 1995, less than a tenth of a percent of NHS research funds were spent on complementary medicine.

Insufficient patient numbers

Without relatively widespread provision of CM it is difficult to study in practice. Recruitment for studies is difficult: private practitioners tend to have small clinic list sizes and tend to see very small numbers of patients with the same clinical condition; private patients may be less interested in the prospect of randomized allocation to different treatments.

Methodological challenges

Complementary treatment is a very diverse and almost unmapped entity. Patient responses to treatment may be unpredictable. As is the case for surgery, speech therapy, and other areas of healthcare, blinding patients or therapists to treatment may sometimes be difficult. Little is known as to which aspects of complementary therapy care are important. This leads to difficulties when setting the boundaries for what package of care is to be evaluated.

The argument for discarding currently used research methods is, however, extremely weak. There has been good and useful complementary medicine research using established methods (Levin *et al.* 1997). Furthermore, research itself has changed over the last few years and should continue to be responsive to perceived needs in healthcare practice. Researchers have taken considerable steps for quite some time to address the concerns of professionals of all sorts who are concerned that the subtleties of their practice will be overlooked. Key research funders are aware that they need to respond to these developments.

The sum effect of the problems outlined in Box 2 is that complementary medicine research to date has tended to be opportunistic and carried out in relative isolation. Practitioners have tended to work outside of the university and NHS systems that are a fundamental support for most healthcare research. Because of a lack of resources of all kinds, research has taken place where it is simplest.

As a result, instead of the chronic, complex problems experienced by those using and practising complementary therapies, research has mainly focused on acute conditions. It has also been carried out where patients are relatively easy to recruit, for example when they are undergoing simple operative procedures. In short, research in complementary medicine has been driven, not by any thought-through programme of research needs, but by whoever happened to have a personal interest, research support, and an available clinical population, when small pockets of money became available.

Improving the evidence-base

There are signs that many of the practical constraints to research in complementary medicine are lessening. Conventional funding bodies are starting to show an interest in complementary therapies and a research ethos is beginning to grow among practitioners. In cancer care, as in other fields, there needs to be greater communication between experienced researchers and those wanting to carry out research. There also needs to be an increased understanding of the practicalities of research. For every research study that reaches the publication stage there are many more that founder because a researcher underestimates the quantity of work and resources involved in managing patient recruitment, data collection, treatments, team working, analysis, and writing up. Box 3 is a list of practical considerations recommended by staff at the RCCM for all those new to research.

Box 3. Advice for individuals who are considering doing complementary medicine research

The RCCM has considerable experience of advising researchers with an interest in complementary medicine, particularly those without previous research experience. We have found the following to be useful:

1. Collaborate. Research has been likened to mountain climbing: first timers rarely make it to the top without the guidance of an experienced individual. Collaboration with someone based in a well-resourced institution, such as a medical school or university is a good idea. Useful institutional resources include libraries, library staff, computing facilities, statistical departments.

Box 3. Advice for individuals who are considering doing complementary medicine research *(continued)*

2. What is your question? Many aspects of research design depend upon the question asked. Interestingly, many of the potential researchers contacting the RCCM find it hard to frame a simple question to illustrate their research interest. For example, 'to investigate the effectiveness of a herbal remedy for cystitis' or to 'investigate massage for cancer patients' might be proffered, but these are clearly not questions.

3. One question at a time. The phrase 'a journey of a thousand miles starts with one small step' is a good metaphor for health research. Overviews such as the one contained in this chapter show that questions such as 'does acupuncture work?' will not be resolved in a single study. Researchers need to break down large, global, questions into manageable stages: a series of questions each associated with a single study.

4. Understand your subject. Research demands an understanding of the subject under study. We would not expect, say, an aromatherapist to design a study of surgery without consulting a surgeon. Researchers without a thorough knowledge of complementary medicine should collaborate with experienced complementary practitioners and should be sensitive to the sometimes subtle differences between therapeutic approaches.

5. Keep things simple. Research almost always turns out more complicated than predicted. Studies involving multiple measures of outcome, complex designs, or large numbers of patients should be avoided by all but the most experienced researchers. Generally speaking, the less data you aim to collect, the better.

6. Get the fundamentals right. Research with basic methodological flaws is as good as worthless, no matter how appropriate it may seem for the special problems of complementary medicine. Researchers should have a thorough understanding of the criteria used to assess methodological rigour for the type of research they wish to undertake. Experts in methodology should be consulted at the very earliest stages of developing a research protocol.

7. Build on existing research. Research is a cumulative enterprise. A literature review can help a researcher to define a study topic, identify appropriate research designs and avoid the mistakes of previous workers. We normally recommend that researchers identify as many studies as possible on both the therapy and the condition under investigation. Since they are often of better quality or better reported, studies of conventional approaches should be examined too. In-depth reading of the research literature may be the single most important preparation for a prospective researcher.

8. Think whether you would prefer to focus initially on clinical audit. Audit is a way of using enquiry to improve care. Where research usually aims to provide information that is relevant to a wide readership, audit focuses on bringing about simple, positive changes to clinical settings or procedures. Examples might include a review of case notes against locally or professionally agreed standards that results in a new case note design. Advice on audit is available from the RCCM.

9. Plan to publish. For scientific work to be of value it must enter the public arena.

Meanwhile, more work to review the research base systematically for the use of therapies is needed urgently. The raw materials for this kind of research are available in the form of published studies. Individuals undertaking systematic reviews can count upon the supportive framework of the Cochrane Collaboration. While research is lacking, there can be considerable value in using formal consensus development methods to decide which complementary approaches to continue using and how (Murphy *et al.* 1998).

Ultimately a planned approach to research is required. It should not be driven merely by the interests of individual therapists or researchers. Prioritization exercises tend to show that health professionals want research to be undertaken on questions that arise in their day to day practice. Because each group of health professionals has a different role in care, each set of priorities will be different. In a recent study by Cawley and Webber (1995) research questions concerning complementary therapies were high on the prioritized lists of palliative care nurses and physiotherapists but absent from those of Macmillan nurses, social workers, and doctors. Patient and carer priorities for research are likely to be different again.

Patient involvement in deciding research priorities might appear at first to be too much to ask, both of users of services and of those developing research programmes. However valuable lessons have been learned from a number of projects (Oliver 1995). A strategic plan for complementary medicine research that takes patient and carer perspectives into account is essential if we are to provide the best and most appropriate forms of therapy for people needing cancer care.

References

Cassileth, B. R. (1999). Complementary therapies: overview and state of the art. *Cancer Nursing*, 22, 85–90.

Cawley, N. and Webber, J. (1995). Research priorities in paliative care. *International Journal of Palliative Nursing*, 1, 101–13.

Downer, S. M. Cody, M. M., McCluskey, P. *et al.* (1994). Pursuit and practice of complementary therapies by cancer patients receiving conventional treatment. *British Medical Journal*, 309, 86–9.

Hammerschlag, R. and Morris, M. M. (1997). Clinical trials comparing acupuncture with biomedical standard care: a criteria-based evaluation of research design and reporting, *Complementary Therapies in Medicine*, 5, 133–40.

Higginson, I. J. (1999). Evidence-based palliative care. *British Medical Journal*, 319, 462–3.

Kite, S. M. Maher, E. J. Anderson, K., *et al.* (1998). Development of an aromatherapy service at a Cancer Centre. *Palliative Medicine*, 12, 171–80.

Kleijnen, J., Knipschild, P., and ter Riet, G. (1991). Clinical trials of homoeopathy, *British Medical Journal*, 302, 316–23.

Levin, J. S., Glass, T. A., Kushi, L. H., *et al.* (1997). Quantitative methods in research on complementary and alternative medicine. A methodological manifesto. NIH Office of Alternative Medicine. *Medical Care*, 35, 1079–94.

Montbriand, M. J. (1997). Abandoning biomedicine for alternate therapies: oncology patients' stories. *Cancer Nursing*, 21, 36–45.

Murphy, M. K., Black, N. A., Lamping, D. L., *et al.* (1998). Consensus development methods, and their use in clinical guideline development. *Health Technology Assessment*, 2 (3).

Oliver, S. (1995). How can health service users contribute to the NHS research and development programme? *British Medical Journal*, 310, 1318–20.

Rees, R., Feigel, I., Vickers, A., Zollman, C., McGurk, R., Smith, C. (2000). Prevalence of complementary therapy use by women with breast cancer: a population-based survey. *European Journal of Cancer.* **36**, 1359–64.

Sackett, D. L., Rosenberg, W. M., Gray, J. A., *et al.* (1996). Evidence based medicine: what it is and what it isn't. *British Medical Journal,* Jan 13, **312**, 71–2.

Seers, K. and Carroll, D. (1998). Relaxation techniques for acute pain management: a systematic review. *Journal of Advanced Nursing,* **27**, 466–75.

Vickers, A. J. (1995). A basic introduction to medical research. Part ii: an overview of different research methods. *Complementary Therapies in Nursing and Midwifery,* **1**, 113–7.

Vickers, A. J. (1996). Complementary therapies in palliative care: the research evidence. *European Journal of Palliative Care,* **3**, 150–3.

Wilkes, E. (1992). *Complementary therapy in hospice and palliative care* Unpublished study available from: Trent Palliative Care Centre, Abbey Lane, Sheffield S11 9NE, UK.

Zollman, C. and Vickers, A. (1999). ABC of complementary medicine: What is complementary medicine? *British Medical Journal,* **319**, 693–6.

Chapter 5

Health service planning issues: the UK perspective

Chris Worth

Chris Worth was formerly a Director of Public Health in Huddersfield, West Yorkshire. For several years he has been an advocate for the NHS to explore the wider integration of complementary therapies more thoroughly.

A number of complementary therapies (notably homoeopathy, acupuncture, osteopathy) have been available within the National Health Service (NHS) since its establishment in 1948. There has been an increasing understanding and usage of these therapies since the 1970s. Equally, there has been an expansion in the number and range of therapies covered by such practitioners (Fulder and Munro 1981). However, a clear distinction between an orthodox medical profession and a 'fringe' of alternative practitioners, which was first given legislative force in the 1858 Medical Registration Act, still exists (Mercer *et al.* 1995). This has been repeatedly confirmed, particularly with the almost complete exclusion of unorthodox, 'alternative' practitioners from the publicly-funded healthcare system when the NHS was established.

The medical establishment's antagonism in the 1980s to the growing public interest in the use of complementary therapies was, perhaps, best illustrated in the 1986 British Medical Association Report, *Alternative Therapy* (BMA 1986). The report was particularly remembered for statements about the lack of scientific research for many therapies. Indeed, there were clearly expressed doubts as to whether these therapies could be evaluated through clinical trials.

The introduction of reforms to the NHS in the early 1990s promoted major organizational change. The establishment of the internal market in healthcare created significant opportunities for the new commissioning organizations (health authorities/boards, general practitioner fundholders) to introduce complementary therapies more broadly into the NHS. In addition, the development of the single market in the European Community in 1993 focused attention on the possibility of greater harmonization *inter alia* over the regulation of, and access to, complementary therapies (Lewith and Aldridge 1991).

In response to the changing political climate, the BMA produced a second report (BMA 1993), very different in its structure and tone to its previous report on the issue (BMA

1986). The later report called for better systems of regulation, including registration, improved professional standards, training, and research.

An independent study carried out for the English Department of Health (Thomas *et al.* 1995) reported that almost 40% of GP partnerships in England provided access to complementary medicine for NHS patients. About one-quarter of practices reported making NHS referrals for complementary therapies. Acupuncture and homoeopathy were the most commonly provided, though the most frequently employed practitioners were osteopaths. The reasons for the growth in the use of these therapies within the NHS are not clear. The climate, world-wide, of rapidly rising health expenditure and the trend towards managed care may have encouraged GPs to hope that non-conventional therapies could be effective and cost-beneficial. Experience by practitioners within the NHS, backed by accepted research methodology, has confirmed that use of certain complementary therapies has resulted in the improved management for chronic inflammatory diseases, stress-related and functional conditions, common musculoskeletal disorders, and pain (Coates *et al.*1998). These are conditions which orthodox practitioners find difficult to manage, but these are the conditions patients also most often take to complementary practitioners.

The changing attitudes to complementary medicine in the 1990s can be summarized thus:

- an estimated 4–5 million people a year in the United Kingdom visit complementary practitioners (RCCM 1997);
- about 14–20% of patients with chronic disease have consulted complementary practitioners (RCCM 1997);
- about three-quarters of the public support NHS access to complementary medicine (RCCM 1997);
- declining public faith in the NHS and its use of drugs (Worth 1999);
- increasing media interest and support for complementary medicine and the role of highly placed 'champions' assigned to complementary therapies (Worth 1999);
- increased public wish to take more responsibility for health choices (Coates *et al.* 1998);
- greater emphasis on consumer choice and patient care (Coates *et al.* 1998);
- the British Medical Association's increasingly positive attitude to complementary medicine with the emphasis on supporting good practice in co-operation, education and research (BMA 1993);
- rising levels of complementary medicine-based research and outcome study publication in mainstream peer-reviewed journals (Coates *et al.* 1998);
- the establishment in the late 1990s of the General Osteopathic Council and General Chiropractic Council as statutory bodies to regulate these professions;
- political will to encourage greater use of complementary therapies (Scottish Office Department of Health 1996) with NHS management in some areas supporting some important pilot initiatives (Cameron-Blackie and Mouncer 1993).

In spite of these changing attitudes in recent years, a number of barriers have persisted. These have led to very variable 'take-up' of complementary therapies within the national health public-sector funded purpose. The barriers include:

- lack of knowledge of practitioners or therapists to whom referral might be appropriate;
- lack of available funds (within the NHS to promote research on efficacy, effectiveness, or appropriate delivery system);
- lack of clarity on the competence of complementary practitioners and, indeed, some of the regulatory organizations;
- frequent assumptions and contradictory views about the amount, availability, and reliability of evidence relating to the effectiveness of complementary therapies.

These barriers have been cited frequently (NHS Confederation 1997; Worth 1999). Healthcare purchasers have been hampered by the lack of credible research-based evidence on complementary therapies (Mercer *et al.* 1995). Indeed, the difficulty of evaluating some therapies and the fact that much research on complementary therapies in recent years has been based on case-studies (as opposed to the 'gold standard' randomized controlled trials) has been acknowledged. The increasing move in the 1990s towards the recognition of purchasing *appropriate* healthcare (be it conventional or complementary) encouraged a greater move by all interested health agencies and organizations to research the literature base of many complementary therapies.

Whether assessing the efficacy, effectiveness, safety, or mechanisms of action, it is acknowledged that research into complementary therapies has tended to be carried out as a collection of isolated studies (Coates *et al.* 1998). Reasons for this include the lack of appropriate infrastructure and funding for research. The lack of effective research methodology and properly trained researchers have also been suggested (Coates *et al.* 1998). In the United States of America, the established Office of Complementary and Alternative Medicine (OCAM) produced a report (Panel Report 1997) on appropriate methods and strategies which identified a number of common failures when a strategic approach was not adopted. The failures included:

- using untested interventions of definitive trials;
- researching the mechanisms of action of a non-pharmacological therapy before establishing whether it was clinically beneficial;
- developing outcome measures at the same time as evaluating a therapy;
- unnecessary replication of negative research. Luff and Thomas (1999) noted that the evidence base for complementary therapies in primary care was limited and had played a small part in the way that services had been set up and operated.

One of the barriers to greater recognition, and perhaps take-up, of particular complementary therapies is the complex issue of regulation. In the United Kingdom, non-medically qualified complementary therapists can practise (under common law) irrespective of their levels of training or clinical knowledge. These practitioners are subject only to the relevant provisions, in the UK, of such statutes as the *Medical, Dental, Professions Supplementary to Medicine and Medicines Acts*. Interestingly, under other legislation, practitioners must not make claims or advertise the treatment of certain diseases which include cancer (Coates *et al.* 1998).

During the 1980s and 1990s, in the United Kingdom, different approaches to regulatory structures by individual professional organizations within a therapeutic area had emerged. Where such organizations had worked closely together (for example, in chiropractic, homoeopathy, osteopathy, acupuncture), improved training and greater public (and wider professional) recognition had followed. This had been seen particularly in the fields of osteopathy and chiropractic where General Councils had been enacted (through Parliament) in the 1990s in a similar way to other 'professional' groups, e.g. doctors (General Medical Council).

A number of commentators have raised the question, however, as to whether there can be a single regulatory system for all complementary therapies, in a way similar to the medical profession. Advocates of this approach argue that a greater acceptance by conventional professional groups, the public, and healthcare purchasers would quickly follow. Given the diversity of complementary therapies it seems unlikely that this would occur as no one over-riding system would be appropriate. The creation of a credible and effective system of voluntary self-regulation would seem to provide the most achievable and desirable way forward (Coates *et al.* 1998).

Subtle Government changes in attitude towards complementary therapies in the 1990s have further developed the debate about the wider use of complementary medicines within the public sector. In Scotland, for example, political will allowed these approaches to be more available within the NHS (Scottish Office 1996).

About one-fifth of patients with chronic disease, e.g. backache, stress, persistent pain, have consulted complementary therapists and approximately one-quarter of the public in a number of surveys have used complementary therapies at some time. The latter is higher in certain European countries. For example, surveys have shown that up to 40% of the French have used homoeopathic remedies for a range of conditions. In the United Kingdom, about 4–5 million people per year visit complementary therapists and about three-quarters of those surveyed say that they would do so if complementary therapies were more widely available within the NHS (RCCM 1997). What, therefore, are the opportunities and possibilities of this happening within the 'new, modern, NHS'?

The publication of *The new NHS — modern, dependable* (Department of Health 1997) created an important change in healthcare policy in the United Kingdom. The deliberately competitive 'internal market' created by the Conservative administration of the early 1990s was replaced by a more partnership-dominated policy. The previous purchaser–provider scenario consisted of healthcare being purchased on behalf of their respective populations, by Health Authorities and General Practitioner Fundholders.

Healthcare was 'provided' by NHS Trusts (consisting of a mixture of acute, community, and mental health service provision) and primary care practitioners (general practitioners, dentists, pharmacists, opticians, primary care nurses). Although GP fundholding prompted a clear drift towards two-tier healthcare provision, it allowed some diversity and innovation to take place with consequent new opportunities to allow wider usage of complementary therapies in public sector primary care (Coates *et al.* 1998). Indeed, a Department of Health-commissioned study (Luff and Thomas 1999) identified that the use of GP fundholding savings provided the most accessible of NHS finance for complementary therapy services in primary care. The study demonstrated that the flexibility afforded by GP fundholding enabled a number of schemes to develop and allowed an overall growth in primary care complementary therapy provision.

The introduction of locality commissioning through Primary Care Groups (PCGs) and their equivalents in Wales and Scotland, will undoubtedly set the context for the survival and the development of complementary healthcare services in primary care in the coming years.

The commissioning groups (and primary care trusts) have been established to respond more quickly than health authorities/boards to changing local demands and needs. Although set within the priorities of the Health Improvement Programme of the local health authority/board (but jointly agreed between it and other non-NHS agencies) and national priorities and policies, there is some scope and potential for complementary therapy provision to develop in this context. Recent reports (Coates *et al.* 1998; Luff and Thomas 1999) have clearly demonstrated the importance that this development be closely linked to meeting some (or many) healthcare needs which had been identified previously. This requirement becomes even more paramount in a largely 'cash-limited' public sector health service where rationing decisions have become more and more evident. Current evidence suggests that complementary therapies are often used with conventional care, as opposed to an 'alternative'. Evidence for the effectiveness and cost-effectiveness of many therapies is still not conclusive. These aspects will increasingly be required by healthcare commissioners. Cancer care provides one clear area where commissioning guidelines should be further developed from clinical research and audit.

Many examples are included elsewhere in this book. For example, evidence exists from sound randomized controlled trials for the use of acupuncture to treat chemotherapy nausea (Lewith *et al.* 1996). Evidence from descriptive studies for the use of iscador (a homoeopathic remedy) in improving certain quality of life measures for cancer sufferers has also been described (Fugh-Berman 1996). Guidelines which may incorporate usage of particular complementary therapies are evidence-based: the need, therefore, for a complementary therapy research base becomes even more paramount.

One of the recent changes in health management policy has been a renewed emphasis on the improvement of clinical quality. Under the concept of *clinical governance*, all NHS organizations are required to implement a range of mechanisms (from clinical audit and professional development through to risk assessment) which, it is intended, will lead to greater clinical accountability and, ultimately, improved healthcare. Within this, two national organizations were created in 1999 to ensure that this policy aim occurs. The first, the National Institute for Clinical Excellence (NICE), in England produced a framework which:

- identifies those new treatments and products which are likely to have a significant impact on the NHS;
- enables evidence of clinical and cost effectiveness to be brought together to inform a judgement on the value of the treatment relative to alternative uses of resources in the NHS;
- will result in the issue of guidance on whether the treatment can be recommended for routine use in the NHS.

It is intended that the second organization, the Commission for Health Improvement (CHI) formally launched in April 2000, will act as a performance monitoring agency and will visit all healthcare institutions every three years or so, or as requested.

It is too early to note how these organizations will impact on the further development of complementary therapies within the NHS sector. However, should any examination by NICE or its equivalent in other countries, of a therapy area (under, for example, a health technology assessment) or clinical guidelines involving one or more complementary therapies be carried out, it should be with the same thoroughness as for a conventional clinical area. The implications, therefore, for all practitioners of complementary therapies and researchers are clear.

The need for more evidence-based, soundly researched information on successful health outcomes from the appropriate use of a complementary therapy, provided as part of a guideline-based package of care, is required. Many service providers of complementary therapies are some way from that. The challenge for those providers and all those interested in the wider integration of these therapies within the NHS is to reach this goal.

Other important issues remain. These include the question of more co-ordinated teaching of all healthcare workers, both conventional and complementary, which includes common elements in the core curriculum. The need for some form of appropriately recognized regulatory body for the complementary therapy professions remains. As important is the sharing of knowledge about the use and effectiveness of complementary therapies between the public, health professionals, and therapists. Mechanisms to establish these, perhaps involving, or supported by, the Departments of Health within the UK, are clearly necessary.

The then Secretary of State for Health, Frank Dobson MP, gave a keynote address at a conference in May 1998 organized by the Foundation for Integrated Medicine and attended by many senior NHS managers and leading conventional clinicians. In his speech, he said, 'It is clear that some people with some conditions do not respond to even the most modern orthodox treatment. It is also clear that some of these people can be and are being helped by forms of complementary (and alternative) medicine'. The work for those involved in health service planning is clearly to identify quickly which people can be helped, to explore how their health can be effectively, appropriately, and measurably improved, and to communicate this knowledge widely and clearly to politicians, NHS, and therapy management and most importantly, to the public.

References

British Medical Association (1986). *Report of the Board of Science and Education on alternative therapy.* British Medical Association, London.

British Medical Association (1993). *Complementary medicine: new approaches to good practice.* Oxford University Press.

Cameron-Blackie, G. and Mouncer, Y. (1993). *Complementary therapies in the NHS.* National Association of Health Authorities and Trusts, London.

Coates, J., Jobst, K., Fielding, S., *et al.* (1998). Integrated healthcare: a way forward for the next five years? A discussion document from the Prince of Wales Initiative on Integrated Medicine. *Journal of Alternative and Complementary Medicine*, 4, 209–47.

Department of Health (1997). *The new NHS — modern, dependable.*

Fugh-Berman, A. (1996). *Complementary therapies: what works?* Odonian Press.

Fulder, S. and Munro, R. (1981). *The status of complementary medicine in the United Kingdom.* Threshold Foundation, London.

Lewith, G. T. and Aldridge, D. (ed) (1991). *Complementary medicine and the European Community.* C. W. Daniel, Saffron Walden.

Lewith, G., Kenyon, J., and Lewis, P. (1996). *Complementary therapies: an integrated approach.* Oxford University Press.

Luff, D. and Thomas, K. (1999). *Models of complementary therapy provision in primary care.* School of Health and Related Research, University of Sheffield Medical Care Research Unit, Sheffield.

Mercer, G., Long, A. F., and Smith, I. J. (1995). *Researching and evaluating complementary therapies: the state of the debate.* Nuffield Institute for Health, Leeds.

NHS Confederation (1997). *Complementary medicine in the NHS — managing the issues.* (Birmingham: The NHS Confederation).

Panel Report from the Conference on Complementary Therapies and Alternative Medicine Research Methodology, National Institute of Health, USA (1997). *International Journal of Technology Assessment in Healthcare.* 13, 111–21.

RCCM (Research Council for Complementary Medicine) (1997). *Public usage of complementary medicine: an overview.* Research Council for Complementary Medicine Information Service, London.

Scottish Office Department of Health (1996). *Complementary medicine and the National Health Service.* The Stationary Office, London.

Thomas, K., Fall, M., Parry, G., and Nicholl, J. (1995). *National survey of access to complementary healthcare via general practice.* University of Sheffield.

Worth, C. (1999). Added value? *Complementary Therapies in Nursing and Midwifery*, 5, 19–21.

Chapter 6

A personal view

Thurstan Brewin

Thurstan Brewin is a Fellow of the Royal College of Physicians who, after war service, trained at Guy's Hospital, London; spent five years in Canada with the Ontario Cancer Foundation; 26 years as a Consultant in Clinical Oncology in Glasgow; and has since worked with three medical charities: Marie Curie Cancer Care, the Sue Ryder Foundation, and Healthwatch. He is the main author of two books: *Relating to the Relatives* and *The Friendly Professional*, and has written in medical journals on various subjects including clinical trials, medical ethics, and complementary medicine.

Mainstream and complementary medicine share many things, but there are important differences in training, emphasis, and attitude.

Like all members of the community who offer a service of any kind, both groups want to help those who seek our help. When anyone comes to us with a problem, we like to be thought of as understanding, trustworthy, and competent and — quite apart from earning a living in this way — to be in demand because of our reputation. For most of us it's not just treatment of the main diagnosis, but treatment of the patient, aiming at such things as peace of mind, greater confidence, a positive attitude and no needless fears. In addition, many *physical* symptoms will respond, at least to some extent, to general non-specific measures such as empathy and encouragement, to what psychologists call 'suggestion', and to all the other elements of a good consultation, leading, we hope, to at least a measure of relaxation (both mental and physical) and mood elevation. And, whether or not we fully deserve to take the credit, it's a great thing to see people improving and recovering.

Since mainstream medicine (unlike most complementary medicine) has always been pragmatic and not based on any particular system or theory, there has never been anything to stop any effective remedy from being incorporated into it. The theories and remedies of complementary medicine are simply those that most medical schools, rightly or wrongly, have never found sufficiently convincing to teach. I've spent most of my professional life treating cancer patients and I find that it surprises people when I tell them that we sometimes used herbal remedies. The reason is simple. More than thirty years ago medical research teams tested countless herbs to see if any showed any anticancer properties. Those that did were immediately adopted. Vincristine, for example, from the periwinkle plant, is for this reason part of mainstream medicine.

There have always been some doctors supporting one or more unconventional remedies and they have always been free to do so (though not free to associate with unqualified practitioners until about 25 years ago). But in this essay I will be thinking of the practice of complementary medicine by those who are *not* qualified doctors. A word is needed here about changing definitions. The USA tends to stick to the term 'alternative' medicine, whether or not this is thought of as being complementary to mainstream medicine. In the UK the word complementary has now virtually replaced not only 'alternative', but also earlier words like 'fringe' (once used by its admirers, but now disliked), 'unorthodox', or 'unconventional'. Meanwhile the word 'holistic' remains ambiguous, representing either the common sense 'whole patient' ideal of mainstream medicine, or the more mystical approach of much complementary medicine.

In this broad and oversimplified personal view I have no choice but to generalize and 1would ask any readers who are supporters or practitioners of complementary medicine to forgive me if I seem unfair to anyone or to cause offence.

The number of different 'complementary' theories and remedies is very large and many healers and counsellors have no qualifications. Nevertheless, in the UK they have always enjoyed almost total freedom to practice as they please, which is not the case in every country, though many turn a blind eye to it. In addition, more and more have some kind of qualification, though this is usually related mainly to a particular method of treatment and does not get anywhere near the much broader education, training, and practical experience offered in medical schools.

Among complementary practitioners there is also a great variation in attitude towards mainstream medicine. Some are totally supportive of what doctors and nurses do, but keen to add to it. Others are very critical, but often fail to make clear whether they are criticizing the teaching and aims of mainstream medicine, or the all too frequent failure to live up to them. Some are in favour of science, admitting its striking benefits, especially in the last hundred years, both in terms of length of life and quality of life. Some attempt the language of science, but without any proper supporting evidence or substance to it ('pseudo science'). Others are to a greater or lesser degree suspicious of all scientific progress, preferring ancient or 'natural' remedies.

There is also a wide spectrum between the more fanciful or magical kinds of complementary medicine and the more realistic aims of, say, present day osteopaths and chiropractors, most of whom have now given up the claims (which they made for many years) that their treatment could cure or greatly ameliorate not just spine, muscle, and joint problems, but almost *any* disease in *any* part the body — and who now each have their own Act of Parliament to regularize their status and training. There had to be separate Acts because, although much of what they do is so similar, they have quite different theories (both of them unconvincing to mainstream specialists) and have always been unwilling to work together. These two Acts are against the spirit of the seminal Medical Act passed by parliament in 1858, which was pragmatic, carefully avoiding any reference to any theory or belief or system, either mainstream or complementary. But there is the advantage that nobody can now call themselves an osteopath or chiropractor without appropriate training.

Reasons for current popularity

Though there does not seem to be any suggestion, even from its greatest admirers, that complementary medicine gets any better results than it did a hundred years ago, there is currently a big increase in demand for it. In my view, dissatisfaction with mainstream medicine, though playing a significant part (so I mention it first) is not the main cause. The main reason is the one least likely to be given in answer to a questionnaire — the pressure to follow fashion, to try remedies that everyone is talking about. Fashion in human affairs is very influential. Many people don't seem to realize that there have been several similar waves of enthusiasm in the past, in particular for acupuncture and for homoeopathy, which have then subsided (Stalker and Glymour 1989).

A third reason is a current cultural change with a renewed interest in the paranormal, in astrology, and in various psychic phenomena, however many times they fail to stand up to objective testing. A fourth reason is the prosperity that many people in developed countries now enjoy, with more money than ever before to spend on their health. In countries with a state subsidized health service more are now prepared to pay out of their own pocket for something extra, perhaps something with a hint of mystery and magic about it — after more conventional measures have failed. This failure may be either because mainstream medicine does not yet have any effective treatment for their problem, or because even the most effective treatment will not help everyone. Another factor is increased anxiety about health. A safer and longer life and the provision of far more health information than ever before seems to have led many people to worry more, not less. There is now a huge market for 'over-the-counter' sales of complementary medicine products of very doubtful value, many of them sold not to remedy symptoms but to 'promote health'.

I would guess that a hundred years ago as much as *two thirds* of what mainstream medicine did was much the same as what complementary medicine did then — and still does now. The doctor's placebos in the old days were cheap and harmless — often a bottle of coloured fluid with an unpleasant taste, containing minuscule amounts of several substances with Latin names — a bit like homoeopathy in fact. This still survived when I was a young doctor in 1950 and of course many patients had confidence in it and said how much it helped them, as happens to some extent with nearly all remedies. Even today, after the big increase in the number of really effective treatments, perhaps as much as *one third* of what mainstream medicine does (I am including general practice) is still not far removed from what complementary medicine does, simply because so far we have nothing better.

Spontaneous improvement

When sham treatment is compared with a treatment of proven effectiveness, and when neither the recipients nor their carers know which they are getting, the sham treatment will often seem to be beneficial, sometimes quite dramatically so. This may be true quite apart from whether or not it turns out to be less effective than the 'real' one. Spontaneous improvement may be just as important as the placebo effect. People who always take a remedy have little idea how frequently improvement or cure occurs without one. And not just in self limiting injuries and infections — temporary remissions are common in most longstanding conditions, whether or not they are curable. The last remedy to be tried may appear to have been by far the best, but the improvement that followed it may have been coincidental.

You could say that when patients *think* that they have benefited from a remedy, then in a sense they have. But faced with limited resources and the need to set priorities, it does not seem right to go too far down that road.

Diagnosis and cause

For an accurate diagnosis it will usually be safer to be seen by a man or woman who has been through medical school, where much time is spent studying this aspect of medicine. This should give a better chance not only of reaching the main diagnosis, but also in chronic or terminal illness of accurately assessing the cause of each separate symptom — and thus knowing how best to deal with it.

What do we do if we are not sure of either the diagnosis or the cause? When, for example, as is so common, someone is 'always tired' and all tests are normal. Some mainstream and nearly all complementary practitioners invariably give the patient a firm diagnosis and a cause for their problem, even if both are based on theories of energy, or hormone balance, or toxins, or stress, or lack of immunity, and so on, which sound plausible, but for which there is no good evidence. All doctors feel the pressure to go at least some way in this direction, rather than just say that they don't know. This is because they soon find that such blunt honesty and humility is appreciated by some patients, but not at all by others who find it depressing and unhelpful.

It seems certain that when it comes to making a diagnosis, such unconventional methods as iridology (Knipschild 1989), reflexology, hair samples, energy waves, and so on — though as popular as palmistry — have no real value. A major source of fallacy is that it takes only an occasional correct diagnosis for some people to be impressed . They forget that to be of any value a method of diagnosis has to get it right more often than would be expected by mere chance, combined with a judicious guess as to what is likely.

A few years ago I was asked to be in the studio audience for the recording of a television program. A woman claiming psychic powers said she could make a diagnosis by 'scanning' a person's body with her hands. A man came on and the question was whether she could detect which part of his body had recently been found to have something wrong with it. She started at the top of his head, holding her hands over him and worked slowly down, tentatively asking at each step if this was where the trouble was — and knowing that sooner or later she would come to it. When she did so, the presenter said he was 'impressed' and asked me, as a doctor, what I thought. When the program was shown my opinion was omitted.

Prevention

Everyone agrees that prevention is better than cure, but for each preventive measure there ought to be some evidence, otherwise money and effort are wasted. There is overwhelming evidence that tens of thousands of us who are alive today would be dead if we had not given up smoking, but when it comes to other factors, such as diet, the position is much more doubtful. There is certainly very little to support the popular (and commercially very profitable) idea that what is sold in high street health shops gives the customers (often 'the worried well') a better chance of staying well.

Ways of preventing cancer (or at least making it less likely) have always had an especially strong appeal both to the public and to doctors like me treating it. Here are two observations that have always intrigued me. First, every type of cancer that is common in one part of the world is uncommon in another. Race has little to do with it. We know this because when people move to another country they soon show the same pattern of cancers as those already living there. Either something in their previous lifestyle or environment was protecting them, or something in their new country is making them more susceptible. It could be either. An example is the low incidence of breast cancer in Japanese women, provided that they don't go and live in the USA. Secondly, nobody knows why cancer of the stomach has become far less common in several countries (including the USA and the UK) where until quite recently it was a major killer. Because this is such good news it seldom appears in the media (scare stories are more popular) and most people are unaware of it. Perhaps artificial food additives or pesticides, often feared as being unnatural, have in this case had a beneficial effect.

These two striking facts, though so far totally unexplained, surely give grounds for optimism. It seems that we don't need to accept any of the common cancers as inevitable.

Comparing results

Arguing too much from theory rather than from results is a failing of both mainstream and complementary medicine. The theories of mainstream medicine usually have a lot more evidence to support them, but that doesn't mean to say that they are always right or relevant. In mainstream medicine there is an unfortunate habit of using the word 'rational' for treatment based on theory, whereas it would be more appropriate to use this word where there is convincing evidence of good results, never mind the underlying theory.

This is where the need for comparisons comes in. Sometimes the benefit of a new treatment is so striking that no formal comparison is needed. But in other cases, few realize how easy it is for an ineffective remedy to look like an effective one, or for harm not to be recognized, unless this is done. Many traditional folk remedies in the shape of local applications for cuts and abrasions used to infect the wound and delay healing, but were thought to be doing good because 'drawing out the pus' was considered evidence of effectiveness, Similarly, in some cultures women welcome heavy menstrual periods and don't want anything done about them because they think that the menstrual flow is getting rid of poisons.

It's surely basic common sense, not just 'science', to compare results carefully in order to see which remedy is generally the best, which is second best, which has the highest number of exceptionally good results, and so on. All the advantages and disadvantages of different remedies or procedures or policies can be compared. You would think that, not just in medicine, but with different agricultural, building, or engineering methods, for example, careful comparisons of this kind would have been done for centuries — perhaps sometimes coming to wrong conclusions due to insufficient understanding of the fallacies of crude statistics, but at least attempting it. But human beings have been surprisingly slow to do this.

Unfortunately, there are snags and here are three of them. First, to make such comparisons reliable we may sometimes need many patients to agree to be randomly allocated either to one policy or the other. Politicians and the media seldom make this clear. When Frank Dobson, UK Secretary of State for Health, spoke in 1998 on the need to test all remedies, whether mainstream or complementary, he did not mention it (Spencer 1998). This, of course, should be done only when ethical committees have approved and when the doctors concerned are satisfied that they would be happy for treatment of themselves or members of their family to be similarly randomized. The point is that if 'like is not compared with like' — and various other sources of bias are not eliminated as far as possible —

it's all too easy to come to false conclusions. In the first half of the twentieth century mainstream medicine's failure to compare results led to needlessly drastic surgery for breast and rectal cancer, while for more than twenty years very high doses of stilboestrol hormone therapy were popular for prostate cancer before a massive randomized comparison in the USA showed that the good done to the cancer was outweighed by harm done to the heart. More recently, when healthy volunteers at the Royal Homoeopathic Hospital, with muscle soreness, took either a homoeopathic remedy, much favoured for this condition, or a sham tablet, the outcome was the same (Vickers *et al.* 1997).

Secondly, small and contradictory differences in different studies (whether in complementary or in mainstream medicine) are common. A difference in outcome that is 'statistically highly significant' means only that the difference is unlikely to be due to chance. It does not mean that the difference is necessarily either a big difference or an important difference. For example, a Medical Research Council randomized study of backache (Meade *et al.* 1995) showed greater patient satisfaction when patients went to chiropractors than when they had routine treatment as a hospital outpatient. But the difference, though unlikely to be due to chance, was very small — 84% compared with 79% . Whichever treatment they got, more than three quarters were pleased with the outcome. And note that this could mean *either* that both treatments were roughly equally effective *or* that neither made much difference. Another point about this study is that it would have been nearer to the ideal of 'comparing like with like' if all patients had been treated in private clinics, half having physiotherapy and half seeing chiropractors.

Thirdly, bias can creep in if both the randomization and the registration of a study are not done independently. One advantage, for example, is that there is then less risk of only favourable results being published. But this adds to costs (Ernst 1999).

Note that such group evidence is an addition to, not a substitution for, the careful consideration of each patient as an individual. There need not be any conflict. Though you can never tell how an individual will react, a markedly higher percentage of success with one remedy than with another in a large number of patients, spells *a better chance* of doing well, other things being equal. To decide on priorities you need to make comparisons — and to make comparisons you need numbers. Even with such things as happiness and satisfaction, it's not quite true that you can't measure them. You can compare which treatment leads to the largest percentage of patients who say they feel better or happier since the treatment.

In life-threatening illness, there is often the hope that some kind of strange or unorthodox therapy might produce a 'miracle cure'. The snag here is that, though the media love to report this sort of outcome after what seemed a hopeless situation, exactly the same welcome surprises are seen in mainstream medicine. The only way to settle the matter is to compare the progress in two groups of patients who are alike apart from how they are treated. What percentage in each group do exceptionally well? Some patients, often those with cancer, take unconventional treatment, but only after a full course of conventional treatment. This policy (which many patients are doubtful about, so they might well be willing to be randomized) could be compared with conventional treatment by itself and we would then find out how much difference, if any, the additional treatment makes.

Progress

For all of us who hate to see either harsh suffering or premature death, progress is a very serious consideration. Mainstream medicine, backed by much hard work (and occasional good luck) by scientists, has achieved far more than would ever have seemed possible a hundred years ago. To name a few — antibiotics, cortisone, surgery, anaesthetics, improved management of wounds and injuries, childbirth that is far safer for both mother and child, a big improvement in childhood cancer, better control of high blood pressure, hip replacements for the elderly, and the virtual eradication of polio, diphtheria, and smallpox. Many deficiency diseases have been finally understood and defeated. Not the imagined deficiencies of the health shops, but real ones, leading, for example. to the terrible long term mental and physical suffering, once common in parts of France and Italy (Johnson 1831), due to pellagra (lack of niacin, one of the B vitamins) or to cretinism (lack of iodine).

How previous generations would envy us. Yet many of us seem to take it all for granted. And it's not just a matter of eradication or cure. Even when it's only improved symptom relief, medicine has made advances that have been of enormous benefit (to myself among many others — people sometimes forget that doctors may have considerable experience of being patients).

Complementary medicine does not make progress of this kind and the interesting thing is that the public don't expect it to It's not just lack of money. Mainstream medicine (like any human activity striving to make real progress) has a long list of problems wholly or partially solved (diagnosis, cause, treatment, and so on) and another long list where such problems have *not* yet been solved and much hard work remains to be done. Complementary medicine doesn't seem to have such lists — or to look at things in quite this way.

Logic and magic

The two powerful instincts of logic and magic seem to coexist in the human brain. I use the word logic as short hand for curiosity, questioning, searching for hard evidence, and trying to solve problems. And the word magic for a fascination with mystery and mysticism, combined with passionately held beliefs and convictions with little or no critical reasoning or demands for more evidence. If two practitioners are heard discussing how they help patients to relax and be more positive, they may turn out to be working in either complementary or mainstream medicine. But if you hear one of them say 'what we then found was a big surprise, which made it clear that our previous thinking had been wrong' you can be fairly sure that the speaker comes from mainstream medicine.

In complementary medicine there is less puzzling over contradictions (to a scientist a contradiction is a challenge) and seldom any talk of remedies that seemed at first hopeful and then turned out to be disappointing. Compared with mainstream medicine there is also much less criticism of the claims of others in the field. Anyone who comes out with some new idea or theory tends to be treated with uncritical respect. In science or in mainstream medicine vigorous debate and criticism is more likely. In these ways — and also in the sense of being upset or angry when claims are doubted or challenged — complementary remedies share some features with the world's religions. Both are concerned not so much with progress as with giving strength, comfort, and hope (especially when individual doctors or nurses in mainstream medicine have failed to do so).

Because a love of magic and miracles is ingrained in our nature, many people very much *want* to believe in such things as astrology and the paranormal. Thus they may fail to see that the evidence is not consistent or convincing; and that there may well be other explanations for what is observed. For the same reason they would in some ways prefer *not to know* the result of medical reasoning and randomized comparisons.

Both mainstream medicine and complementary medicine are fascinated by the way the mind can affect the body, but complementary medicine seems to go beyond the evidence. There is no doubt about effects on quality of life, but there is much less evidence for the popular belief that the mental state can make a big difference to whether a person lives or dies from cancer or other serious illness. Personally I have always found it unattractive when patients who have recovered from a serious situation congratulate themselves on their fighting spirit rather than just being grateful. I have seen too many die when there was nothing wrong with their fighting spirit or their will to live. This idea may also rather cruelly suggest to those who relapse that this is in some way their own fault.

'Natural' or 'ancient' remedies also appeal strongly to something in human nature, but faith in them is often illogical and lacking in good evidence. The death of young children or young animals — so common in natural surroundings — is much less common when civilization does unnatural things like putting chemicals into drinking water to reduce its bacterial content. Nature is not always gentle. She is often violent and cruel. Certain plants and animals may have survived in the course of evolution only because of the poisons they have developed as a defence against predators.

Finally, love of magic and miracles can lead to double standards. With complementary medicine it seems more likely than with mainstream medicine that either the speed or the completeness of recovery will be exaggerated. Secondly, if in a particular kind of cancer, either surgery or radiotherapy achieves an overall cure rate of, say, 50% (as is seen, for example, in cancer of the cervix in women) some critics will stress the failure to cure half the patients — and at the same time be impressed by a very occasional instance of healing after unconventional treatment.

Harm from treatment

The incidence of harm from treatment is much higher in mainstream medicine than in complementary medicine, but this is because of the much higher incidence of cure and other benefits. Unfortunately any really effective treatment seems capable on occasions of doing harm. This is not a dogma. It is a fact. Would it were not so.

In serious illness it may well be that a treatment is far from being completely safe, but that, because of the dangers implicit in *not* having it, it is safer to have it. Whenever there are difficult decisions to be made, not just in medicine, but with other problems such as politics or economics, there will always be 'hawks' and 'doves'. Hawks fear failure if they are not sufficiently bold and drastic. Doves want to be gentle at all costs and dread making things worse.

It should be remembered that complementary medicine can do indirect harm when there is a failure to make the correct diagnosis due to lack of training in this area.

A very different kind of harm is more likely to occur today than in the old days, whether in mainstream or complementary medicine. To 'comfort always' is one of the most precious traditional aspects of mainstream medicine, but you can have too much of a good thing. Concern and sympathy need to be mixed with brevity and humour. A patient dying of acute leukaemia said to me, 'I appreciated it the first time someone asked me if anything was worrying me, or if there was anything I'd like to talk about, but after the third or fourth time it just depressed me'. This patient was my wife and she added, 'the staff all look so sad — if only they would brighten up a bit — the person who helps me most is the man selling newspapers who asks me how I can possibly expect him to earn a living if my husband brings them in to me.'

Pros and cons of integrating

At first sight there are some attractive reasons to integrate complementary medicine with mainstream medicine. We all like to patch up old quarrels where possible and it sounds more positive and friendly to integrate. Doctors, especially hospital consultants, are anxious to lose the old image of being somewhat arrogant and superior. But any more integration than there is already might prove to be not a step forward but a step backward to the years before the Medical Act of 1858 when the public was not clear who was medically qualified and who wasn't.

Since mainstream medicine is pragmatic and not based on any fixed belief or theory, you could argue that as much time ought to be spent testing complementary remedies as more orthodox ones. In an ideal world this would be true. A remedy is a remedy. But how much money can we afford to take away from other needs, in order to do independent assessments and trials in cases where outcomes seem to be no better than those seen after almost *any* treatment — and where the underlying theory for the treatment is not supported by any convincing evidence? Whether mainstream or complementary, when dozens of totally different remedies and theories are all followed by roughly the same outcome it seems unlikely that any are having any significant, measurable effect on the underlying state of the disease.

Here is another factor. My impression is that many in complementary medicine, whether patients or practitioners — though they might not say so when filling up a questionnaire — would actually prefer complementary medicine and mainstream medicine to remain separate. Both healers and those seeking their help get a certain satisfaction from the special relationship when the patient chooses and pays. And complementary medicine might lose some of its special semi-magical power if it became more orthodox. Sometimes the disapproval of doctors and the practitioner's lack of qualifications seems to boost the placebo effect.

Finally, if practitioners from both camps are to sit round a table and discuss health and disease, where do we draw the line between the professional and the amateur, the qualified and the unqualified, the mystic and the scientist? Should astronomers, constantly seeking new knowledge about the universe we live in, integrate with astrologers, who use old maps of the stars that we now know to be as wrong as old maps of the world or old maps of the human body? They think differently. They don't speak the same language. Are there areas where a rational approach, based on the weighing of evidence, is not appropriate? Maybe — but it doesn't lead to problem solving or progress. We are back to the tension in our nature between logic and magic. Basic human nature and current cultural trends seem to need both, but perhaps it's best they are kept a little apart.

References

Ernst, E. (1999). Commitment to complementary medicine: politically correct lip service or coordinated strategy? *Journal of the Royal College of Physicians*, **33**, 114–15.

Johnson, J. (1831). *Change of air: through France, Switzerland & Italy in the year 1829*. Highley and Underwood, London.

Knipschild, P. (1989). Changing belief in iridology after an empirical study. *British Medical Journal*, **299**, 491–2.

Meade, T. W., Dyer, S., Browne, W., Frank, A. O. (1995). Randomized comparison of chiropractic and hospital outpatient management for low back pain: results from extended follow-up. *British Medical Journal*, **311**, 349–51.

Spencer, W. (1998). A critique of an official UK view of complementary medicine. In *The scientific review of alternative medicine*, 2, 45–7.

Stalker, D. and Glymour, C. (1989). *Examining holistic medicine*. Prometheus Books, New York.

Vickers, A. J., Fisher, P., Smith, C., *et al.* (1997). Homoeopathy for delayed onset muscle soreness: a randomized double blind placebo controlled trial. *British Journal of Sports Medicine*, 31, 304–7.

Part II

Selected therapies

Chapter 7

Acupuncture

Jacqueline Filshie and Adrian White

Jacqueline Filshie is a Consultant in Anaesthesia and Pain Management at the Royal Marsden NHS Trust, Sutton, Surrey and London and Honorary Senior Lecturer, Institute of Cancer Research, Sutton, Surrey, UK. Adrian White is Senior Lecturer, Department of Complementary Medicine, University of Exeter, UK.

History

Acupuncture is a form of therapy in which needles are inserted into skin and underlying tissues in special sites, known as acupuncture points, either as a treatment or in order to improve health. It may have evolved from massage therapy, the points being sites of particular tenderness. By the time of the first written records, the Yellow Emperor's *Classic of Internal Medicine* dating from about 150 BC, acupuncture was already an established and systematic therapy in which clinical observations and deductions were interpreted according to the philosophy of the age, Taoism. However, acupuncture may not have originated in China: it has been suggested by some authors that tattoo markings on the Tyrolian Ice Man, Ötzi, dating from about 5200 BC, could indicate a similar form of therapy (Dorfer *et al.* 1999). The marks are found in sites that are recognized as acupuncture points in Chinese charts, and are appropriate for medical conditions that Ötzi is known to have suffered, i.e. arthritis of the lumbar spine and legs, and intestinal parasites.

Acupuncture developed in China over several centuries, and the practice spread first to other Eastern countries, especially Japan, and then to the West. The first reports reached the West through the descriptions of Willem ten Rhijne (1647–1700) a doctor employed by the Dutch East India Company. In China, acupuncture became overshadowed by western scientific medicine in the 19th century, but was re-established in the 1950s under the Communist regime as part of traditional medicine with the purpose of providing affordable medical care to the massive population. In the West an explosion of interest started in the 1970s when American physicians visiting China described their experiences of seeing acupuncture practised, particularly witnessing major surgery performed apparently with only acupuncture for anaesthesia.

Philosophy

The unique experience of acupuncture, and in particular the strange sensations that arise when needles are inserted and manipulated, have been interpreted in different ways at different periods of history, depending on the prevailing culture and philosophy. Fundamental to the Eastern interpretation is the concept of Qi (pronounced 'chee' as in cheese) which is loosely translated as 'energy'. It is considered a vital force, and disturbances in Qi are associated with mental and physical conditions. The aim of ancient physicians was to use the history and examination, particularly changes in the tongue and radial pulse, together with knowledge of the patient's character, to decide the pattern of disturbance. This was regarded as more fundamental therapy than simply treating symptoms. The disturbance was then corrected by placing needles in chosen acupuncture points. Acupuncture was often combined with nutritional advice, herbs, manipulation, and treatment with moxa (see below).

Patterns of disturbance might also be identified in terms of imbalances of Yin and Yang: these are fundamental properties of all matter, and can be thought of as opposite extremes such as light and dark, or heat and cold. Other fundamental concepts include five 'elements' (or 'phases') which represent five different aspects of the person's physical and mental make-up. Adverse effects of the weather would be incorporated in the pattern of disturbance, an example being wind-cold which is associated with upper respiratory infections. During the restoration of acupuncture in China in the 1950s, a major effort was made to combine the different strands of traditional acupuncture and, strongly influenced by western diagnosis, to produce a unitary system of diagnosis and treatment that involves identifying 'syndromes'; this is the system known as Traditional Chinese Acupuncture.

The western, (bio) medical approach, sometimes also called 'scientific', emphasizes that there is little evidence supporting any of the traditional concepts in a physical sense, and works from the premise that acupuncture is more likely to activate standard physiological mechanisms. With this approach, a diagnosis is made in conventional western terms, on the basis of standard history, examination and investigations. Treatment with acupuncture is seen as one of a range of therapies including drugs, surgery, counselling, and so on. Treatment is directed towards stimulating nerves, muscles and other tissues. The sites used are chosen partly according to the (spinal) segment which requires attention, and partly according to traditional use. For example, some points in hands and feet seem empirically to be useful in treating particular symptoms, even though the precise neurological basis for this effect is still uncertain. When a point below the knee is needled, for instance, there is a clear effect on the stomach even though it is not in the appropriate segment (Tougas *et al.* 1992). (Bio)medical acupuncturists also use needles to treat muscle trigger points, which are areas of muscle that have become hypersensitive after injury and produce pain which can be very severe and prolonged. Trigger points tend to occur at a constant site within each particular muscle and have only been described relatively recently in the west. It is fascinating to learn that the sites of trigger points are virtually identical to many of the acupuncture points which were described by the ancient Chinese.

Mode of action

There is now considerable evidence for acupuncture's actions from a wide range of physiological experiments (see Table 7.1). Acupuncture can produce local effects on the tissue surrounding the needle, as may be guessed at from the fact that a flare is often seen directly

Table 7.1 Clinical relevance of some of acupuncture's probable modes of action

Physiological action of acupuncture	Probable clinical relevance
Local release of calcitonin gene-related peptide (CGRP)	Powerful vasodilator
Stimulation of A delta nerve fibres	Analgesia. Acupuncture ineffective unless nerve supply is intact
Local action on dorsal horn	'Closing the gate' to incoming pain signals
Stimulation of ascending and descending pain inhibitory pathways	Produces heterosegmental pain relief, i.e. throughout the body
Endogenous opioid release: β-endorphin, met-enkephalin, dynorphins	Some effects can be blocked by naloxone (but not at kappa opioid sites)
Opioid gene up-regulation, e.g. preprometenkephalin, preprodynorphin	May explain sustained beneficial effects of treatment
Releases cholecystokinin (CCK)	Endogenous opioid antagonist, can contribute to acupuncture tolerance. Anti-epileptic
Releases ACTH	Anti-inflammatory
Releases oxytocin	Analgesic and sedative
Releases serotonin	Analgesic and mood enhancing
Releases nerve growth factor (NGF)	Has a trophic effect on sensory and autonomic nerves
Widespread autonomic effects	Normalizes blood flow, BP, gastric motility etc. Contributes to pain relief

(Filshie and White 1998 and Ernst and White 1999 — these textbooks contain numerous references to the neurophysiology of acupuncture.)

around the needle. Some of these local effects have been shown to depend on the release of local transmitters such as calcitonin gene-related peptide, CGRP. Acupuncture is also known to stimulate nerve endings, particularly A delta fibres: this can be shown by the fact that injecting local anaesthetic into the point before inserting the needle can prevent the effects of acupuncture. Acupuncture thus acts on the dorsal horn of the spinal cord to 'close the gate' to incoming pain signals. It probably does this both by a local effect and by stimulating the brain-stem's inherent system of pain control, so-called descending inhibition. This inhibition operates throughout the spinal cord to reduce the sensation of pain anywhere in the body, which goes some way towards explaining how a needle in the hand, for example, can treat a pain elsewhere such as the chest. The action of acupuncture in the central nervous system involves the release of three types of endogenous opioids, β-endorphin, met-enkephalin, and dynorphins. Up-regulation of opioid genes may be responsible for the sustained, analgesic effects of acupuncture. However, when acupuncture stimulation is prolonged, it can lead to raised levels of cholecytokinin (CCK), which antagonizes endogenous opioids. Acupuncture has been shown to act at other important CNS structures such as the hypothalamus and other brain-stem centres, causing the release of hormones such as ACTH and oxytocin, and other active substances such as serotonin, which have both analgesic and mood enhancing properties. Through the hypothalamus, acupuncture could have powerful effects on autonomic balance and on the immune system.

Administration

Standards for training vary from country to country and, in the USA, from state to state. Practitioners may be doctors, physiotherapists, or non-medically qualified acupuncturists, and established training programmes and qualification standards exist for each group. In some countries, the practice of acupuncture is totally unregulated. Details of treatment vary enormously between practitioners, depending on their own teaching, experience, and beliefs.

Between 1 and 30 pre-sterilized, disposable needles may be inserted at each treatment. The needles may be stimulated by hand, which causes an odd sensation known as 'deqi' (pronounced 'der-chee'). This was originally believed to signal the 'arrival of qi' but now many people believe it indicates that the appropriate nerves have been stimulated. Needles are left in for varying periods up to about 20 minutes. The needles may also be warmed by burning moxa, a traditional aromatic herb which looks like brown cotton-wool and can be used to warm either the needle or the skin directly. Other forms of stimulation include electroacupuncture using a battery operated apparatus attached to the needles with clips, and stimulation with 'cold' laser apparatus, directly on the skin with no needle.

Clinical application to cancer patients

The subspecialty of palliative medicine has revolutionized the treatment of both pain and other symptoms in cancer patients over the last 15 years. By using the latest analgesic ladder developed by the World Health Organization and judiciously adding co-analgesics, most patients in pain with advanced cancer can either be pain free or have significant pain relief without recourse to other treatment. However, a significant minority are either very sensitive to conventional medicine or particularly prone to side-effects, or are resistant to high doses of analgesia, and therefore non-drug treatments for cancer pain are still very much sought after. A further group of patients with pain and emotional problems, either through denial, or from anger about their diagnosis, can be particularly challenging. Acupuncture treatment may be suitable for these three groups of patients. Nevertheless, much of the available data on the use of acupuncture for pain and symptom control are observational, and more formal testing with randomized controlled clinical trials is necessary. Acupuncture has an increasing role in the treatment of pain and also for many non-pain symptoms in the cancer population.

Pain symptoms

Pain in a cancer patient can be caused by either primary or secondary cancer, or due to cancer treatment with surgery, radiotherapy, or chemotherapy, or may be totally unrelated to the cancer e.g. osteoporosis. It can have nociceptive or neuropathic components, or both.

The best approach to treatment is the use of segmental, paravertebral needling, using points corresponding to the segments where the pain arises, together with a selection of traditional 'strong' acupuncture points. These are often sited in the hands and feet (examples are L14, TE5, ST36, SP6, and LR3). Lundeberg has shown that the combination of distal and segmental points is most effective for pain control (Lundeberg et al. 1988). Some patients appear to be more sensitive to acupuncture than others — so called strong reactors (Mann 1992). As cancer patients often appear to be more sensitive to treatment than non-cancer patients, it seems wise to give a gentle treatment initially, in case of a strong response. The strength of treatment can then be increased or reduced on subsequent occasions. The optimal timing of the treatment is weekly for four to six weeks, or twice weekly for three weeks. Depending on the duration of the response, the treatment intervals can then be increased.

Filshie and Redman (1985) and Filshie (1990) summarized two audits on 339 patients with a heterogeneous group of cancers who were treated in a cancer hospital after full investigations and staging, and who had failed to respond to conventional analgesic treatment. Between 52% and 56% had pain relief for a worthwhile duration after 3 treatments, a further 30% and 22% had analgesia for only up to 2 days. The remainder failed to respond. Patients with treatment related pain, such as post-surgical syndromes or post-irradiation pain, had more prolonged benefit than patients with metastatic disease. Pain relief was often accompanied by increased mobility. Analgesic medication could often be reduced or even tailed off completely if the course of treatment was successful. Two further audits by Aung in Canada and Leng in a hospice setting describing one year's acupuncture experience showed similar results (Aung 1994; Leng 1999).

Myofascial pain is common in both cancer and non-cancer patients, and deactivation of trigger points is a vital part of treatment for both (Baldry 1993). Muscle spasm mostly melts away with acupuncture treatment. Paravertebral needling at the levels of C7, T1, and T2 together with suprascapular trigger point treatment is recommended for pain in the head, neck, upper arm, and chest region. This often produces a temporary sympathetic blockade resulting in beneficial vasodilatation in discolored limbs. Paravertebral needling at the levels of L1 to L5, together with superficial needling over sacroiliac joints, is used to treat low back pain and for vascular problems in the lower limbs. Points in the sacral segmental levels can be added for perineal or pelvic pain. Additionally, 'strong' traditional distal points can be used in each treatment. A local treatment with needles encircling the area of pain, a treatment called 'surrounding the dragon', is useful for treating scar pain, areas of postherpetic neuralgia, and ulcers including radionecrotic ulcers.

Pain relief may be incomplete with acupuncture and may need supplementing with analgesics and co-analgesics, chosen according to an individual's response and the clinical situation.

Tolerance

In the first two audits described above, patients with a greater tumour burden were noticed to have a shorter duration of analgesia following acupuncture treatment. Indeed, tolerance to treatment may be due to a recurrence of cancer, so patients who responded well initially but then suddenly become unresponsive to acupuncture may well need reinvestigating. If metastatic disease is found and treated, these patients may again respond to acupuncture.

There are numerous ways in which one can try to increase the duration of analgesia with acupuncture in cancer patients. Electroacupuncture treatments can be repeated several times a day initially, reducing rapidly to once or twice daily, for patients in late stage cancer with opioid toxicity and inadequate analgesia (Wen 1977). However this is labour intensive. Dillon and Lucas showed a statistically significant pain reduction in 28 patients, in a hospice setting, using minute press needles (semi-permanent indwelling needles) in the ear, which patients could massage if pain became intense (Dillon and Lucas 1999).

Transcutaneous electrical nerve stimulation (TENS) is another form of sensory stimulation which is commonly used and can often give relief when the analgesia from acupuncture wears off before the next 'top up' treatment is due. TENS stimulates Aβ nerve fibres and therefore has a different mechanism from acupuncture, but can be a useful adjunct.

Although acupuncture is rarely used as a substitute for operative anaesthesia, acupuncture given before and during cancer surgery can reduce analgesic requirements both per- and postoperatively, as shown in two studies by Poulain in patients having major abdominal cancer surgery (personal communication 1993; Poulain *et al.* 1997).

Non-pain symptoms

Nausea and vomiting

Needling at the traditional point PC6 on the inner aspect of the forearm, several centimeters from the wrist (Fig. 7 1), has been tested against numerous control interventions for nausea and vomiting due to a variety of causes. A systematic review by Vickers of 33 such trials showed 27 out of 33 to be positive (Vickers 1996). The trials included patients with anticipatory chemotherapy-induced nausea and vomiting as well as postoperative nausea and vomiting and that associated with pregnancy. Five of these studies, involving 151 subjects with nausea due to chemotherapy, found acupuncture or acupressure better than various controls. Transcutaneous electrical stimulation can be used to prolong the effects in patients with chemotherapy related symptoms and can be a useful alternative to needling in patients with clotting dysfunction (McMillan and Dundee 1991). Massaging semi-permanent indwelling needles inserted high in the sternum was found to reduce nausea in patients who already had the studs inserted for treatment of dyspnoea or anxiety. The outcomes of several more recent trials using PC6 acupuncture have been mixed but are predominantly positive (Vickers 1999 personal communication).

Anxiety and shortness of breath

In an open pilot study, 20 cancer patients with breathlessness at rest, due to primary or secondary cancer, were treated at two upper sternal acupuncture points (Fig. 7.2a) and at L14 on each hand. Seventy per cent (14/20) reported statistically significant symptomatic benefit, using two subjective dyspnoea scoring scales, supported by measured improvement

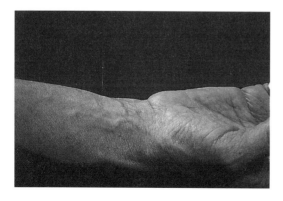

Fig. 7.1 Acupuncture at PC6 for treatment of nausea and vomiting.

(a)

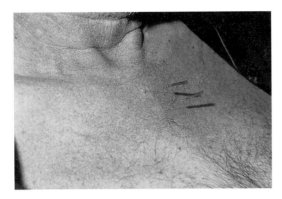

Fig. 7.2a Two needles in the upper sternum for dyspnoea related to advanced cancer.

(b)

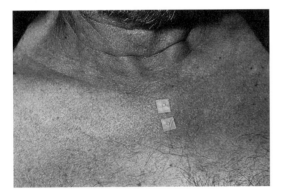

Fig. 7.2b Two semi-permanent indwelling needles for patients to massage if anxious or dyspnoeic.

in respiratory rate. There was also a significant sense of relaxation and relief of anxiety after treatment for at least six hours, the limit of close observation. Part way into the pilot study, in an attempt to prolong the symptomatic relief of the dyspnoea, two tiny, indwelling acupuncture stud needles were placed in the sternal points in eight patients who had reported global relief of breathlessness with the treatment (Fig. 7.2b). Patients were encouraged to massage the studs for two to three minutes before exercise such as going to the toilet, or in the event of a 'panic attack'. All reported some benefit which lasted for up to two weeks, although this was not formally assessed. These studs are now used routinely in our own unit and in many others. The studs are secured and covered by a clear plastic dressing, and can be left for up to four weeks before needing to be changed. The points have been renamed 'ASAD' points or Anxiety, Sickness And Dyspnoea points, as they can be used for all these symptoms.

Xerostomia

Lundeberg and colleagues have performed several controlled studies on acupuncture to increase salivary flow in patients after radiation damage to the salivary glands as well as patients with Sjögren's syndrome (Lundeberg 1999). They have demonstrated that release of the neuropeptides, calcitonin gene related peptide and vasoactive intestinal peptide may contribute to the increased salivary flow. This effect can be very beneficial clinically. However, if the salivary glands have been destroyed completely by radiotherapy, rather than partially damaged, acupuncture is ineffective.

Cancer related hot flushes

In addition to helping to reduce hot flushes due to the natural climacteric (Wyon *et al.* 1995), acupuncture has helped to reduce Tamoxifen induced hot flushes (Towlerton *et al.* 1999). These side effects of therapy can be particularly debilitating and result in 10% of patients giving up treatment. If patients failed to respond to a four-week course of treatment, semi-permanent indwelling studs were inserted bilaterally at SP6, a traditional acupuncture point on the medial side of the leg above the ankle. These could be massaged daily by patients, increasing their sense of autonomy. Preliminary results have also shown benefit using somewhat different stimulation in men undergoing hormone manipulation for prostate cancer (Hammar *et al.* 1999).

Miscellaneous

In clinical trials of acupuncture for depression, acupuncture gave relief equal to anti-depressant drugs, but it has not been formally tested in depressed cancer patients. With the availability of so many new, successful, specific antidepressants on the market, formal testing of acupuncture for this group of patients probably becomes less of a priority.

Acupuncture has been observed to reduce or abolish symptoms of radiation rectitis, oesophageal obstruction, hiccup, and pruritus and to heal radionecrotic ulcers (summarized by Thompson and Filshie 1997).

Enhancement of well-being

Although acupuncture is used to control specific symptoms such as pain or dyspnoea more often than to enhance well-being, patients often do describe an improvement in their general well-being during and after a course of treatment. As acupuncture stimulates endogenous opioid release, it can help well-being in a similar way to the endogenous opioid release that occurs with moderate exercise in a gym. Also, a course of treatment that increases endogenous endorphin output and up-regulates expression of endogenous analgesic genes might be expected to produce a prolonged sense of well-being. Acupuncture releases serotonin which has antidepressant activity as noted above. Acupuncture also releases oxytocin which is increasingly recognized as having anxiolytic effects, another theoretical basis for the improvement of morale with acupuncture. An audit on the psychological profile of breast cancer patients given acupuncture treatment for pain control for one month has shown not only a statistically significant reduction in 'average' and 'worst' pain, but also a decrease in distress levels and interference with lifestyle (Filshie *et al.* 1997). Further more specific work in this area is recommended.

Sense of control

Acupuncture has no role in controlling disease progression, but patients who are given indwelling acupuncture studs for dyspnoea, anxiety, nausea, or treatment for hot flushes can, and do, feel the benefit of having some control over those symptoms. This is particularly reassuring in the case of dyspnoea, when the studs can be massaged prior to exercise, or in the event of panic attacks. Very anxious patients can give themselves a burst of anxiolysis after massaging the ASAD studs. Patients with hot flushes can be given needling packs for self administered treatment every ten days or so, at the SP6 point on the leg, after clear instructions.

Adjustment to illness

Acupuncture is not used to help patients adjust to illness. However, the consultations often give sufficient time for patients to benefit from the 'therapeutic interview' which accompanies a course of treatment. This can give an opportunity for the patient to express fears and emotions freely and patients may benefit from this support, in addition to the support from their oncology team and general practitioners.

Complications and contraindications

There are few serious adverse effects associated with acupuncture therapy and only 300 serious complications were reported world-wide over a 30 year period (Rampes and Peuker 1999). They classified the effects as follows:

- Delayed or missed diagnosis;
- Deterioration of disorder under treatment;
- Pain;
- Vegetative reactions;
- Bacterial and viral infection;
- Trauma of tissues and organs;
- Miscellaneous.

Any delay in diagnosis in a cancer patient of either the primary condition or metastatic disease is obviously counter productive. As already mentioned, any failure to respond in a patient who was previously responsive may be due to disease progression and it is valuable to have patients treated by suitably qualified medical practitioners with some oncology knowledge, or at least closely supervised by them at almost every clinic treatment, to know when to reinvestigate patients. Serious post-needling pain and somnolence happen very rarely, and any patients with prolonged sleepiness after treatment should be advised not to drive themselves home. The use of disposable needles should be mandatory, to reduce the chance of infection from needles. Any patient who has valvular heart disease should not be treated with semi-permanent indwelling needles. Serious anatomical damage, e.g. pneumothorax, should be preventable by good knowledge of anatomy. Particular caution must be used needling areas overlying lung in cachectic patients. Electroacupuncture should not be used in patients with a pacemaker. Acupuncture should not be used in the area of any spinal instability, as it may remove protective muscle spasm around the vertebral column with risk of cord compression. It is contraindicated to needle patients with a moderately or severely lymphoedematous limb, and contraindicated in patients with severe clotting dysfunction.

Acupuncture given by trained personnel appears to be very safe, although minor side-effects are common, including pain from the needles, local bleeding, drowsiness after treatment, and a temporary exacerbation of symptoms. Improvement or even resolution of other symptoms, such as migraine, prostatism, or psoriasis, may occur coincidentally as a side-effect of acupuncture treatment—and a welcome one!

Effect on the cancer process

There is a small body of literature which suggests that acupuncture has immunomodulating properties, much like exercise (Jonsdottir 1999). However, the clinical evidence is still scant, and until further substantial clinical research has been carried out in this population, acupuncture should not be offered as an alternative to conventional treatment in any circumstances. It is, currently, a matter of conjecture whether acupuncture's immuno-enhancing effects will be beneficial alongside conventional anticancer treatment.

Compatibility with conventional treatments

Acupuncture is rarely contraindicated in cancer patients, but would probably be inadvisable in pancytopenia immediately following bone marrow transplantation when high dose chemotherapy has been given. Some knowledge of the treatment regimens is therefore helpful to a practitioner, and the nadir of the response to chemotherapy courses may not be the ideal time to commence therapy. Semi-permanent indwelling stud needles should not be used in patients who are likely to suffer neutropenia associated with anticancer treatment, in case resistance is low; septicaemia could result. Otherwise, acupuncture can be given quite safely at most stages of cancer therapy.

The evidence base for acupuncture

Acupuncture's popularity is an indication of its acceptability and perceived effectiveness. For example, it is now available in 86% of UK pain clinics (CSAG, 2000). There are numerous experiments in a variety of clinical conditions that have shown the benefits of acupuncture compared to an untreated control group, for example in back pain, neck pain, and dysmenorrhoea. However, as with many interventions, there is a relative shortage of rigorous evidence that acupuncture is better than placebo. Research is hindered by lack of funding and research facilities, often being practised away from the mainstream of medicine. A large number of early studies were marred by poor quality. Moreover, it has been difficult to devise a suitable placebo control for clinical studies, since nothing else is quite like a needle.

One solution for the control procedure has been to insert needles just beneath the skin in inappropriate sites, but even this has its drawbacks as it does produce a physiological response. Despite this, rigorous randomized controlled trials of good quality have shown that acupuncture is superior to this form of needle placebo for the treatment of migraine headaches, facial neuralgia, fibromyalgia, sports injury, and lateral epicondylitis, for example. Similarly, acupuncture was shown to be as effective as steroid injection for the treatment of osteoarthritis of the hip. In contrast, acupuncture was not superior to placebo needling for osteoarthritis of the knee, which is surprising since this is one of the conditions that seems to do particularly well in normal clinical practice.

Systematic reviews have been performed for acupuncture in a number of treatment areas, but have often been hampered by lack of good quality studies. The most reliable reviews with a positive outcome (i.e. greater effect than placebo) have been for dental pain (which includes both experimental and clinical pain) (Ernst and Pittler 1998) and in nausea and vomiting from several causes (Vickers 1996 — see above). A meta-analysis of acupuncture for chronic headache found a significant effect of acupuncture for migraine but insufficient evidence for tension headache (Melchart *et al.* 1999). The evidence in back pain is contradictory with one positive meta-analysis (Ernst and White 1998) counterbalanced by one negative review (van Tulder *et al.* 1999).

The evidence from other systematic reviews shows that acupuncture has no effect in smoking cessation (White *et al.* 1999) or in weight loss (Ernst 1997). Evidence for its effect in treating neck pain and osteoarthritis in general is contradictory so no firm conclusions can be drawn and further studies are awaited: these are areas in which clinical experience suggests considerable benefit. Acupuncture is used routinely in the East for stroke rehabilitation and several studies have shown promise; notably Johansson *et al.* (1993); however a subsequent rigorous, placebo-controlled trial could find no effect (Gosman-Hedstroem *et al.* 1998).

Clearly, once methodological problems are overcome in acupuncture research, further evidence will determine the place of acupuncture in cancer pain and symptom control.

Case history

Patient's Viewpoint

In 1983, almost 17 years ago, I discovered a lump in my neck which was removed at our local hospital. Ten days later I received a phone call telling me it was cancer, and I required further surgery. I was fortunate to be referred to the Royal Marsden, where I had a total thyroidectomy; the tumour was in fact quite a rare type! No further treatment was needed. I went for regular check ups over the following years. We knew there were elevated levels of calcitonin in my blood, which acts as a marker to the tumour, and so this was always carefully monitored.

During 1994 — eleven years later, I was aware of something seriously wrong with my throat and neck. It wasn't too much of a shock when, in November, after various investigations, I was told there were two tumours on the left side of my neck. An operation to remove them turned out to be far more extensive than expected. I had a neck resection, and the consequences were quite devastating: my vocal cords were damaged, the nerves to the left side of my face and tongue were affected, removal of muscle restricted use of my left arm and I was in **constant** pain.

I couldn't sleep; I had a croaky little voice, felt utterly miserable, and was in never-ending pain. To begin with I had quite mild tablets to ease the pain, which were useless; these progressed in strength. Over the forthcoming months things didn't improve.

In May 1995 I saw a physiotherapist, who showed my husband various exercises to help the mobility of my arm and shoulder. I also had the use of a TENS machine, which was no help, unfortunately.

One bright spot during this time was that, due to the skill of the head and neck surgeon and a procedure using Teflon, my vocal chords were healed.

Something I wasn't prepared for was depression, my 'black hole'. Still unable to sleep, feeling utterly useless, with never ending pain. My GP arranged for me to see a psychiatrist, as a result I spent two weeks in our local hospital. With the help of anti-depressants, I slowly improved.

In July 1996 I had six weeks of radiotherapy in hospital. As a result, I had various, not unexpected, after-effects, such as burnt skin, great difficulty swallowing, and tiredness. These improved — but the pain never diminished, and when I went back for a check up, I was told it could take anything up to a year to fully recover. So I soldiered on optimistically.

By this time, I was taking MST 60 mg a day, plus antidepressants and sleeping tablets. Not only my life, but my husband's wasn't easy or pleasant. Constant pain takes over your whole life — it blots out everything. (I fully understand and sympathize when I have read about people committing suicide because they are in severe pain.) I couldn't see my life improving!!

In March 1997, the consultant asked if I would like to 'try acupuncture'. Of course I said 'yes'. Then I was referred to the pain clinic and I had the first session of acupuncture. The doctor asked me to come back the following week, and so I saw her weekly to begin with, then this interval increased to every five or six weeks.

I must be honest, and say my expectations were not optimistic — of course, I knew a little of how acupuncture works, but I really didn't think it could help me.

I'm not certain when I realized the pain was easier, it was a gradual realization that I felt so much better. The MST was reduced, and then I wondered — do I need to take it? So I just decided to stop it altogether, with drastic results: I quickly felt very ill, shivering, shaking uncontrollably, I really thought I was going to die, I spent a very miserable weekend. Fortunately we were seeing Dr F that week, who soon realized what had happened and explained that it was withdrawal symptoms of stopping the MST suddenly. Looking back, I realize I was rather naïve. After this hiccup, I really did begin to feel much better, more alert, and just feeling — normal — I had almost forgotten what it was like to feel normal.

I am so grateful that I was asked if I would like to 'try acupuncture' I'm sure my husband will agree with everything I have said, both of us have so much to thank Dr F and her team for.

Additional notes

A 64 year old lady, diagnosed with thyroid cancer 14 years previously and needing a left block dissection of neck nodes two and a half years previously, was referred for treatment of severe pain in the left shoulder, suprascapular area, and neck. The pain had been inadequately controlled on moderate opioids. She was taking a morphine preparation (MST), carbamazepine and diazepam. On referral, this lady had average pain scores of 70/100 on a visual analogue scale. On examination, she had a left accessory nerve palsy and almost concrete-like muscles in the posterior triangle of the suprascapular area, with numerous trigger points. Treatment was given to trigger points on the both suprascapular areas (in order to cover any compensatory strain on the muscles of the right side). Also, the lateral side of the spinous processes T1 and T2 were needled on the left in order to achieve a sympathetic blockade. In addition, the traditional point LI4, on the left hand, was used. With four weekly treatments of 10 minutes, her average pain scores reduced to 10/100 and she managed to drive a car for the first time in 8 months. During the next three months, she took herself off the morphine (experiencing a slight 'cold turkey' reaction which she did not realize may happen). She then maintained extremely low pain scores, using only occasional dihydrocodeine tablets and 100 mg carbamazepine a day. She felt her life had been transformed as her activity had increased so much. Her pain was satisfactorily controlled on four-weekly acupuncture 'top up' treatments.

A few months after referral, she developed one small concentrated area of muscle pain which became unresponsive to acupuncture treatment and so she was given baclofen 2.5 mg three times a day with good relief.

She remains well controlled over two years later but still requires monthly treatments, as the analgesic effects of the acupuncture treatment seem to wear off after four weeks, which was discovered by trial and error. She appears to be eternally grateful for the prolonged relief she obtains and heartily recommends acupuncture to all her friends!

References

Aung, S. (1994). The clinical use of acupuncture in oncology: symptom control. *Acupuncture in Medicine*, XII, 37–40.

Baldry, P. E. (1993). *Acupuncture, trigger points and musculoskeletal pain.* 2nd edn. Churchill Livingstone, Edinburgh.

(CSAG) Clinical Standards Advisory Group (2000). Services for patients with pain. Department of Health Publication.

Dillon, M. and Lucas, C. F. (1999). Auricular stud acupuncture in palliative care patients: an initial report. *Palliative Medicine*, 13, 253–4.

Dorfer, L., Moser, M., Bahr, F., *et al.* (1999). A medical report from the stone age? *Lancet*, 354, 1023–5.

Ernst, E. (1997). Acupuncture/acupressure for weight reduction? A systematic review. *Wiener Klinische Wochenschrift*, 109, 60–2.

Ernst, E. and Pittler, M. H. (1998). The effectiveness of acupuncture in treating acute dental pain: a systematic review. *British Dental Journal*, 184, 443–7.

Ernst, E. and White, A. R. (1998). Acupuncture for back pain: a meta-analysis of randomized controlled trials. *Archives of Internal Medicine*, 158, 2235–41.

Ernst, E. and White, A. (ed.) (1999). *Acupuncture: a scientific appraisal.* Butterworth-Heinemann, Oxford.

Filshie J. (1990). Acupuncture for malignant pain. *Acupuncture in Medicine*, VIII, 38–9.

Filshie, J. and Redman, D. (1985). Acupuncture and malignant pain problems. *European Journal of Surgical Oncology*, 11, 389–94.

Filshie, J., Scase, A., Ashley, S., and Hood, J. (1997). A study of the effect of acupuncture on pain, anxiety and depression in patients with breast cancer. Pain Society Meeting. Abstract.

Filshie, J. and White, A. (ed.) (1998). *Medical acupuncture: a western scientific approach.* Churchill Livingstone, Edinburgh.

Gosman-Hedstroem, G., Claesson, L., Klingenstierna, U., *et al.* (1998). Effects of acupuncture treatment on daily life activities and quality of life. *Stroke*, 29, 2100–8.

Hammar, M., Frisk, J., Grimas, O., *et al.* (1999). Acupuncture treatment of vasomotor symptoms in men with prostatic carcinoma: a pilot study. *Journal of Urology*, 161, 853–6.

Johansson, K., Lindgren, I., Widner, H., Wiklund, I., and Johansson, B. B. (1993). Can sensory stimulation improve the functional outcome in stroke patients? *Neurology*, 43, 2189–92.

Jonsdottir, I. H. (1999). Physical exercise, acupuncture and immune function. *Acupuncture in Medicine*, 17, 50–3.

Leng, G. (1999). A year of acupuncture in palliative care. *Palliative Medicine*, 13, 163–4.

Lundeberg, T. (1999). Effects of sensory stimulation (acupuncture) on circulatory and immune systems. In *Acupuncture: a scientific appraisal* (ed E. Ernst and A. White), pp. 93–106. Butterworth-Heinemann, Oxford.

Lundeberg, T., Hurtig, T., Lundeberg, S.and Thomas, M. (1988). Long-term results of acupuncture in chronic head and neck pain. *The Pain Clinic*, 2, 15–31.

Mann, F. (1992). *Reinventing acupuncture: a new concept of ancient medicine.* Butterworth-Heinemann, Oxford.

McMillan, C. M. and Dundee, J. W. (1991). The role of transcutaneous electrical stimulation of Neiguan antiemetic acupuncture point in controlling sickness after cancer chemotherapy. *Physiotherapy*, 77, 499–502.

Melchart, D., Linde, K., Fischer, P., *et al.* (1999). Acupuncture for recurrent headaches: a systematic review of randomized controlled trials. *Cephalalgia*, 19, 779–86.

Poulain, P., Pichard Leandri, E., Laplanche, A., *et al.* (1997). Electroacupuncture analgesia in major abdominal and pelvic surgery: a randomized study. *Acupuncture in Medicine*, XV, 10–13.

Rampes, H. and Peuker, E. (1999). Adverse effects of acupuncture. In *Acupuncture: a scientific appraisal* (ed E. Ernst and A. White), pp. 128–52. Butterworth-Heinemann, Oxford.

Thompson, J. W. and Filshie, J. (1997). Transcutaneous electrical nerve stimulation (TENS) and acupuncture. In *Oxford Textbook of Palliative Medicine*, (2nd edn) (ed D. Doyle, G. Hanks, and N. Macdonald), pp. 421–37. Oxford Medical Publications, Oxford.

Tougas, G., Yuan, L. Y., Radamaker, J. W., *et al.* (1992). Effect of acupuncture on gastric acid secretion in healthy male volunteers. *Digestive Diseases and Sciences*, 37, 1576–82.

Towlerton, G., Filshie J., O'Brien, M., and Duncan, A. (1999). Acupuncture in the control of vasomotor symptoms caused by tamoxifen. *Palliative Medicine*, 13, 445.

van Tulder, M. W., Cherkin, D. C., Berman, B., *et al.* (1999). The effectiveness of acupuncture in the management of acute and chronic low back pain. *Spine*, 24, 1113–23.

Vickers, A. J. (1996). Can acupuncture have specific effects on health? A systematic review of acupuncture antiemesis trials. *Journal of the Royal Society of Medicine*, 89, 303–11.

Wen, H. L. (1977). Cancer pain treated with acupuncture and electrical stimulation. *Modern Medicine of Asia*, 13(2), 12–17.

White, A. R., Resch, K.-L., and Ernst, E. (1999). A meta-analysis of acupuncture techniques for smoking cessation. *Tobacco Control*, 8, 393–7.

Wyon, Y., Lindgren, R., Lundeberg, T. and Hammar, M. (1995). Effects of acupuncture on climacteric vasomotor symptoms, quality of life, and urinary excretion of neuropeptides among postmenopausal women. *Menopause*, 2, 3–12.

Chapter 8

Aromatherapy and massage

Sheila Hallissey

Sheila Hallissey writes: 'The decision to specialize in oncology nursing led me to look at medicine in a different way. The importance and necessity of true holistic care became evident very quickly. Realizing this I undertook a combined counselling certificate, a diploma of holistic aromatherapy, and the study of kinesiology. I firmly believe that treating the whole person is the best medicine.'

For many patients the diagnosis of cancer is received with a dread and fear akin to being given a death sentence (McIntosch 1974). In spite of huge advances in treatment, many people still regard cancer as a fatal disease. The diagnosis of cancer, combined or not with treatment, produces a vast range of emotions which affect well-being and quality of life. Intense emotional responses to threatening news are entirely natural. Each person has to cope with cancer in their individual way, mobilizing individual coping strategies according to their personality type. Cancer can produce varying physical symptoms but let us never forget that the human being is more than a physical being, thus cancer and its diagnosis also affects the psychological, social, and spiritual aspects of the patient's life. In order to address cancer and its effects, both the psychological and physical problems must be considered. An integrated package of care, stemming from a thorough initial assessment together with constant reviews, is vital if we are to improve the quality of life of cancer patients.

To appreciate how aromatherapy and massage fit within this package, one has to look at a four-dimensional model comprising cognitive, sensory, psychological, and emotional aspects. The cognitive aspect involves counselling and listening skills.

Aromatherapy and massage can play an important role in facilitating communication. No two people are alike, and the individual's coping mechanisms must be considered and facilitated. One-to-one interaction where time and undivided attention is given to the patient is a valuable means of developing a therapeutic relationship. This relationship plays an important part in the overall benefit of the treatment (Penson 1998) but it is also one of the factors which makes research into the effectiveness of aromatherapy and massage difficult. The provision of a safe environment and facilitating discussion of fears and anxieties, when and if the patient wishes, is akin to the philosophy of person-centred Rogerian psychotherapy. The sensory aspect involves the senses of touch and smell. Touch is a basic human need, the amount and type varying at different stages of lifestyle and in different cultures, but it is a powerful means of non-verbal communication. Odour can be interlinked with the psychological and emotional benefits of aromatherapy, the effects of essential oils occurring through two routes, inhalation and dermal absorption, which will be discussed later in the chapter.

Descriptions

'Massage is a systematic and scientific manipulation of body tissues performed with the hands, for therapeutic effect on the nervous and muscular systems and on the systemic circulation' (Encyclopedia Britannica 1984). It has also been described as 'the systematic manual or mechanical manipulations of the soft tissues of the body by such movements as rubbing, kneading, pressing, rolling, slapping and tapping, for the purpose of promoting circulation of the blood, lymph, relaxation of the muscles, relief from pain, restoration of metabolic balance and other benefits both physical and mental' (Beck 1988).

Holistic aromatherapy is 'a hands-on therapy employing essential oils for treating a wide range of disorders which may involve both mind and body. Other factors such as nutrition and subtle energy imbalances are usually taken into consideration too' (Tisserand 1988). Aromatherapy within an oncological or palliative care setting is used primarily in combination with gentle massage and for this reason effleurage is the movement of choice. This is a slow gentle rhythmic movement of the whole hand. The more pressure that is applied, the deeper the effect on the blood circulation and muscular tissue; the lighter, the greater the reflex effect on the nervous system. Shiatsu massage although generally fairly vigorous, can be incorporated very successfully into the treatment, as the pressure does not have to be deep. It is the application of what the Chinese call C'hi and we call energy, rather than physical force. Its purpose is to charge the patient's C'hi and to affect the energy flow of the meridians in the body, in order to stimulate and activate the body's self-healing and self-regulating abilities. Aromatherapy and massage are natural therapies whose philosophies encompass the concepts of life force and yin and yang. All living things have a life energy that is not physical, and it is because of this belief that complementary therapies treat the person as a whole, believing that mind, body, and spirit are interlinked. The concept of yin and yang relates to the way things function in relation to each other and are used to explain the continual and natural process of change. Medical science does not embrace this philosophy as it cannot be scientifically measured and analysed.

The essential oils

There are approximately 400 plants that yield essential oil. The odoriferous materials are found in the chloroplasts of the leaf where they combine with glucose to form glucosides, which are transported around the plant structures. The oils are present in tiny droplets and occur in different parts of the plants, e.g. leaves, bark, root, resins, flowers, and the rind of some fruits. Essential oil is 'a fragrant, volatile liquid, extracted by distillation or expression from a single botanical source' (Tisserand 1985). Essential oils, which must be distinguished from fatty oils, are odoriferous and highly volatile and have a consistency more like water than oil. They are soluble in alcohol, ether, and fixed oils, but insoluble in water, where nevertheless they impart their odours. Most oils are clear although a few are distinctively coloured, for instance vetiver (brown), german chamomile (blue), benzoin (red), lemon (yellow), and bergamot (green). Most oils are liquid although a few are solid. Their chemistry is quite complex with between 30–500 compounds present in each. They can be divided into two main categories, terpenes which are hydrocarbons and the terpenoids which are their oxygenated compounds. The terpenoids are further subdivided into alcohols, phenols, esters, aldehydes, and ketones depending on their chemical structure. The scope of this chapter prohibits deeper investigation into the chemical compositions of the oils, suffice to say that they are powerful natural medicines with a wide range of effects. As with any medical treatment a full medical history of the patient is essential, as is a thorough knowledge of the medicine you are administrating.

Ancient times

Aromatherapy and massage today provides us with a contemporary version of an ancient healing art. The use of aromatic essences and what are today known as essential oils goes back to ancient times in the same way as the history and use of massage. Archaeological findings show that some 5000 years ago the ancient civilizations of China, Egypt, and India were using aromatic essences and practising some form of touch therapy or massage. Inscriptions found in the temples of Aescupapium and Aphrodite also tell us that aromatic medicine was practised widely in Greece during these ancient times. Aromatic massage is one of the principle aspects of Ayurvedic medicine which dates back to 1800 BC, as confirmed in the classic Indian herbal texts called the 'Ayurvedic'. Oils used at this time were not essential oils but some form of infused oils. It was not until 1000 AD that an Arabian physician, known in the West as Avicenna, developed the process of distillation. This huge advance enabled essential oil to be extracted from plants and is a process used to this day. Much was written during these early days about benefits of aromatics and herbs. We know that during the Great Plague, every aromatic substance available seems to have been used in one form or another. Aromatics were the best antiseptics of the time and it was noted that those in closest contact with them, especially the perfumers, were largely untouched by the disease. Growth in the knowledge of herbal medicine continued and by the turn of the eighteenth century essential oils were comprehensively being used in medicine.

However, herbal medicine become so popular that 'quacks' soon took advantage and herbal medicine began to lose respect, especially among the medical profession. By the end of the nineteenth century, experiments into the antibacterial properties of plants clarified the chemical composition and the potential healing power of essential oils. With advancement in laboratory technology and testing, attempts to mimic the oils' properties with synthetic chemical equivalents were employed more and more. This research was principally conducted by chemists and pharmacists. Today, aromatherapy is recognized as a therapy in its own right. In France, many physicians use essential oils therapeutically to treat their patients. This is due to the research of Rene Maurice Gattefosse, Dr Jean Valnet, and Marguerite Maury. During the 1950s Maury discovered that by using the oils in massage both the mind and body could be stimulated or relaxed, complementing the body's natural healing ability. She conceived the notion of individual prescription, blending oils to affect the whole person. It could be said that she was the instigator of modern holistic care. Until she reintroduced the concept, essential oils had not been used in combination with massage for almost 1000 years. The importance of massage became evident following the World

Wars where it was used to treat injuries. This developed into physiotherapy, particularly where rehabilitation was the treatment and as a result massage diminished within the broader healthcare setting.

Modern times

Are we today seeing another milestone in the use of aromatherapy and massage? They are part of what is commonly known as complementary medicine, the practice of which has increased dramatically in recent years. It was described as the growth industry of the 1980s and was predicted to become even more popular (Downer *et al.* 1994). The 1993 report on complementary therapies published by the BMA (British Medical Association) recommended more research into the area, and the development of postgraduate education to inform doctors about techniques and benefits. The report represents an important development of communication between general practitioners, the BMA and complementary therapists. In 1997, HRH the Prince of Wales delivered the first King's Fund President's Lecture to an audience of over 250 people from all areas of medicine. He introduced the discussion document '*Integrated healthcare — a way forward for the next five years*'? This document was the result of the endeavours of four working parties and the most comprehensive review of complementary medicine. The document addressed what was wrong with the current situation and proposed action in the areas of research, regulation, education and training, and the delivery of integrated healthcare. This reiterates the BMA report of 1993. Both reports set out a positive agenda for increased harmonization and discussion rather than the acrimonious debate that occurred after the 1986 report. The challenge is to integrate aromatherapy and massage safely into the present healthcare system as a therapeutic intervention, at appropriate times in the management of the patient's condition, and to prove the benefits by research.

Aromatherapy and massage are presently offered to patients in many cancer centres and hospices, and still more patients seek private treatment. In spite of its growth there is a lack of substantial clinical evidence of its efficacy and also difficulty in defining outcomes. Most practitioners outside the clinical setting rely on anecdotal evidence, whereas orthodox medicine uses empirical evidence to evaluate a therapy's success. In spite of the lack of this empirical evidence patients do say they feel better and the reasons for this are complex. Reviewing published literature it appears that the benefits of stress reduction, reduced anxiety, the length of time of the treatment, interaction with the therapist and communication, be this verbal or non-verbal, all play a part in improving the quality of life of the patient (Sims 1986; Farrell-Tory and Glick 1993;Corner *et al.* 1995; Wilkinson 1995). Benefits may also be due in part to the release of neurochemicals during the treatment.

Mode of action

Aromatherapy works by intervening on both physical and mental levels. Physically, this involves the therapeutic properties of the oils as they are absorbed through the skin: the mucous membranes and skin absorb essential oil by passive diffusion (Tisserand and Balacs 1995). Buchbauer (1993) states that there is evidence to prove that a good to excellent resorption takes place through the mucosa of mouth, nose, pharynx, gastrointestines, and intact skin. Molecules which pass through the epidermis to the dermis are transported around the body by the capillary blood circulation. Systemic absorption of the oil is increased by warmth and massage, which enhances the normal blood flow of the skin. The condition of the skin also affects the degree to which oils are absorbed. Well-hydrated skin is more permeable, as is damaged or irritated skin, while absorption is reduced in congested skin states. These are important factors to consider as patients often have altered skin conditions. The liver is the main organ involved in the metabolism of essential oils, as with all fat-soluble molecules, and once metabolized the kidney is the organ of excretion. The chemical composition of the oil can also affect the rate and degree of absorption, 'oils containing ester possibly being metabolized within the skin by esterase enzymes' (Balacs 1992a). While comparing essential oil behaviour to that of drugs he also expects the large essential oil molecules such as terpenes to be filtered more slowly than the very small molecules like alcohols and aldehydes. Also since ketones, esters and aldehydes tend to hydrogen bond with plasma albumin, it is expected that these ingredients in essential oils would react in the same way, thus slowing filtration (Balacs 1992b). This aspect should be considered when treating patients with altered plasma protein levels as it results in an increased concentration of oil in the bloodstream. However, the quantity of the dose of essential oil used in a treatment is minute when compared to orthodox drug dosage.

Essential oils are highly scented and as the sense of smell has a great impact on emotion, this plays an important role in the benefit of aromatherapy. The stimulation of receptor cells in the olfactory mucosa of the nose sets up an action potential and nerve impulses are carried to the area for the perception of smell in the temporal lobe of the cerebral cortex. There are also connections with the hypothalamus and the limbic system which is concerned with learning, memory, and emotion.

A study by Klemm (1992) demonstrated that odours can produce cortical brainwaves whereas Balacs (1992c), reported that lavender and alpha-pinene increased alpha brainwave activity while jasmine increased beta-wave activity.

Clinical application

As cancer treatments become more successful in extending life, evaluation of the quality of this extended survival has increased. Quality of life in healthcare is usually defined in terms of four dimensions; physical, psychological, social/role functioning, and symptoms. It is a term frequently used by patients and carers as they discuss the impact of cancer and its treatments on lifestyle. Over 1000 articles have been published relating to the quality of life of cancer patients and although several different tools have been developed to measure this quality, symptom experience is a common variable. The main symptoms experienced by cancer patients are pain, anxiety, depression, fatigue, changes or loss of body image and self-esteem, sleep disturbances, alteration in taste, mucositis, nausea, accompanied or not by vomiting, loss of appetite, constipation, and diarrhoea. This list is by no means exhaustive, but illustrates the many problems with which an individual may be faced.

Pain

Pain is one of the most common and most feared symptoms: 30–50% of cancer patients receiving active treatment and 60–80% of patients with advanced cancer suffer from significant pain (Elliott and Elliott 1991). The ISNCC (International Society of Nurses in Cancer Care) issued a position statement on cancer pain based on the premise that all individuals with cancer pain have the right to obtain optimal pain relief (RCN 1999). Studies show that the associated social, cultural, spiritual, emotional, bureaucratic, and financial challenges have a significant impact on the patient's perception of physical pain (Portenoy 1988; Welk 1991). The pathophysiology of nociception and pain is well documented and many theories exist which provide a basis for understanding pain management. Approaches to pain management must therefore be directed not only towards the sensory input, but to all the factors which influence the patient's response. It is vital to identify the cause(s) of the pain, whether related to the malignancy, secondary to treatment, or unrelated to the illness. In today's over-stretched healthcare system many patients are being treated by ineffective pharmacological means, as the cause of pain is not being addressed.

Acute pain is commonly associated with fear and anxiety, while chronic pain may be associated with anxiety, depression, anger, or acceptance. Employing interventions which affect these factors can contribute significantly to pain management (Farrell-Torry and Glick 1993). The activation of pain receptors also excites several autonomic reflexes producing effects that contribute to a general feeling of malaise and weakness (Rutishauser 1994). Enhancing the psychological well-being of patients is empowering and is associated with perceived changes of symptom distress and mood (Sims 1986). Attention must be paid to issues which have been proven in research to have an impact on the patient's perception of pain, if improvement in pain control is to take place.

Anxiety, depression, loss of self-esteem, fatigue

The impact of bad news consultations is well documented. The reduction of stress and relief of tension, combined or not with expression of fears and anxieties, modifies the stress response and may allow the patient to cope better with their disease and its treatment. It is accepted and well documented that conventional medicine fails in one aspect of care, that is the giving of time. Taking into account the stress response of patients diagnosed with cancer, time is one element of their total care that is of the utmost importance. Aromatherapy and massage are therapies where time is given individually to each patient, if included in care it would give patients a sense of control and may contribute to improvement in symptoms they suffer. Control over some aspects of life is important to the health of people with potentially fatal diseases (Fryback and Reinert 1997). Lidell (1984) identified groups who would benefit from touch: people with altered body image, lowered self-esteem, and those who are depressed, anxious, or dying. Allowing the patient to smell and choose the oils has a dual effect. It gives them a sense of control, and if they have commenced treatment, it takes into account the side-effects of nausea and altered smell they may be experiencing, which are common side-effects of chemotherapy. Secondly, it addresses their likes and dislikes, an important factor when stimulating the emotional response to smell, which plays an important part in the overall benefit of the treatment. Aromatherapy massage can be soothing and revitalizing. On occasions patients sleep, but relaxation does not have to lead to sleep, it can lead to an increase in energy as blocked energies are allowed to flow. This is an important consideration in aromatherapy massage when one considers the fatigue that such patients suffer. A study by Hilfinger Messias et al. (1997) indicates that fatigue is often singled out as the greatest concern that patients undergoing chemotherapy encounter. The data also suggested that fatigue was intertwined with other physical and emotional experiences. Patients often experience their worst fatigue around the time of their nadir blood count. The use of essential oils may therefore be of benefit as Tisserand (1994) suggests that all essential oils stimulate leucocytosis. It is also commonly cited that the oils have a stimulating effect on the immune system. This is an area where research, if proved positive, would greatly benefit patients. Increased secretion of catecholamines, adrenaline, and nor-adrenaline is related to stress and any strategy that reduces the secretion of these hormones has a beneficial effect, which may not be solely physiological as the state of mind can influence activity in the viscera through the autonomic nervous system and through the release of hormones.

Possible effects on the cancer process

The effect on the cancer process itself is much less clear. An interesting paper (Tisserand and Balacs 1989) covers the possible uses of aromatherapy in cancer care and the anti-tumoral action of various aromachemicals and essential oils. Another factor that may influence the cancer process is the negative effect stress has on the immune system. Lambley (1987) states 'that people who experience anxiety and stress on a routine day to day level tend to have persistently lower natural killer cell activity measures than people who do not experience high levels of anxiety'. Thus, reducing stress levels could have a therapeutic effect on the cancer process. The second aspect to consider is the release of endorphins and enkephalins during massage. These have a dual effect, the 'feel good factor' and their action as natural pain-killers, both important aspects of cancer care. Much more research is needed to prove the benefits of aromatherapy and massage, but looking at the published material and the mode of action of the therapies it appears there is scope for their inclusion in the care of cancer patients.

Indications and contraindications

The positive psychological benefits of aromatherapy and massage are indications for their inclusion in the treatment of patients diagnosed with cancer. They may also be indicated in the relief of physical problems, especially pain. So far, there is no evidence to prove that massage might cause cancer to spread. It appears that it can be used safely within an oncological setting, provided certain precautions are considered. However it is widely accepted that massage is contraindicated in the following conditions:

- infectious or contagious skin conditions or diseases, as it may spread the infection from one area of the body to another, as well as to the therapist and to anyone else the therapist treats;
- during pyrexial episodes;
- deep vein thrombosis, as there is a possibility of producing pulmonary embolus;
- over recent scar tissue or open wounds.

Within an oncological setting special consideration has to be given to each patient's history, disease and its staging, treatment, and blood profile, in order to carry out aromatherapy and massage safely. The consent of the medical team and the patient must be obtained. If the patient is unable to give consent for any reason then the consent of the next of kin should be sought and the purpose and aim of the treatment must be understood by the patient so that no misunderstanding occurs. The treatment and its effects should also be recorded and evaluated.

Cancer patients receiving massage, combined or not with essential oils, require special consideration. When treating patients with low platelet counts the massage must be extremely gentle, otherwise bruising will occur. Where oedema exists, massage will move this extracellular fluid into the lymphatic system, from which it drains into the circulation. This extra volume can put an increased load on the heart, and caution is needed if the heart is already overworked or damaged. Lymphoedema massage is a specialist technique and should only be performed by therapists who are specially trained in this area. In this situation the oxygenation and nutritional status is minimal due to stagnation of fluid and the cells are more prone to damage. Patients with bone involvement often suffer severe pain and fractures. The gentlest of strokes should be used so as not to cause physical injury and to gain the greatest pain relief through reflex action on the nervous system. If fractures are present, working over the fracture is contraindicated but massaging on proximal areas can be useful. This also applies to any area of inflammation and to tumour sites where working on the area may be contraindicated, however therapeutic touch, which is simply placing the hands on the area, can be incorporated into the treatment. In fatigued patients the system is already overburdened and massage must be extremely light and superficial to encourage rest and relaxation. Areas of blocked energy can be unblocked, revitalizing and balancing the patient. These patients cannot tolerate the drainage of excess toxins into their systems, which puts additional strain on the already overloaded liver. When working with essential oils the therapist must pay particular attention to the state of the patient' skin, their blood profile, especially the kidney and liver functions and also inquire if the patient suffers any skin sensitivities or allergies. The blood pressure has to be taken into consideration as some oils are hypotensive, for example lavender and marjoram, whereas others are hypertensive, such as rosemary. Oils which have an oestrogenic action , for example fennel, need to be used with caution and thus it is important to be aware of tumours that are hormone sensitive. A full history is vital with all treatments, special note being taken of a history of epilepsy or any contributing factor which may trigger seizures with the use of stimulating oils.

An experienced therapist will have in-depth knowledge of the chemistry of the oils, know their properties and contraindications, and be aware of the importance of choosing high quality oils. A recognized training course, clinical knowledge, and the effect that massage and essential oils have on cancer patients in the various stages of their disease is paramount, to ensure the safety of the patient.

Conclusion

In conclusion let us hope that with knowledge and research the importance and need for holistic care is appreciated and that it becomes readily available to all patients in the near future. Massage possibly has the greatest benefit, but the oils can also be used in baths, as inhalations, in compresses, infusions, and in skin care preparations.

Finally some words of thought from Doyle (1993): 'At one time, all cure of those with cancer was palliative, as there were no treatments. As medical science advanced the emphasis of care became treatment. It could be said, we lost sight of the need to provide comfort care in the midst of an environment focused on cure'.

From a patient: Anthea

In early 1995 I began to feel increasingly over-tired. Unconsciously I paced my days in order to achieve things I had to do. I am an artist and therefore work most days, including the weekends, standing in my studio for up to five hours a day. When my illness began my family had grown up, I am a mother of six children — my youngest at the time of my illness was 24 and I was 63. I am by nature and habit an energetic, rather 'driven' type. I enjoy my work and organizing my home. However, I saw to it that as my tiredness increased I did less and less outside my home and in a sense we did not lead an active life. I tried to go to bed reasonably early around 9.00 or even 8.00 pm. In March '96 it suddenly became quite plain that I was very ill. My son-in-law, a doctor, took one look at me and said I should get my GP along. Reluctantly, I asked my GP to call. He had a blood test done immediately and within a few hours I was settled in hospital. The diagnosis was acute myeloid leukaemia. When I was told I had leukaemia, my feelings clicked into a gear of resolution and determination, like one might have, say, in going into battle.

I was extremely confident in my specialist as soon as I met him. The reason for this was quite obscure. My instincts were spot-on as it turned out. Treatment started within a few hours of being admitted to hospital. A central line was inserted into my chest to give the chemotherapy through and for taking bloods. This was followed by the first session of chemotherapy. The suddenness and shock of all this was extreme. No amount of warning can alleviate the shock. I felt I was in a strange and terrible dream but determined to be as cheerful and amenable as I possibly could. After the second chemotherapy at the end of the first month, I was pronounced to be in remission. The chemotherapy lasted 30 hours each session, a painless but rather depressing ordeal. I then had four more sessions, six in all, with intervals between each for my platelets and white cells to recover before the next. After five days of each I went down into a dark valley of weakness. I could walk no more than a few faltering steps and I became more or less bed-bound for 18 months. There were some very severe side-effects to the treatment, one after my second dose. My body reacted to the antibiotic ciproxin. I developed a terrible rash, becoming bright red all over my face, torso, legs, and arms. This was extremely painful. It was alleviated by special cream created for me by Sheila, a sister on the oncology unit. With her training in aromatherapy and great knowledge of the science, she created a mixture of chamomile, lavender, tea-tree, sandalwood, and rose essential oils in a base of aqueous cream. I found this, spread over my skin, soothing and very helpful for the three to four weeks I was in this condition. This was my first encounter with aromatherapy.

The second occasion was when one of the drugs in the chemotherapy cocktail affected my lumbar region. I think the pain on that occasion was the most violent I had ever encountered. It was shortly after this that it was suggested I might have some regular aromatherapy. I had by now lost three stone in weight, being only eight stone. My skin and indeed entire body was feeling very fragile, like a bruised leaf. My resistance was getting weaker with each chemotherapy session. My taste buds had been so affected by the drugs, I could not eat and had to be drip-fed.

The first aromatherapy session was a revelation. Sheila was so gentle that my body felt quite rejuvenated. During the next four months not only were the physical symptoms reduced, but I was also helped with the ups and downs that anyone going through cancer has to undergo.

To sum up I would say that I believe my recovery was thanks to several threads at work throughout the illness. I was fortunate to have an outstanding haematologist. The prayers, love, and confidence of friends and family were and still are of help beyond words. When I had finished with the chemotherapy, I underwent a monthly regime of acupuncture. I still have acupuncture and aromatherapy and imagine I will continue to do so into the future. The aromatherapy oils that are rubbed into one's skin are clearly a huge assistance. The regular relaxation and feeling of well-being from a positive and gentle massage cannot be overestimated.

I am now three years into remission. I would like to add a post script. Seeing the whole illness in retrospect, I feel it was a cathartic and worthwhile experience. Not only did it give me a huge insight into the suffering of others, the wonders of modern medicine, and the commitment and kindness of the medical staff, it was also cathartic for my husband and family. It enabled us to come together in a different way as a family unit, and for my husband in particular, it gave him the opportunity of really looking after me.

References

Balacs, T. (1992a). Dermal crossing. *International Journal of Aromatherapy*, **4**, 25.

Balacs, T. (1992b). Well oiled pathways. *International Journal of Aromatherapy*, **4**, 5–16

Balacs, T. (1992c). Research reports. *International Journal of Aromatherapy*, **4**, 28.

Beck, M. (1988). *The theory and practice of therapeutic massage*, p3. Milady Publishing Company, New York.

British Medical Association (1993). *Complementary medicine: new approaches to good practice*. Oxford University Press, Oxford.

Buchbauer, G. (1993). Biological effects of fragrances and essential oils. *Perfumer and Flavorist*, **18**, 19–24.

Corner, J., Cawley, N., and Hildbrand, S. (1995). An evaluation of the use of massage and essential oils on the well-being of cancer patients. *International Journal of Palliative Nursing*, **1**, 67–73.

Downer, S. M. Arnott, S. J. Cody, M., *et al.* (1994). Pursuit and practice of complementary therapies by cancer patients receiving conventional treatment. *British Medical Journal*, **309**, 86–9.

Doyle, D. (1993). *Oxford textbook of palliative medicine*. Oxford University Press, Oxford.

Elliot, T. E. and Elliot B. A. (1991). Physician acquisition of cancer pain management knowledge. *Journal of Pain and Symptom Management*, **6**, 224–5.

Farrell-Torry, A. and Glick, O. J. (1993). The use of therapeutic massage as a nursing intervention to modify anxiety and the perception of cancer pain. *Cancer Nursing*, **16**, 93–101.

Fryback, P. B. and Reinert, B. R. (1997). Alternative therapies and control for health in cancer and AIDS. *Clinical Nurse Specialist*, **11**, 64–9.

Hilfinger Messias, D. K., Dibble, S. L., Dodd, M. J., and Yeager, K. A. (1997). Patients' perspectives of fatigue while undergoing chemotherapy. *Oncology Nursing Forum*, **24**, 43–8.

Klemm, W. R. (1992). Topographical EEG maps of human responses to odors. *Chemical Senses*, **17**, 233–44.

Lambley, P. (1987). *The psychology of cancer*, p63. Macdonald & Co, London

Lidell, L. (1984). *The book of massage*. Ebury Press, London.

McIntosch, J. (1974). Process of communication information seeking and control associated with cancer. A selective review of the literature. *Social Science in Medicine*, **8**, 167–87.

Penson, J. (1998). Complementary therapies: making a difference in palliative care. *Complementary Therapies in Nursing and Midwifery*, 4, 77–81

Portenoy, R. K. (1988). Practical aspects of pain control in patients with cancer. *CA: a Cancer Journal for Clinicians*, 38, 327—52.

RCN (Royal College of Nursing) (1999). *Cancer Nursing Society Newsletter*, 3, 6.

Rutishauser, S. (1994). *Physiology and anatomy, a basis for nursing and healthcare*, p. 539. Churchill Livingstone, London.

Sims, S. (1986). Slow stroke back massage for cancer patients. *Nursing Times*, Occasional Paper, 82, 47–50.

Tisserand, R. (1988). *Aromatherapy for everyone*. p. 2. Penguin Books, London.

Tisserand, R. (1985). *The essential oil safety data manual*. Tisserand Aromatherapy Institute, Brighton.

Tisserand, R. (1994). *The art of aromatherapy*. The C. W. Daniel Company, Saffron Walden.

Tisserand, R. and Balacs, T. (1995). Essential oil safety: a guide for healthcare professionals. Churchill, London

Tisserand, R. and Balacs, T. (1989). Essential oil therapy for cancer. *The International Journal of Aromatherapy*, 2, 20–5.

Welk, T. (1991). An educational model for explaining hospice services. *American Journal of Hospice and Palliative Care*, 8, 14–17

Wilkinson, S. (1995). Aromatherapy and massage in palliative care. *International Journal of Palliative Nursing*, 1, 21–30.

Chapter 9

Beyond the image: art therapy and a note on poetry

Camilla Connell

Camilla Connell introduced and developed the art therapy service at the Royal Marsden from 1988 until 2000. In 1998 she published a book entitled *Something understood: art therapy in cancer care* (Wrexham Publications).

Historical background

Art therapy, or art psychotherapy, is in brief the use of art materials for the purpose of image-making in the presence of a trained art therapist.

Art therapy has its roots, on one hand, in art and art education, and on the other, in psychology and psychoanalysis, as it is based on the notion that visual image-making is an important part of mental functioning, and that individuals may project their internal world, both consciously and unconsciously, into visual forms (Waller 1992).

Art as therapy began in Europe in the 1940s with artists such as Adrian Hill working in a tuberculosis hospital, and Edward Adamson who opened his studio at Netherne in 1946 to psychiatric patients. As artists, both understood the healing properties of the creative process and its value as a means of communication. 1964 saw the establishment of the British Association of Art Therapists bringing together a group of practitioners working largely in psychiatric hospitals. They recognized that their transactions with their patients were something other than technical instruction, other than the interpretation of images, and other than counselling or advice giving. It was something else, something unique. They saw themselves offering an essentially 'alternative' form of treatment and thus they were outsiders in a scientific environment (Woddis 1998).

Formal training in art therapy began in the 1970s, and with it the recognition that art therapy is a psychodynamic process, where 'the elements of transference, projection and fantasy are manifested in imagery as well as in discourse and behaviour. They sought to integrate these in a triangular relationship of therapist, client, and image and began to draw on the theories of psychoanalysis and developmental psychology. In 1982 the then department of Health and Social Security recognized the profession and established a structure for its clinical practice' (Woddis 1998). State Registration followed in 1997 through an extension to the Act of Professions Supplementary to Medicine.

Now, from early practice, and one which is still largely based in psychiatry, art therapy has moved to include a much wider range of patient and client groups. Approaches have been adapted accordingly although the overall aim of enabling the client to change and grow on a personal level remains true to all settings. By the 1980s a small number of art therapists were being employed to work with people with life-threatening illnesses and now services are being developed in hospitals, hospices and in the community around the UK. In 1993, with interest growing in this area, the art therapists concerned formed a special interest group within the British Association of Art Therapists entitled 'The Creative Response'. Participants are able to meet and offer mutual support and exchange of ideas through study days. They have worked towards raising the profile of art therapy in oncology through organizing conferences for other health professionals. In 1998 the group published a book entitled *Art therapy in palliative care; the creative response* which contains contributions by nine art therapists working in cancer, AIDS, and palliative care. It gives a more comprehensive account of work in this area than is possible in this short chapter. A database of arts therapies available nationwide for all those with life-threatening illness was published in 1999.

What is an art therapist?

Art therapists hold a postgraduate diploma in art therapy. The training usually follows a first degree in fine art or art and design, or in other relevant subjects such as psychology or social sciences. The student is also required to have had at least one year's relevant work experience. Usually they are mature people often having worked in education or healthcare prior to training. The duration of the course is from 2 to 3 years, full or part time and includes the consideration of theories in psychiatry, psychology, psychotherapy and art therapy. Appreciation of the art process through personal artwork is supported, and awareness of interpersonal dynamics is gained through experiential group-work. Practical experience is offered through placements in art therapy settings. Due to its demanding nature students are required to undertake their own personal therapy for the duration of the course.

The role of the art therapist in cancer care

Art therapy in cancer care can offer a range of psychological benefits on different levels but it is subject first and foremost to the exigencies of the illness of cancer. Inevitably the primary and over-riding concern of the patient is for the body and the events which are taking place within and around it. Patients have come to the hospital not for psychotherapy, but for the treatment and hopefully the cure of their cancer. However, man being both psyche and soma, an interrelation which is intensely real and intimate even when viewed from the most basic physiology, means that the emotional impact of such an illness is inestimable. Every aspect of life and lifestyle may feel threatened. This can lead not only to distress but also to serious reflection and questioning such as has never before been experienced. It is here for some people that art therapy can find a place. The role of the therapist is crucial before and during treatment. From the outset the method of introduction and presentation of the art therapy service has to be extremely 'user friendly' in order to pave the way into a treatment modality which is viewed with a certain incomprehension. Perhaps when the healing arts have been accepted as fully as the healing sciences and integration has become a reality in the minds of more than a few, the starting point will be easier.

The therapist's initial task is to offer a safe and confidential environment, being aware of any physical limitations of patients so that materials are appropriately organized. They must be able to convey a sense of openness and flexibility in order that the patient may work as they wish. Often the spectre of schoolroom art still lingers, having been the last experience of art for many people, and their first concern is whether they will do the 'right' thing. An atmosphere of exploration and experimentation is then encouraged to help the patient to tell their story on whatever level they wish. The therapist needs to provide a holding and containing atmosphere through their presence, so that strong emotions such as anger and distress can be safely expressed. They should also be open to entertaining the unanswerable questions that frequently arise.

The resulting artwork needs to be acknowledged and the therapist will encourage the patient to reflect upon it if it seems appropriate. They will try not to impose their own interpretation on the images, but rather wait for the arising of the patient's own insight.

The confidential nature of the work is always respected unless negotiated otherwise with the patient, although many sign their names on the work with a flourish. Patients are at liberty to choose what they wish to do with their work. Some are quite clear that it remains where it was made, in the art room. For others it is evidence of their achievement or reminder of their experience on that occasion and it goes with them, maybe to become a gift for someone. The artwork can hold enormous significance in different ways and the therapist becomes custodian of an ever-increasing body of work.

Mode of action

The mode of action of art therapy is well expressed by Luzzatto (1998) as the 'externalization of the mental content of the patient into visual images'. This approach is further described by a tripolar field of patient, therapist, and image with the possibility of acting in a range of communicative dimensions which are continually in movement. (Fig. 9.1) The three dimensions are: expressive-creative, cognitive-symbolic, interactive-analytic (Fig. 9.2). These three dimensions are always present in the art therapy field, but they may be activated at different times. This gives a great flexibility to art therapy, which may be used as a supportive, as a cognitive, or as a psychoanalytic form of psychotherapy. 'Cancer patients do not constitute a homogeneous population: some of them may need to find a new form of

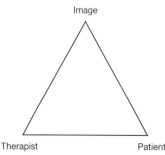

Image

Therapist   Patient   **Fig. 9.1** The tripolar field of art therapy.

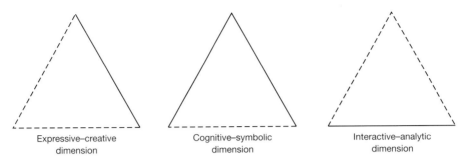

Expressive–creative
dimension

Cognitive–symbolic
dimension

Interactive–analytic
dimension

Fig. 9.2 The three communicative dimensions in art therapy: expressive–creative; cognitive–symbolic; interactive–analytic.

relaxation; others may need to explore their way of coping with the traumatic experience of cancer diagnosis and treatment; others may need a psychodynamic approach to deal with unresolved conflicts and resentments which precede their illness' (Luzzatto 1998).

Ways of working

The mode of action described by the tripolar figure above provides a very useful theoretical structure to demonstrate the interactions which can take place in an encounter with art therapy. It is a starting point from which to understand the inner processes. The art therapy service can be offered in a number of ways to meet the needs of patients, taking into account the practical constraints of their situation (Fig. 9.3).

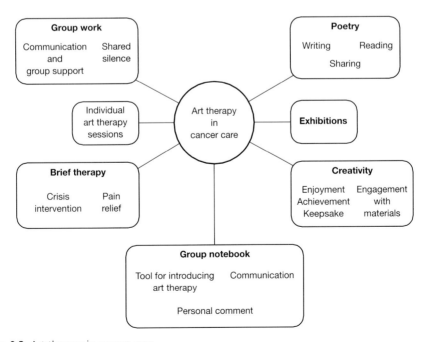

Fig. 9.3 Art therapy in cancer care.

Individual sessions: these can take place in a designated room and last for up to an hour depending on the condition of the patient. The therapist remains present having organized the space and appropriate materials. The content of the session will depend on the patient who may wish to engage immediately with the materials, or talk, or both, the essence of it being that it is their time to use as they wish. The therapist will respond by showing that she is open and accepting of anything which may occur, facilitating and supporting the patient in the art-making at the beginning if necessary. Verbal reflection on the work will often conclude the session if the patient feels able or wishes to do so. The privacy of a one-to-one contact often seems more possible for a patient who is feeling emotionally fragile and needing to find release from some of the pressures to which they feel subject.

Group art therapy: the group setting shares some aspects of individual treatment, but has the additional benefit of sharing work and of talking with other patients who have undergone similar difficult experiences. Much can be given and received by members of a group in an atmosphere of mutual understanding. For some patients this is the preferred choice from the beginning, while others feel ready to come after one or two individual sessions.

Working at the bedside: it is possible to organize materials on a trolley or in a bag to take to patients in the wards. It is here that many people first become aware of the art therapy service, although they may not wish to pursue it at this stage, or indeed have much opportunity during a short admission. However, some people feel underoccupied or overanxious; they may dislike television and be unable to concentrate on reading, so they welcome a chat and the possibility of borrowing something from the art trolley for the duration of their stay. When and if they use them is their decision, sometimes in the middle of the night if sleep proves difficult. Much can happen and if the therapist is able to revisit the patient the work can be acknowledged, even without her physical presence she is still the invisible witness of the process.

The group notebook: a useful tool that I have developed is a 'group notebook'. It is entitled *Memories, dreams, reflections*, the title of Jung's autobiography which seemed best to describe what I envisaged would be the nature of its contents. It now extends to 5 volumes and contains not only images, but poetry, prose, quotations, messages, and comments. This is shown to other patients on different wards at different times and serves as a means of communication as in a group. Having left A4 drawing pads and crayons with patients I suggest that if they would like to make something for the book it would be very welcome and appreciated by many, and indeed it is so. It is a useful way of introducing art therapy and of showing that most people are not experts at art, a frequent concern for many people.

Brief art therapy: art therapy can be used in crisis intervention and in pain relief. Only one opportunity may present itself, but the effects of a single session can be dramatic and/or cathartic depending on the situation. For the therapist the keynote here is flexibility and availability to respond to the immediate situation as appropriate.

Poetry: the use of poetry as another art-form has seemed a natural step to take when a patient does not wish to engage in art, or when their circumstances make it too difficult for them to do so. Poetry reading and writing can equally offer a path for exploration and expression of feeling. A good anthology of poetry has been very useful as it can be offered to a patient for them to choose something that they know or remember from the distant past and then read it aloud, either themselves, or if they prefer, by the therapist. This is an intimate experience and can be very rewarding and psychologically nourishing for the patient, and incidentally the therapist.

It seems that when all a patient's needs have been addressed on the physical and even psychological level, they can still be left bored and in a vacuum, starved of the sort of impressions which feed the need for meaning and provide material for thought. The influences that can be transmitted by art, literature, and music can be of profound help in arousing the patient's capacity for responding to an innate and finer area of perception within himself, so that he can touch a deeper understanding of the direction his life is taking.

Poetry reading can also stimulate imagery in the art group, so sometimes a poem is chosen or brought by a member to be read aloud at the beginning. The silent listening involved brings patients together which is helpful at the start of a group even if their own imagery predominates over the poem when they come to paint.

The 'poetry box' is a precious collection of short verses written on index cards and stored in a box. It began with a collection of Haiku, which are a traditional form of Japanese poetry stemming from several cultures. They usually consist of a limited number of syllables, around 14 to 18, so only the essence of the matter is conveyed. Now the collection has grown with the addition of contributions from patients who have written out favourite quotations or composed their own short verses, even in Haiku style.

On writing Haiku
To fold a poem like a paper boat
Sent a-sail to unknown harbours.
Radiotherapy
The rising morning moon —
I am a planet
Bathed in its sterile waves.
Pearl
I will bear this pain
As the oyster its grain of sand
To make a pearl.
Breath
Air stream —
I try to trap it in my chest cage
Oh! I can't contain it.

These were written by a woman in her 60s. They convey her experiences with accuracy, economy, and poignancy. They were greatly appreciated and a source of inspiration to other members of the art therapy group.

Exhibitions: are an unusual aspect of an art therapy service because great emphasis is placed on the confidential nature of artwork which is created in a therapeutic setting. It is the type of client group in this case which makes the additional aspect of exhibiting a valuable element for the patients themselves. Patients come to a cancer hospital for treatment of a physical illness. The nature of the illness is such that it can precipitate many losses in an individual's life and style. These may increase, and greatly diminish many of the factors which were formerly an affirmation of that person's existence. Art therapy can find a very important role here in offering someone the means to be creative, in itself a vital necessity. However, outcomes of therapy, that is the artwork, can be displayed for all to see and admire.

This shows the world and the artist themselves, that they exist, they can make something of worth, of beauty, even with a message. The message, frequently present and clearly stated, is an indication of the search that person has been undertaking through their work. Initially made only for themselves and maybe the group, there was no intention of exhibiting, but when the time comes and if the opportunity is offered it is accepted, even to the extent that the maker's name is signed with a flourish. For some it is not anonymity that is sought, but recognition and acknowledgement. Even if the exhibition is limited and low-key, there is great satisfaction for the patient in seeing their work well mounted and hanging on the wall. Sometimes they can add their own explanatory titles which makes the content of the picture additionally meaningful for the viewer. For the therapist in her struggles to promote the service it is of course valuable to display the artwork, both to attract future patients to venture into art therapy and to educate other professionals in the multidisciplinary team.

Clinical application to cancer patients

Art therapy in cancer care is patient-led. It is the patients' decision as to whether they wish to engage with art therapy and their level of involvement is their choice, although this may change as experience and confidence are gained. It is one of very few therapies which invite the patient to be active rather than passive. What is more, both the words 'art' and 'therapy' can evoke a certain anxiety which also has to be overcome. So the agenda is set by the patient, knowingly or not, and it can change as they are able to change. For example someone makes in the first instance a respectable, traditional, acceptable painting such as a country cottage, or a vase of flowers. Then their agenda may change dramatically as a result of the experience and a realization of the potential of this non-verbal medium. Given a second sheet of paper they then will use the materials with a freedom and an energy that surprises even themselves, to discharge deep-seated pent-up feelings of totally different import. So nothing can be prepared, pre-planned, other than the time, the space, the materials, and not least the therapist!

However a wide range of outcomes is demonstrated by the work itself and some of these can be anticipated or hoped for on the part of the therapist. She can offer her services with a view to relieving pain, nausea, headache, tinnitus, tension, anxiety, anger, fear, feelings of isolation, meaningless, boredom and so on, because from patient accounts all these can be affected.

Art therapy can promote self-affirmation, hope, delight and a feeling of community. It can also assist patients in their need to externalize an inner call for help from different realms, including the transcendent. So aims are many, but it is largely a matter of discovering them.

The relief of physical pain

Physical pain naturally combines with tension and stress, often heightening the levels of suffering. Art therapy through its emotional and cognitive impact can address a number of situations here. Firstly, and most directly, by imaging the pain, its location, distribution, intensity within the body and through opening to it, rather than resisting, depict its colour, shape, and effect. Secondly by an attempt to integrate it through image-making with an existential dimension which can confer meaning and reduce the isolating effect of pain. Thirdly, pain which is exacerbated by high levels of stress can be worked through in art therapy, either rapidly through catharsis, or gradually as the patient is able to relax and describe their situation.

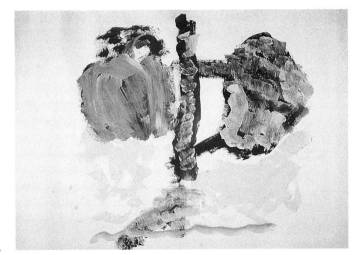

Plate 1 Case history 1. See p. 101 for details.Painted by a man with chest pain.

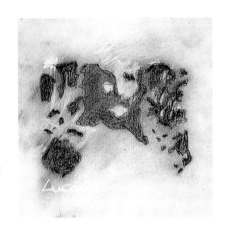

Plate 2 Case history 2. See p. 101 for details. 'The face of suffering of Christ'

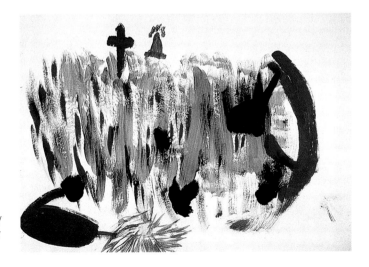

Plate 3 Case history 3.See pp. 101–2 for details.

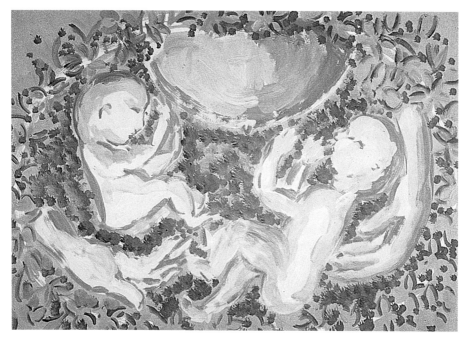

Plate 4 Painted by a woman awaiting chemotherapy. See p. 103 for details.

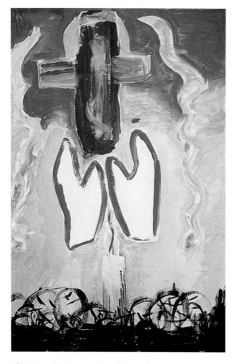

Plate 5 Jill.See p. 104 for details.

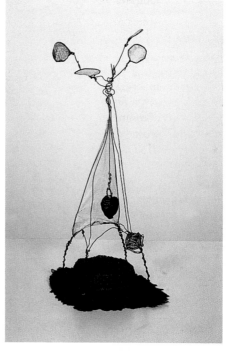

Plate 6 Julie.See p. 105 for details.

Three case examples

1. (PLATE 1) A retired successful businessman came to the art therapy group whilst recovering from recent surgery, the latest intervention of many over a number of years. Wanting to make a birthday card for his grandson, he started to make a charming picture of a running deer-like creature. After a while he began to experience considerable pain in his chest and it became difficult for him to continue. I asked if he would be willing to try an experiment and placed a clean sheet of paper in front of him. I suggested that he try to be open to the pain instead of resisting it and to see if he could then let it take on a colour and shape in his body and to put the image on the paper. With little hesitation he chose the red paint, saying that the pain was very hot, and made a ragged red patch on the sheet. As he focused his attention on the pain it diminished, so he then covered the red with cooling blue. The pain moved to the other side of his chest, and a second red area appeared on the paper. From then it moved to his spine, the area of his recent surgery, but again it diminished in the chest and he covered it with blue. Suddenly he began to have breathing difficulties and walked to the window for air. I encouraged him to relax and after a difficult moment he found himself overcome by uncontrollable weeping. He soon recovered himself, explaining that this was nothing to do with the pain but was connected with the love that he felt from his wife and family. The pain however had gone and with it the breathing problem. A moment later he was called to see his doctor and I learned subsequently that he had recounted the event to this doctor, saying what a tremendous release he had found in the experience.

2. (PLATE 2) A young man in his 30s with cancer of the lymphatic system had undergone much treatment in the previous months and was confined to bed in pain. He asked to borrow a pad of paper and some crayons from my trolley. On my next visit he showed me his work. The first piece was a strangely fragmented black and grey drawing, part of which began to reveal itself as a face or mask, the rest was shattered and blown apart. Describing it as 'the face of the suffering Christ', he began to talk about his suffering, the impossibility of communicating it to anyone and the isolation he felt as a result. He then showed me a second drawing; the same image but enlarged and reinforced being drawn this time in red. He talked at length of what he was going through. By identifying his suffering with the sufferings of Christ it seemed as if he could alleviate his sense of isolation and pain. Here it seemed as though a certain integration had taken place as to relate his condition to something of an higher order was vitally important to him. I hoped he had found a direction akin to the statement of Simone Weil; 'no pain, however great, up to the point of losing consciousness, touches that part of the soul which consents to a right orientation' (Weil 1968).

3. A young woman in her early 40s had just been admitted and was sitting cross-legged on her bed in the ward, frightened and in pain. She had been struggling for a year to treat her cancer with complementary methods; in spite of her fear of hospital and treatments she had eventually acknowledged that she needed more help. She was so distressed from pain and anxiety that sedation had had little effect; at this point someone suggested calling the art therapist.

When I found her in this state I cut introductions to a minimum and suggested that we immediately embark on some painting. Choosing a large brush and loading it with paint, she began covering the paper in an energetic disorganized manner. After a while she remarked that it was 'chaotic' and asked for a second sheet of paper. Already something had changed because she began by painting a blue spiral at the bottom left with a care and concentration that had been absent from the first painting. The paper was again covered and she asked for a third sheet. (PLATE 3) She began again in yet a different frame of mind, this time depicting the dreaded treatment of chemotherapy combined with all the protective symbols significant to her. All was now no longer just pain and despair, healing elements were being discovered. Her pain had abated and she was composed and more at peace in her situation. Her medical attendants were impressed with this change that had taken place through her encounter with art therapy.

These examples illustrate the three ways in which pain can be relieved when art therapy is used as an intervention. More work is required in this area so that it can be assessed for concrete evidence as to its effectiveness.

Patients need to find a safe way of communicating, articulating, sharing their responses and reactions to the different conditions which are imposed on them by their illness. Some are due to the material aspects of hospitalization and treatment and there is often a strong need to comment on these conditions. However many responses are of an emotional or existential nature and these require careful attention so they are allowed to develop as fully as seems necessary. In addition a diagnosis of cancer will re-awaken past events and experiences and many people who come to art therapy bring their whole life history with them. So there is an infinite variety of stories waiting to be told if the opportunity should be there, and crucially for some while there is yet time. However it is frequently only in periods of crisis as with diagnosis or recurrence that pressure for such reflection appears, quite naturally the need passes if and when life resumes its normal pattern.

The first and overriding concern of any patient is for the body. In the usual militaristic terms which seem to be employed, it has been invaded by an alien force, origins unknown and unseen, a sinister presence with which battle has to be done. Every attempt is made to rationalize it 'I know why I got my cancer'… and once it is there and has been investigated it can be classified by science in great detail, but … neither the cause nor the cure are fully known so the patient is thrown into a turmoil of uncertainty as to where the assaults on their body will end. Following tests which lead to the diagnosis, invasive treatments will follow. Most people realize that through these treatments lies the road to health and recovery and they have little choice but to submit. If they refuse what is offered they will do so at their own peril. So the body is subject to change, first by the illness and then by treatment before normal life can resume. At first the fear of the illness is greater than fear of the treatment; maybe if a later stage ensues, that orientation will change. A procedure such as surgery for example must be approached with extraordinarily ambivalent feelings. The curative/palliative versus debilitating effects of radiotherapy and chemotherapy are less immediately obvious. All this is encountered, faced, and survived with great courage by most people, but not without considerable stress for the duration. What can art therapy offer here? It is not easy to voice the feelings arising at the loss of a breast, of womanhood, of manhood, at visible disfigurement whether through surgery or illness, hair loss, speech loss, loss of function, of mobility, perhaps never to be regained. In a cancer hospital it is all seen to happen in a concentrated fashion for those working in the medical professions. Where is there time, space, and opportunity for such concerns to be stated and re-stated? In a good hospital perhaps many places, and not least through the creative therapies. In art therapy for example there occur images of the severed breast, the diseased breast, the celebrated breast which has been bid farewell, the metaphorical loss of a breast (PLATE 4). So not only has some of the pain of loss been externalized into the picture, but it can be spoken of via the image which is less immediate, less personal than pointing to one's own chest and attempting to say what it means. In addition it is easier to voice these painful issues in a safe and impartial setting with others in a group who know from experience what it means, away from those whom the patient wishes to protect for whatever reason. Anatomical images arise frequently, particularly of the unseen areas of the abdomen and even genitals. Pictures appear depicting ascites, chemotherapy, tumours, X-rays, scans, and also coffins. So fears and emotional concerns are externalized, sometimes unconsciously to the amazement of the patient when they realize what they have done. They are now visible to others and hence shared and acknowledged, not least by the art therapist. Thus the instinct to survive is in some way served and given a voice. The body is central to us. On one level it has a beginning and an end; on another, it is a vehicle for another body of a different materiality, which, according to religious tradition can have no beginning nor end. As we are now it is the visible evidence of our existence — we see, hear, touch, and sense our own body and that of another. It is as precious to us as life itself, being the bearer of life. What is currently known as 'body image' is a deeply felt support for us as social, sexual human beings, so when it is altered (especially when the effects are visible exteriorly) the consequences are sharply felt by the patient. Hence it is not surprising that images concerning these events should appear in the artwork as the patient searches to accept and come to terms with what has happened to the body.

However beneath a thin veneer there is a deep feeling of unfulfilled longing in all of us which is hard to define. It is this that having been aroused by the illness, combined with the need for meaning prompts the appearance of another group of images communicating through myth and symbol what is being experienced.

We grope for meaning and although that need is unsatisfied we continue to search, often investing time and energy into things which bring no real nourishment. So life passes, until with the onset of a life-threatening illness we wake up in quite a new way to what has been happening. Repeatedly patients have told me how their scale of values has changed dramatically, that life will never be the same again. Alongside the concern for the body arises a deep concern to forge a link with the transcendent which could be a source of succour and of meaning.

When it comes to attempting to forge this link through visual imagery the methods chosen are often very simple. For example one young woman with a brain tumour, and in hospital to receive radiotherapy, spent 3 or 4 weeks painting one sheet of paper various shades of yellow to try to give an impression of light streaming forth from the centre. She succeeded. It was a powerful statement of need and of faith.

Some pictures express a sense of uncertainty and not knowing. One posing the question 'why?' enshrines the word in a golden flower flanked by two fishes reminiscent of her Catholic childhood. Another shows an empty rudderless boat adrift on an empty sea; this is a frequent image. A young woman's picture entitled '*Cloud of unknowing*' depicts three large question marks which are also spirals in the form of clouds in a blue sky. In another, two conjoined solar bodies seem to revolve around a sun in a deep blue firmament.

Again a small matchstick figure is seen in the centre of a starry universe, this time the title was 'We reach for the universe'.

Balloons appear, in two paintings the bunches strain upwards on the end of strings like envoys waiting to be released to continue their ascent. In each case they are held by a single human figure, one alone on a beach, another a clown with one hand on hip, saying 'Oh well, what next then?' Kites also, and there are many, which impart the same feeling. The call for help appears more directly in the Christian symbol of the cross which has been depicted often, sometimes accompanied by a church or a praying figure. Here it would help to describe in some detail one encounter when these elements appeared.

Jill was determined to reach the art therapy group in the Rehabilitation unit from her ward. She arrived in a wheelchair with a friend in close attendance, already tired but glad to be there. She had been suffering from metastatic breast cancer for some time, the disease was widespread and her bones were in a very fragile condition, she could barely walk and her neck was in a collar as the onset of spinal cord compression was a possibility. She had suffered more than one fracture. She was very thin and debilitated but her spirit was strong! I felt quite anxious at what might happen. Jill knew what she wanted to paint and began immediately on a large sheet of paper. (PLATE 5) Starting at the top she drew a large cross, then moving down she drew a pair of supplicant hands. She had worked on hands on a previous occasion, making cut-outs of them in various attitudes of prayer. Then she depicted the candle at the bottom of the page with a flame leaping up between them and then she began to paint. At this point fatigue overcame her and she asked to lie down on two broad cushioned chairs which were pushed together. This was quite difficult as we had to help her all the way down and very carefully. However, once settled, I thought it would be worth suggesting that if she could tell me what she wanted on the painting I could fill it in for her. Jill agreed readily and we resumed work she telling me the specific colours and how she wanted everything to be surrounded with light. At the bottom I was instructed to paint in some barbed wire to indicate how she was trapped in her diseased body on an earthly level. Otherwise the forms were all hers. I was glad to have been able to assist in what was for her an enormous effort and she was happy to have been able to give form to her desperate need for help and comfort from a higher level.

Some people express a certain conflict between their two natures, depicting two images side by side, representing inner and outer or higher and lower. Yet others in varying ways seem to find the possibility of an integration between the body and its affliction and support or energy from a higher realm. Images of the body appear with the tumours in symbolic form and a healing energy present. I have described the art to some extent but an important part of the session is to allow for the content of the work to be explored verbally. Some people are reluctant to find words for what may well have been a powerful experience for them, this is always respected, the statement has been made in the painting and need not be spoken about. For others it is an unusual situation where they feel safe enough to voice their deep fears, hopes, and aspirations and are ready to share them with other members of the group. The therapist has no answers here, she can only respect what she hears and try not to be the cause for inhibiting anything that might be said. On the other hand she shows her willingness to enter in and face the unanswerable questions.

Albert Kreinheder, a Jungian analyst for 25 years, when himself dying of cancer, said; 'We serve our patients best when we are able to bring them again and again to the place where the mundane ego and the sacred archetype meet and touch' (Kreinheder 1991).

If this our task it is an extraordinarily sensitive one, as we are not there to force insights or destroy icons, but to 'attend, witness, and wait.'

From a patient: Julie

I believe art therapy saved my life by giving me the opportunity to get in touch with my authentic self. This part of me is now allowed to have a life. The part that existed in the world before was a highly developed false self. Every year it became harder and harder to do everything I thought I should do. I felt as though I was running to stay still. My will power forced me to go on and my body forced me to slow down. But I had no respect for my body even though I had had breast cancer. I continued to ignore my body's messages until one day I scattered into tiny pieces and my self-sufficiency, my bravado, my achievements trickled out of my body as I sobbed and shivered. I could not hold in any more suffering.

I was having psychotherapy, creating images with my mind, but in art therapy my mind was not in charge. It did not control the paint or the glue. I interacted with it by relating to whatever materials I had chosen. It was like meeting someone new. The materials would have their say, be whatever they were, show their qualities and I would make a connection, engage with them. Images emerged from an inner world that I had lost touch with. It was here that I discovered my values, my priorities and came to understand that I had sacrificed them for the more urgent demands of life. As time went on it was here that I examined the parts of myself that had been scattered, and I reclaimed those that I recognized as authentic.

These fragmented and lost parts appeared week by week on the paper. It was a process of gathering — my grief, my desolate childhood, my feminine qualities, divinity. They were brought to my centre, later I mixed a pulse of light and leaps of joy.

Art therapy is not for producing a picture for anyone else, it is about being spontaneous, allowing something deep inside to express itself, to make its mark. I believe that the body knows how to heal itself, redress the balance. Feelings are processed and expressed without the involvement of the ordinary mind. So I mix, glue, tear, and fix together. I construct sculpture and structures which represent me as I change. Recently I made the 'well' of my being which reached down into the watery depths and stretched up higher than a spire to bubbles of joy. (PLATE 6)

From a patient: Mary

I first came to art therapy three weeks after my mastectomy, 18 months ago. I had left hospital a week after the operation but still felt I was emotionally stuck at the hospital. I realized this was because I had not said goodbye to my breast. There had been no ceremony attached to losing so important a part of my body, but I felt that maybe I could paint something to represent a ceremony.

When I found the art therapy room, it was like an Aladdin's cave of colourful poster paints, crayons, and tissue papers. I felt inhibited to start with, although I had done lots of art training in the past. However I tried to forget my training, knowing that this was not important, and concentrate on expressing my feelings rather than making a nice picture. I painted the breast in a ceremonial way surrounded by my children as babies, and flowers. It really worked so well for me that I quickly became 'hooked' on coming up to the hospital for the weekly sessions. It worked in different ways for me, sometimes expressing fears. I painted a demonic crab (representing cancer) on a moonlit beach, which was playing with us patients like a cat with mice, alternately attacking and letting us go. Sometimes it was a visual affirmation. I painted a large strong tree with roots reaching down to the water beneath the soil. In the water were the words of all the strengths and positives I wanted to draw in and falling from the tree's branches were all the weaknesses and negatives I wanted to lose. Sometimes I didn't know what I was painting and would just enjoy the paint or tissue paper and allow the picture to emerge intuitively. I painted a picture in the style of Van Gogh. It was of a ripe cornfield to which the 'Sower' had returned to shoot the crows (i.e. omens of death that appeared in Van Gogh's last painting). We always put the pictures up on the wall at the end of the session and talk about each others' work and it is interesting to hear comments. There is a lot of empathy, tears, laughter, and a nice cup of tea!

Sometimes I have felt like running up to the hospital when I have had a picture in my mind that had to be put down. When I had a recurrence six months ago and had to have chemotherapy, I wanted to be positive about it. Before the first session, I began to see a picture in my mind of a 'chemo cocktail' with the words 'Love Your Chemo' across the bottom. There was always something that needed to be expressed to help with different aspects of the disease, treatment, and how it affected me. Sometimes I would come to the hospital thinking 'Why am I dragging myself up here when I feel so tired', but would soon be lost in making a picture, the tiredness would be gone and I would feel invigorated by the end.

Coming to art therapy also helped in that it gave me very good associations with the hospital. It is a very nice hospital anyway with some wonderful people there and a pleasant atmosphere, but I had memories of a very traumatic time at hospital when I was a child to overcome. The Marsden just doesn't feel like a hospital to me anymore. It is a place I go to where sometimes I paint, sometimes I have my hair done, and sometimes I have treatment. But I never have that feeling of dread and fear about coming to the hospital for treatment because it is also the place where I paint.

Evaluation

In 1998 the first two books relating solely to the practice of art therapy in cancer, palliative care, and AIDS were published in the UK. These two books are the best sources of information for the practice of art therapy in these areas.

Art therapy in palliative care; the creative response (1998). ed. Mandy Pratt and Michele J. M. Wood. Routledge

Something understood; art therapy in cancer care (1998). C. Connell. Wrexham Publications.

Art therapy research in the UK is focused mainly on professional development and the exploration of clinical practice using case-study based research. Training into research methodology is only available on the advanced art therapy course. There is much scope for work to be done in this direction.

Useful addresses

The Creative Response
AIDS. Cancer and Loss
The Old Coal House
Station Road
Ardleigh
Colchester CO7 7RR

British Association of Art Therapists
Mary Ward House
5, Tavistock Place
London WC1H 9SN

Training establishments

City of Bath College
1 Avon Street
Bath BA1 1UP

Edinburgh University
Wilkie House
31 Guthrie Street
Edinburgh EH1 1JG

Goldsmith's College
University of London
New Cross
London SE14 6NW

University of Sheffield
16 Claremont Crescent
Sheffield
South Yorkshire S10 2TA

University of Hertfordshire
Art and Design Building
Manor Road
Hatfield
Herts AL10 9TL

References

Kreinheder, A. (1991). *Body and soul.* Inner City Books, Canada.

Luzzatto, P. (1998). In *Psycho-oncology.* (ed. Jimmie Holland)., New York.

Waller, D. (1992). *Becoming a profession.* Tavistock, London.

Weil, S. (ed. Richard Rees 1968). *The love of God and affliction.* Oxford University Press, Oxford.

Connell, C. (1998). *Something understood: art therapy in cancer care.* Wrexham, London.

Woddis, J. (1998). Art therapy: the professional context. In *Something understood: art therapy in cancer care* (ed. C. Connell) pp. 133–35. Wrexham, London.

Chapter 10

The role of nutrition

Sandra Goodman

Sandra Goodman, PhD, is Editor and Director of *Positive Health*, a monthly magazine and substantial internet site — **www.positivehealth.com** — providing authoritative information across the entire range of complementary medicine disciplines.

Nutrition ought to be an integral part of conventional cancer care

This chapter explaining the role of nutrition in relation to cancer prevention and treatment does not rightfully belong in a book devoted to complementary approaches to cancer care; it should be part of mainstream medical care for cancer patients. Health-promoting nutrition, recognized by leading epidemiologists, oncologists, and molecular biologists alike to be a factor in reducing cancer risk by some 30–40% (WCRF 1997), should form a major part of the curriculum for medical students, be taught to all children from primary school age, practised within our daily lives, and should form an integral part of cancer treatment for all cancer patients.

Yet perversely, the opposite situation prevails. The commercial messages beamed out via the media promote the consumption of manifestly unhealthy foods high in fats, sugar, and salt, and the 'sexy' consumption of alcoholic, caffeinated, sugary, and carbonated beverages. Negative messages pervade the media, criticising and ridiculing the consumption of healthy and organic foods, dietary supplements and natural remedies, while physicians and holistic centres for cancer patients recommending dietary regimens fight desperately for survival, let alone for professional legitimacy.

I didn't always feel this stridently. Until the mid 1980s I was a molecular biology scientist working in the field of agricultural biotechnology, endeavouring to find ways to increase agricultural yields of crops such as soybeans. Since I moved from that field to explore the health-enhancing benefits of nutrition, I have written books and scientific articles (Goodman 1988, 1991, 1995; Goodman and Daniel 1994; Goodman *et al.* 1994), compiled databases relating to cancer and nutrition (BCHC 1993) as well as many aspects of complementary medicine (*Positive Health*).

During the past 15 years, I have witnessed the almost total marginalization of nutrition in cancer treatment, despite the existence of many thousands of high quality published research papers in the most highly respected scholarly journals attesting to the important role of nutrition in all stages of cancer aetiology and development (WCRF 1997). Furthermore, having read widely from the huge literature attesting to the massive environmental contributions to cancer (Epstein 1998), I have realized that there has also been an almost total separation of the knowledge bases of these three integrally-linked disciplines — nutritional research, environmental research, and oncology care.

It is incomprehensible to me as a research scientist, as well as a scandal to the medical profession, that nutrition does not play a central role in cancer care, given the massive body of published literature documenting the important role played by nutrition both in the prevention and the treatment of cancer (BCHC 1993; Goodman 1998; WCRF 1997; Wheatley 1998).

The wider general public has become much more aware than have physicians of the role of environmental carcinogens as well as the benefits of healthful nutrition in the fight against cancer. It is my hope to attempt to activate an acute interest in nutrition among physicians by providing a flavour of the findings of this research and in directing the reader to the massive body of research within the literature sources appended.

Nutrition's vital role in cancer prevention and treatment

The extent of the published scientific evidence regarding the role of food and nutrition in cancer prevention and treatment is considerable. The initial database compiled for the Bristol Cancer Help Centre (BCHC 1993) consisted of 5000 records during the previous decade alone! The database compiled for *Positive Health* numbers some 1000 references since 1993, and the World Cancer Research Fund's epic tome (WCRF 1997), cites more than 3000 references covering:

- patterns of diet and cancer;
- diet and the cancer process, including the genetic and molecular processes of cancer initiation, promotion, and progression;
- the types of scientific evidence published;
- 18 distinct types of cancer and how they are affected by food and nutrition;
- dietary constituents, i.e. carbohydrates, energy factors, fats, proteins, alcohol, vitamins, minerals;
- foods and drinks, i.e. grains, vegetables and fruits, pulses, nuts and seeds, meat, poultry, fish, eggs, milk, coffee, tea, and other drinks;
- food preparation, including contaminants, additives, processes such as curing, salting, and other cooking methods.

The evidence is graphically illustrated with charts, colour drawings, and tables listing, in great detail, the scientific literature from which the text is drawn.

Some 15 distinguished international scientists assembled this massive amount of evidence which, in short, concluded the following with regard to cancer prevention:

- That 30–40% of all cancers, representing the prevention of some 3–4 million cancer cases each year, could be prevented using appropriate diet, physical activity, and maintaining proper body weight;

Table 10.1 Guidelines on diet

Foods and substances to avoid, or take in minimal amounts:

Tobacco

Alcohol

Tea, coffee, caffeine drinks

Excessive salt, chemical preservatives and processed foods

Sugar

Saturated fat

Hydrogenated margarine

Red meat, smoked and cured meats

Foods to eat in moderate amounts:

Eggs

Dairy produce

Fish, preferably deep-sea oily fish (salmon, tuna, mackerel, herring, pilchards)

White meat and poultry (preferably organic)

Foods to eat liberally:

Whole grains (brown rice, barley, oats, millet, rye, wheat, corn, quinoa)

Vegetables

Fruits

Legumes (peas, beans, legumes)

Seeds (sesame, sunflower, pumpkin)

Nuts

Water (filtered)

Suggested daily supplement levels:

Nutrient	Active cancer	Maintenance level
Vitamin A	10 000 IU	7500 IU
Beta-carotene	25 000 IU	10 000 IU
Vitamin B complex	50 mg	50 mg
Vitamin C	6–10 g	1–3 g
Vitamin E	200–400 IU	100 IU
Zinc (elemental)	15–25 mg	15 mg
Selenium	200 mcg	100 mg
Chromium GTF	100 mg	50 mg
Magnesium	100–200 mg	100–200 mg

Adapted from: Goodman *et al.* (1994) Nutrition and lifestyle guidelines for people with cancer. *Journal of Nutritional Medicine* **4** 199–214.

- That diets with substantial and varied amounts of fruits and vegetables could prevent 20% or more of all cancer cases;
- That if alcohol consumption were maintained within recommended limits, up to 20% of aerodigestive tract, colon, rectal, and breast cancer cases could be prevented;
- That appropriate diet could prevent most stomach cancers and that colon and rectal cancers are mainly preventable by diet, physical activity, and appropriate body weight.

Given the paltry attention and resources currently expended upon nutritional methods for the prevention and treatment of cancer, and considering the mammoth implications of the above projections, along with its respectable documentation of scientific literature, a great deal needs to change in order to accommodate nutritional methodologies into cancer care.

However, very few physicians can afford the luxury of reading the entire research literature for cancer, or neoplasms as it is categorized within *MedLine*. Hence, here are a few examples of published research from the literature illustrating the extent of progress in nutritional cancer research.

Evidence from epidemiological and clinical trials

Although there is a vast literature on nutrition and cancer, few studies addressed supplemental nutrients directly. Patterson *et al.* (1997) compared the results of 7 clinical trials, 16 cohort and 36 case-control studies and demonstrated the effects of nutrients which are distinguishable from the effects of biologically active compounds in foods.

Randomized clinical trials have not demonstrated significant protective effects of beta-carotene, but have found protective effects of vitamin E against prostate cancer, vitamin A, zinc, beta-carotene, vitamin E, and selenium against stomach cancer, and selenium against total, lung, and prostate cancers.

Cohort studies provide scant evidence that vitamin supplements are associated with cancer. Case-control studies have demonstrated an inverse association between vitamin C and bladder cancer, several supplemental vitamins and oral/pharyngeal cancer and vitamin E and several cancers. Inverse associations between vitamin E and colon cancer have been found by a randomized clinical trial, a cohort study, and a case-control study.

In conclusion there is, overall, modest evidence regarding the protective effects of nutrients from supplements against a number of cancers. Future studies of vitamin supplement use and cancer are justified, however methodological problems which impede the ability to assess supplement use, and statistical modelling of the relation between cancer risk and supplement use, require ironing out.

Zhang *et al.* (1999) studied the associations between dietary intakes of carotenoids, vitamins A, C, and E, consumption of fruits and vegetables and breast cancer risk. The authors conducted a large, prospective study to evaluate long-term intakes of these nutrients and breast cancer risk, in a cohort of 83 234 women, aged 33–60 years in 1980, who were participants in the Nurses' Health study. During 1994, the authors identified 2697 incident cases of invasive breast cancer (784 premenopausal; 1913 postmenopausal).

There was a weak, inverse association between intakes of beta-carotene from food and supplements, lutein/zeaxanthin and vitamin A from foods and breast cancer risk in premenopausal women. There were strong inverse associations for increasing quintiles of alpha-carotene, beta-carotene, lutein/zeaxanthin, total vitamin C from foods and total vitamin A in premenopausal women with a positive family history of breast cancer. There was also an inverse association for increasing quintile of beta-carotene in premenopausal women who consumed 15 g or more of alcohol daily. Additionally, premenopausal women consuming 5 or more servings per day of fruits and vegetables had modestly lower risk of breast cancer than women who consumed fewer than 2 servings per day (relative risk (RR) = 0.77). The latter association was stronger in premenopausal women with a positive family history of breast cancer (RR = 0.29) or those women consuming 15 g or more of alcohol per day (RR = 0.53). The authors concluded that the consumption of fruits and vegetables high in specific carotenoids and vitamins may reduce the risk of breast cancer in premenopausal women.

La Vecchia and Decarli (1996) noted that following early increases, mortality rates from oesophageal cancer have levelled off in Italy over the past two decades and are now inter-mediate on a European scale: 4.7/100 000 men; 0.8/100 000 women. The authors say that this reflects trends in consumption of tobacco and alcohol, major risk factors for this type of cancer. Within Italy there is considerable variation in rates of oesophageal cancer, with high mortality areas in the North-East. The relative risk (RR) of oesophageal cancer was 4.3 in heavy smokers and 3.5 in heavy drinkers, based upon a case-control study in northern Italy. A diet poor in fresh fruit and vegetables was also related to risk (RR = 2.5).

Regarding population attributable risk, 71% of cases in men and 32% in women were accounted for by tobacco smoking, 45% in men and 10% in women by alcohol drinking, 40% in men and 29% in women by a diet poor in fresh fruit and vegetables. Altogether, these 3 factors — tobacco, alcohol and poor diet — accounted for 90% of cases in Italian men and 58% in women (83% in both sexes combined).

A case-control study of lung cancer incidence among women in Shenyang, China explored the relationship between diet and lung cancer risk, with emphasis upon the potential effects of specific dietary nutrients in being able to modify lung cancer risk (Zhou et al. 1999). Dietary information regarding 290 cases and population-matched controls was obtained using person-al interviews. There was a significant difference between cases and controls with respect to intake of beta-carotene, vitamin C, and fibre, all of which reduced the risk for lung cancer in a dose-dependent manner, with calculated odds ratio (OR) of 0.84, 0.75, and 0.46, respectively. The apparent effects of these nutrients persisted after adjusting for cigarette smoking. The authors' conclusions were that beta-carotene, vitamin C, and fibre may function as protective factors to reduce the risk of lung cancer in women in China.

Breast cancer is a serious health problem, accounting for almost one-third of cancer-related deaths in women in America (Kimmick et al. 1997). As the prevention of breast cancer using dietary modification is an active area of clinical and epidemiological research, it has been proposed that vitamin E supplementation may reduce a woman's risk of devel-oping breast cancer. The authors review (60 references) the available evidence regarding vitamin E and breast cancer.

Vitamin E has decreased incidence of carcinogen-induced breast tumours in animal studies. However, there have been conflicting results in human epidemiological research. Further study is warranted, particularly regarding its interactions with other antioxidants and to the duration and timing — pre- versus postmenopausal — of vitamin E use to determine its use in the treatment and prevention of breast cancer.

Nutritional evidence at the cell and molecular level

The potential antiproliferative effects of tocotrienols, the vitamin E component in palm oil, upon human breast cancer cell growth have been studied by Nesaretnam et al. (1998). Both oestrogen-responsive (ER+) MCF7 and oestrogen-unresponsive (ER-) MDA-MB-231 human breast cancer cells were used in this study. The effects of the tocotrienol -ich fraction (TRF) of palm oil were compared with those of alpha-tocopherol (alphaT).

TRF inhibited growth of MCF7 cells (ER+) both in the presence and absence of oestradiol; the dose-response was nonlinear, and complete suppression of growth was achieved at 8 μg/ml. MDA-MB-231 (ER-) cells were also inhibited by TRF; there was a linear dose-response and complete growth suppression was achieved with 20 μg/ml. Fractionation of the TRF into individual tocotrienols revealed that all the fractions inhibited the growth of both ER+ and ER- cells, and of ER+ cells both in the presence and absence of oestradiol. The most highly inhibitory were the gamma- and delta-fractions; complete inhibition of MCF7 cell growth was achieved at 6 μg/ml of gamma-tocotrienol/delta-tocotrienol (gammaT3/deltaT3) in the absence of oestradiol and 10 μg/ml of deltaT3 in the presence of oestradiol. Complete suppression of growth of MDA-MB-231 (ER-) cells was not achieved even at concentrations of 10 μg/ml deltaT3. In contrast to the inhibitory effects of tocotrienols, alphaT had no inhibitory effect upon MCF7 nor on MDA-MB-231 cell growth either in the presence or absence of oestradiol.

These data confirm results from other studies using other sublines of human breast cancer cells and demonstrate that tocotrienols exert direct inhibitory effects upon breast cancer cell growth. Studies of the effects of the tocotrienol-rich fraction (TRF) upon oestrogen-regulated pS2 gene expression in MCF7 showed that tocotrienols do not act via an oestrogen receptor-mediated pathway and must therefore act differently from oestrogen antagonists. Also, tocotrienols did not increase levels of growth-inhibitory insulin-like growth factor binding proteins (IGFBP) in MCF7 cells, implying a different mechanism from the one proposed for retinoic acid inhibition of oestrogen-responsive breast cancer cell growth.

The inhibition of breast cancer cell growth by tocotrienols may have important clinical implications not only because tocotrienols inhibit the growth of both ER+ and ER- cells types, but also because ER+ cells could be growth-inhibited in the presence as well as in the absence of oestradiol. Future clinical applications of TRF may arise from potential growth suppression of ER+ breast cancer cells which are resistant to growth inhibition by anti-oestrogens and retinoic acid.

The antitumour effect of the herbal medicine sho-saiko-to, and its mechanism of action upon a murine malignant melanoma cell line (Mel-ret) was studied by Liu *et al.* (1998). Sho-saiko-to induced apoptotic cell death of Mel-ret cells with a definite increase of cell surface Fas antigen and Fas ligand (FasL). [Fas is a protein recognition/signalling pathway.] Sho-saiko-to arrested Mel-ret cells in G1 phase (a phase during cell division) by decreasing the expression of cyclin-dependent kinase (cdk) 4 and its homologue cdk6. Kinase activities of cdk4 and cdk6 were shown to be downregulated by sho-saiko-to. Ingredient analysis revealed that baicalin is likely to be the main active constituent in the upregulation of Fas antigen and Fas ligand, while glycyrrhizin is the main constituent in the inhibition of cyclin-dependent kinases.

Zheng *et al.* (1997) recognized that various naturally occurring substances from vegetables and herbs exert chemopreventive properties against cancer. The authors reviewed two such compounds, isolated from garlic and from a traditional Chinese medicinal herb, elemene, isolated from the herb Rhizoma zedoariae.

Elemene was shown to exhibit antitumour activity in human and murine tumour cells both *in vitro* and *in vivo* and has shown substantial clinical activity against various tumours. Analysis by MTT assay of the effect of elemene upon the growth of leukaemia cells showed that the IC50 for promyelocytic leukaemia HL-60 cells and erythroleukaemia K562 cells were 27.5 μg/ml and 81 μg/ml respectively, and the IC50 for peripheral blood leukocytes PBL) was 254.3 μg/ml. Inhibition of elemene upon the proliferation of HL-60 cells was associated with cell cycle arrest from S to G2M phase transition, and with the induction of apoptosis. The apoptosis of tumour cells was confirmed by DNA ladder formation using gel electrophoresis and ultrastructural alterations.

The results also demonstrated that the inhibitory effects of allicin, a natural organo-sulphide from garlic, upon the proliferation of tumour cells were associated with the cell cycle blockage of S/G2M boundary phase and the induction of apoptosis.

These results suggest that the induction of apoptosis may contribute to the mechanisms of antitumour activity of elemene and allicin, which deserve further investigation as potential chemoprevention agents in humans.

The mechanism by which vitamin A prevents or delays carcinogenesis is still unclear (Maziere *et al.* 1997). Vitamin A, in addition to antimutagenic and antiproliferative pro-perties, also appears to be able to induce programmed cell death (apoptosis). The authors studied the role of vitamin A regarding in vitro apoptosis induction in a rat colon tumour cell line. Retinyl palmitate in varying concentrations were added to the culture media. Cell proliferation was measured via (3H)thymidine incorporation, cell differentiation via intestinal alkaline phosphatase expression and apoptosis induction by DNA fragmentation and morphological evolution of adherent and floating cells.

Vitamin A decreased (3H)thymidine incorporation following one day of treatment, induced alkaline phosphatase expression and increased cells undergoing apoptosis. This study confirms the role of vitamin A regarding proliferation and demonstrates the capacity of vitamin A to induce apoptosis. These results may be useful to prevent development of colon cancer by supplementation of the diet with vitamin A.

Roles of individual nutrients and foods

Proposed mechanisms of vitamin C (ascorbic acid, ascorbate) for cancer treatment and prevention were reviewed by Head (1998). They include immune system enhancement, stimulation of collagen formation for 'walling off' tumours, inhibition of hyaluronidase to keep intact the ground substance around the tumour and prevent metastasis, prevention of oncogenic viruses, correction of ascorbate deficiency frequently observed in cancer patients, speeding up of wound healing following cancer surgery, enhancement of various chemotherapy drugs, reduction of toxicity of chemotherapeutic agents such as Adriamycin, prevention of damage from free radicals, and neutralization of carcinogenic substances.

Published studies from Scotland and Japan have reported the potential benefit of high dosages of vitamin C in the treatment of terminal cancer. Studies from the Mayo Clinic disputed those findings, resulting in acrimonious accusations of methodological flaws from both sides. Numerous epidemiological studies have demonstrated the importance of dietary and supplemental vitamin C in the prevention of numerous cancers, including bladder, breast, cervical, colorectal, oesophageal, lung, pancreatic, prostate, salivary gland, stomach, leukaemia and non-Hodgkin's lymphoma.

Clinical research studies with animals

The effect of diet treatments with soy flour and rye bran upon prostate tumour develop-ment in rats was investigated by Landstrom *et al.* (1998). 125 rats with transplanted R3327 PAP prostate tumours were divided into five groups. Tumour development was studied for

24 weeks during treatment with diets containing: 1) 33% soy flour (SD); 2) rye bran (RB); 3) heat-treated rye bran (HRB); 4) rye endosperm (RE); 5) control, fibre-free dietary (FF).

Compared with the control (FF), there were significantly fewer palpable tumours and lower tumour volume detected 14 and 16 weeks following transplantation in the SD (soy), RB (rye bran), and HRB (heat-treated rye bran) groups. Compared with the control, body weight was lower 16 weeks after transplantation in the RB and HRB groups. There was a significantly lower energy intake in the RB and HRB groups, compared with the controls during the 3–6 weeks following tumour transplantation, whereas energy intake was the same in all groups 13–16 weeks following transplantation. Even following adjustment of tumour volume for body weight, there were still significantly lower tumour volumes in the SD, RB, and HRB groups compared with the FF controls. There was a significant increase in daily urinary excretion of the isoflavonoids daidzein, O-desmethylangolensin, equol and Genistein in the SD group, and of the ligands enterolactone and enterodiol in the RB and HRB groups. There were no differences in testosterone levels between the groups.

These data show that soy flour inhibits implanted prostate cancer growth. Rye bran and heat-treated rye bran had a protective effect; however further studies are required to exclude the possibility that a low energy intake may have played a role in this regard. These results also suggest that phytoestrogens, isoflavonoids, and ligands may be responsible for the delayed prostate tumour growth.

Kishimoto et al. (1998) studied the effectiveness of vitamin E in the prevention of lung cancer in mice. NNK (4-(methylnitrosamino)-1-(3-pyridyl)-1-butanone was the chemical agent used to induce lung tumours. High doses of vitamin E suppressed NNK-induced increased activity of ornithine decarboxylase, a key enzyme of polyamine biosynthesis, in the lungs of mice 4 weeks following injection. Vitamin E, in contrast, increased the NNK-induced decrease of spermidine/spermine N1-acetyltransferase activity, a key enzyme of polyamine biodegradation. Vitamin E treatment suppressed NNK-increased levels of proliferating nuclear cell antigen, a marker of cell proliferation, and high doses of vitamin E suppressed NNK-induced lung tumourigenesis, i.e. inhibiting the development of lung tumours. The mechanism of inhibition is in part due to the regulation of polyamine metabolism.

Beta-carotene (BC) has been found to possess potent antitumour activity in liver carcinogenesis chemically induced by diethylnitrosamine (DEN) in rats (Sarkar et al. 1997). The authors studied the basic cytogenetic and molecular mechanisms of the antitumour effects of beta-carotene. They monitored the effect of beta-carotene upon rat liver chromosomal aberrations (CAs) and DNA chain breaks in the early precancerous stage of liver cancer in rats. Even one DNA strand break per chromosome can be detected. A BC supplement, 120 mg/kg was fed to rats 15 days prior to challenge with a carcinogenic chemical.

Beta-carotene provided a unique protection against chromosomal strand breaks 96 hours following injection of DEN. Long-term treatment also afforded a protective effect on induction of CAs 15, 30 and 45 days following DEN treatment. Beta-carotene treatment for 15 days prior to DEN injection offered significant protection in the generation of single-strand breaks compared with DEN control. Beta-carotene ranks as a potential chemopreventive agent regarding rat liver carcinogenesis.

Clinical research studies in humans

A cross-sectional study of postoperative non-small cell lung cancer (NSCLC) patients looked at the possible effects of vitamin intake and folate status upon disease-free survival (Jatoi et al. 1998). Supplemental vitamin usage, dietary vitamin intake, red blood cell (RBC) folate, and serum folate concentrations were assessed in 36 patients with a history of NSCLC. Exclusion criteria included factors altering folate status or associated with altered nutritional habits: 1) evidence of cancer on history, physical, or chest radiograph; 2) tobacco, alcohol ingestion (>2 drinks/day) or cancer treatment within 3 months; 3) the use of folate antagonists; and 4) age <60 years.

The median disease-free censored survival was 24 months (range 4–41 months). 19 of 36 patients (53%) reported vitamin supplementation. Compared with non vitamin supplement users, vitamin users had a longer median censored survival (41 months versus 11 months, P = 0.002). Following adjustment for stage of cancer, the association between RBC folate and censored survival (r = 0.35) and serum folate and censored survival (r = 0.32) approached statistical significance. Thus those patients with NSCLC who took vitamin supplements were more likely to be long-term survivors. A similar trend toward long-term survival was seen in patients with higher circulating folate concentrations.

Sixty cancer patients with secondary lymphoedema, with particular reference to the development of the incidence of erysipelas (acute, streptococcal inflammation of the skin and subcutaneous tissues, infection accompanied by fever and constitutional disturbances) took part in a randomised, double-blind study to determine the efficacy of sodium selenite in combination with physical therapy to relieve congestion (Kasseroller 1998). All the patients in this study had erysipelas infection of the skin. Selenium was administered in pharmacological doses. Physical therapy was for 3 weeks and patients were observed for a further 3 months.

The incidence of erysipelas among the patients was 11%. During the 3-week period of intensive treatment, there was not a single case of erysipelas in the treatment, compared to a single case in the placebo group. During the follow-up period of 3 months, there was not a single case of erysipelas in the treatment group, compared to 50% of the patients in the placebo group. Despite the higher doses, the selenium level did not rise above normal values. Patients under long-term antibiotic therapy suffered no relapse when the antibiotic therapy was stopped and selenium was administered instead. Additionally, the administration of a single high-dose of sodium selenite could immediately bring the inflammation under control.

In another trial, 974 men with a history of either basal cell or squamous cell cancer were randomized to receive a daily supplement of 200 μg of selenium or a placebo to test whether supplemental dietary selenium is associated with changed incidence of prostate cancer. The men were treated for a mean of 4.5 years and followed for a mean of 6.5 years (Clark *et al.* 1998).

Selenium treatment was associated with a significant (63%) reduction in the secondary endpoint of prostate cancer incidence during 1983–93. There were 13 prostate cancer cases in the selenium-treated compared with 35 in the placebo group (relative risk RR = 0.37). If the analysis is restricted to the 843 patients with initially normal levels of prostate-specific antigen (PSA), there were only 4 cases diagnosed in the selenium-treated group compared with 16 in the placebo group following a 2 year treatment lag (RR = 0.26). Other significant health benefits were observed for the secondary endpoints of total cancer mortality and incidence of total, lung, and colorectal cancer. There were no significant changes in incidence for primary endpoints of basal and squamous cell skin cancer. In the light of these results, the 'blinded' phase of this trial was stopped early. In conclusion, selenium treatment was associated with substantial reductions in the incidence of prostate cancer and total cancer incidence and mortality. Selenium did not show a protective effect against squamous and basal skin cancers.

Peng *et al.* (1998) analysed the plasma concentrations of 10 micronutrients in cervical tissue from cancerous, precancerous, and noncancerous women. Paired blood and cervical tissue samples were taken from 87 patients, aged from 21–86 years who had a hysterectomy or biopsy due to cervical cancer, precancer (cervical intraepithelial neoplasia I, II and III), or noncancerous diseases. The samples were analysed for 10 micronutrients (lutein, zeaxanthin, beta-cryptoxanthin, lycopene, alpha-carotene, beta-carotene, cis-beta-carotene, alpha-tocopherol, gamma-tocopherol and retinol).

In the three patient groups, the mean plasma concentrations of all micronutrients except gamma-tocopherol were lowest in the cancer patients; however, the mean tissue concentrations of the two tocopherols and certain carotenoids were highest in the cancerous tissue. Among the 10 micronutrients, only the concentrations of beta-carotene and cis-beta-carotene were lower in both the plasma and tissue of cancer and precancer patients than in those of noncancer controls. These data suggest that not all the micronutrient concentrations in plasma reflect the micronutrient concentrations in cervical tissue. In some cases, it may be necessary to measure the tissue micronutrient concentrations in order to define the role of the micronutrients in cervical cancer. An adequate plasma and tissue concentration of beta-carotene should be maintained for the prevention of cervical cancer and precancer.

To investigate whether dietary supplements of selenium (Se) reduce the risk of cancer 312 patients with histories of basal/squamous cell carcinomas, recruited from 1983–1990 were randomly assigned in double-blind fashion to daily oral supplements of either Se-enriched yeast (200 μg/Se/day) or a low-Se yeast placebo (Combs *et al.* 1997). Patients were followed with regular dermatological examinations through to 1993, representing 8269 person-years of observation. Skin cancer diagnoses were confirmed histologically, plasma selenium concentrations were determined at 6–12 month intervals, and deaths and patient illnesses were recorded, confirmed, and documented in consultation with medical care providers. Although selenium did not significantly affect the primary endpoints, incidence of recurrent basal/squamous cell skin cancer, selenium treatment was associated with reduction in a number of secondary endpoints: total mortality from all cancers, combined incidence of all cancers, combined lung cancer, colorectal cancer and prostate cancer.

These results strongly demonstrated the benefits of Se-supplementation, supporting the hypothesis that supplemental selenium can reduce cancer risk. Despite the lack of protective effects against non-melanoma skin cancer, the reductions in risk of other frequent cancers demand further evaluation in controlled clinical intervention trials.

Conclusions

There is no doubt from the few examples cited above that much research has already been conducted and is ongoing regarding the application of nutrition in both the prevention and treatment of cancer. However, more concerning is the virtual non-translation of these findings into either medical or people's lifestyle practices. Considering the ageing of the developed world's population and the rising incidence of cancer, associated with lifestyle, environmental, and dietary factors, and the human and monetary costs of cancer, social, environmental and lifestyle issues need to be addressed. It would help if the medical professional appeared to be cognisant of the huge body of evidence already amassed, rather than always attempting to deride and denigrate the use of nutritional approaches to cancer treatment.

Today there are also a variety of non-mainstream nutritional therapeutic practices — various dietary regimes such as Gerson, macrobiotics, Vries, wheat grass, fasting, colon cleansing, herbal regimes — espoused by a variety of practitioners which may be scorned by the general medical community, but which, if subjected to serious and concerted research, may reveal significant therapeutic efficacy. Today's marginal practice may become tomorrow's mainstream clinical protocol. There is an urgent requirement for research regarding the efficacy of these nutritional and dietary cancer regimes in treatment of cancer patients, and the decriminalization of nutrition as a cancer treatment methodology.

A few selected areas of education, policy and research requiring urgent attention include:

- The addition of nutrition into the medical school curriculum;
- The improved communication of published research to physicians and the systemic and comprehensive integration of published findings into clinical practice;
- The requirement of open and vigorous debate about fundamental precepts such as RDAs (recommended daily allowances), balanced diet, and the use of supplements;
- The necessity for serious research about the many and varied dietary regimes currently being advocated and used by many tens of thousands of people, who claim efficacy, particularly for cancer — vegetarian, frugivore, raw food, macrobiotic, Gerson diet, fasting;
- The identification and research of components within vegetables and other foods which appear to protect against cancer;
- Research of anti-oestrogen foods such as soybeans and their preventive effects in cancer.

References

Bristol Cancer Help Centre (BCHC) Cancer and Nutrition Database. (1993–present). Database of some 5000 published records compiled by the author for the Bristol Cancer Help Centre, Bristol UK.

Cancer Research Campaign. (1999). *CRC Cancerstats: survival: England and Wales 1971–95.* Available from Cancer Research Campaign, 10 Cambridge Terrace London NW1 4JL.

Clark, L. C., Dalkin, B., Kongrad, A., *et al.* (1998). Decreased incidence of prostate cancer with selenium supplementation: results of a double-blind cancer prevention trial. *British Journal of Urology,* **81**, 730–4.

Combs, G. F. Jr., Clark, L. C. and Turnbull, B. W. (1997). Reduction of cancer risk with an oral supplement of selenium. *Biomedical and Environmental Sciences,* **10** (2–3), 227–34.

Epstein, S. S. (1998). *The politics of cancer revisited.* East Ridge Press, NY, USA.

Goodman, S. (1988). *Germanium the health enhancer.* Thorsons, UK.

Goodman, S. (1991). *Vitamin C the master nutrient.* Keats, Connecticut, USA.

Goodman, S. and Daniel, R. (1994). *Cancer and nutrition: the positive scientific evidence.* Bristol Cancer Help Centre.

Goodman, S. (1995, 1998). *Nutrition and cancer: state of the art.* Positive Health Publications Ltd., Bristol, UK.

Goodman, S. (1997). Nutrition — pivotal in prevention and treatment of disease. In: *Mind-body medicine: a clinician's guide to psychoneuroimmunology.* Churchill Livingstone.

Goodman, S., Howard, J., and Barker W. (1994). Nutritional and lifestyle guidelines for people with cancer. *Journal of Nutritional Medicine,* **4** (2), 199–214.

Head, K. A. (1998). Ascorbic acid in the prevention and treatment of cancer. *Alternative Medicine Review,* **3** (3), 174–86.

Jatoi, A., Daly, B. D., Kramer, G., *et al.* (1998) A cross-sectional study of vitamin intake in postoperative non-small cell lung cancer patients. *Jouranl of Surgical Oncology*, **68** (**4**), 231–6.

Kasseroller, R. (1998). Sodium selenite as prophylaxis against erysipelas in secondary lymphedema. *Anticancer Research*, **18** (**3c**), 2227–30.

Kimmick, G. G., Bell, R. A. and Bostick, R. H. (1997). Vitamin E and breast cancer: a review. *Nutrition and Cancer*, **27** (**2**), 109–17.

Kishimoto, M., Yano, Y., Yajimas, S., *et al.* (1998). The inhibitory effect of vitamin E on 4-(methylnitrosamino)-1-(3-pyridyl)-1-butanone-induced lung tumorigenesis in mice based on the regulation of polyamine metabolism. *Cancer Letters* 126 (**2**), 173–8.

Landstrom, M., Zhang, J. X., Hallmans, G., *et al.* (1998). Inhibitory effects of soy and rye diets on the development of Dunning R3327 prostate adenocarcinoma in rats. *Prostate*, **36** (**3**), 151–611.

La-Vecchia, C. and Decarli, A. (1996). Esophageal carcinoma. *Annali Dell Instituto Superiore Di Sanita*, **32** (**4**), 551–6.

Liu, W., Kato, M., Akhand, A. A., *et al.* (1998).The herbal medicine sho-saiko-to inhibits the growth of malignant melanoma cells by upregulating Fas-mediated apoptosis and arresting cell cycle through downregulation of cyclin dependent kinases. *International Journal of Oncology*, 12 (**60**), 1321–6.

Maziere, S., Cassand, P., Narbonne, J. F., *et al.* (1997). Vitamin A and apoptosis in colonic tumor cells. *International Journal of Vitamin and Nutrition Research*, **67** (**4**), 237–41.

Nesaretnam, K., Stephen, R., Dils, R., *et al.* (1998).Tocotrienols inhibit the growth of human breast cancer cells irrespective of estrogen receptor status. *Lipids*, **33** (**5**), 461–9.

Patterson, R. E., White, E., Kristal, A. R., *et al.* (1997). Vitamin supplements and cancer risk: the epidemiological evidence. *Cancer Causes Control*, **8** (**5**), 786–802.

Peng, Y. M., Peng, Y. S., Childers, J. M., *et al.* (1998). Concentrations of carotenoids, tocopherols, and retinol in paired plasma and cervical tissue of patients with cervical cancer, precancer, and non-cancerous diseases. *Cancer Epidemiology, Biomarkers and Prevention*, 7 (**40**), 347–50.

Positive Health (1994-present). Monthly publication specializing in authoritative information regarding all aspects of complementary medicine and also extracting research relating to complementary approaches to all illnesses, including cancer and nutrition.

Sarkar, A., Basak, R., Bishayee, A., *et al.* (1997). Beta-carotene inhibits rat liver chromosomal aberrations and DNA chain break after a single injection of diethylnitrosamine. *British Journal of Cancer*, **76** (**7**), 855–61.

Wheatley, C. (1998). Vitamin trials and cancer: what went wrong? *Journal of Nutritional and Environmental Medicine.* **8**, 277–88.

World Cancer Research Fund (WCRF) in association with American Institute for Cancer Research (1997). *Food, nutrition and the prevention of cancer: a global perspective.* World Cancer Research Fund, 105 Park Street, London W1Y 3FB. Tel: 0171 343 4200; Fax: 0171 343 4201.

Zhang, S., Hunter, D. J., Forman, M. R., *et al.* (1999) Dietary carotenoids and vitamins A, C, and E and risk of breast cancer. *Journal of the National Cancer Institute*, **91** (**6**), 547–56.

Zhang, S., Yang, H., Zhang, S. *et al.* (1997). Initial study on naturally occurring products from traditional Chinese herbs and vegetables for chemoprevention. *Journal of Cell Biochemistry Supplement*, **27**, 106–12.

Zhou, B., Wang, T., Sun, G., *et al.* (1999) A case-control study of the relationship between dietary factors and risk of lung cancer in women of Shenyang, China. *Oncology Reports*, **6** (**1**), 139–43.

Chapter 11

Healing the whole person

Tony and Ann Neate

Tony Neate is a healer, transpersonal counsellor and nutritional adviser. He offers help in these areas as a support to other forms of treatment being received by the patient. Ann Neate is a healer and counsellor, trained in the transpersonal and humanistic traditions. She is particularly interested in psychological causes of illness.

'The cure of a part should not be attempted without treatment of the whole' Plato *c.* 480 BC

A brief history of healing

Healing has existed throughout history. There is evidence among early civilizations dating back to 3000 BC in Mesopotamia; the Egyptian healer Imhotep who founded the tradition of healing in the temples; and around 1200 BC, the famous Greek healer Asclepius who founded healing temples throughout the Greek states and subsequently in various parts of the Roman Empire. In the latter, the patients were clothed in white and slept near the statue of Asclepius. In dream-state, the patient saw the spirit of the healer appear at his side and prescribe appropriate treatment. History shows that cures were frequent (Jones 1983).

In this list, we must include the Shamans, the Medicine Men, the Essenes, and the Druids. In the early 15th century AD, the Swiss doctor, Paracelsus wrote: 'Medicine is not merely a science but an art; it does not merely consist in compounding pills and plasters and drugs of all kinds but it deals with the processes of life which must be understood before they can be guided. A powerful will may cure where a doubt will end in failure'.

As science and religion began to develop in different directions, the care of the body and mind became separated with the mind and spirit designated to the exclusive care of religion. This lead to healing outside the Church becoming outlawed and the persecution, torture, and death of many healers. So the baby was thrown out with the bath water!

It was not until the middle of the 20th century in the UK, when the Witchcraft Act was repealed in 1951, that healing once again became increasingly acknowledged as a powerful source of help to rebalance the human soul and body.

The authors' journey

Following the death of his mother from stomach cancer in the early 1970s, Tony became interested in nutrition and its possibilities as a support system in the treatment of cancer. Through this interest, he became acquainted with Dr Alec Forbes, a senior consultant physician at Plymouth Hospital, who was also interested in the nutritional aspects of treating disease; and who subsequently took early retirement to become the first Medical Director of the now famous Bristol Cancer Help Centre.

In pursuit of the nutritional approach, Alec and Tony visited and studied the work of Dr Hans Moolenburg in Holland and Dr Hans Nieper in Germany, both internationally renowned doctors involved in the complementary treatment of cancer. Alec then needed a reliable source of nutritional supplements which were free of any known carcinogenic excipients which would also provide active ingredients that offered a high bio-availability to the body's systems. Tony together with a friend, Eric Llewellyn, started a company called Nature's Own Limited to provide these products.

Along with this development, Alec and Tony were also interested in energy healing and quickly saw that healing would ideally complement the nutritional approach and that together, these two therapies could have a powerful healing effect.

Tony and his wife Ann both studied counselling in depth as an adjunct to healing, realizing that healing the subtle energies of the body could easily be undermined if a person's mental/emotional attitude remained in a negative state. Counselling skills help patients to understand the aspects of their lives that might have contributed to the development of cancer, a realization and acceptance of which can not only transform their outlook, but sometimes assist a progressing cancer to retreat.

Tony and Ann kept in close contact with Bristol Cancer Help Centre, studying their approach, which included counselling, healing nutrition, various forms of relaxation techniques, and a doctor's consultation. In the early 1980s, together with Dr John Cosh, a retired consultant, they ran a Cancer Help Centre in Cheltenham for three years.

The late Penny Brohn, another founder of Bristol Cancer Help Centre, on discovering that she had breast cancer, walked out of the hospital in which she was a patient. She felt that there had to be some other way than having her breast removed. A lady of independence and determination, she objected to being told that there was nothing she could do for herself. She became famous as a pioneer of the complementary approach and for her statement, 'I'm glad I have cancer!' She found it enabled her to appreciate life and to see it in a much deeper and more integrated way.

So a trio of skills was developed: energy healing, counselling, and nutrition — a combination of spirit, mind, and body therapies. Over the years, this has proved to be very effective in helping cancer sufferers.

Healing: its definition

What is energy healing and how does it work? First of all, let us look at some definitions. The Confederation of Healing Organizations (CHO) is the main body representing healing organizations in the UK and it has authorized the following definitions of healing:

For the purpose of the CHO generally, and of the Healing Research project in particular, the following definition applies: 'Healing is the beneficial effect which healers in CHO terms are believed to have on patients when, motivated by their own beliefs and following their normal practices, they administer healing in contact through the hands or at a distance by thought (or prayer) transference or by radionic instrument.'

For general use by members in relation to their own beliefs: 'A dictionary definition of healing is "to make well". To the extent that it occurs, healing is the transference of harmonizing paraphysical energies. What energies are transferred depend upon the needs, beliefs, capabilities, and procedures of the persons involved. Every living being is maintained by these energies which may be transferred in the presence of those concerned or at a distance'. 'Healing may be of one individual by another, or a group by one person, or of a group, by a group or of one person by a group, or it may be self-induced.'

It goes on to state that every member is free to define healing further in their own terms in relation to their own beliefs without in any way detracting from the above Code.

Our own definition

Healing is the channelling of universal energy to a patient by thought processes to bring about an overall state of energy balance and harmonization on all levels, thus stimulating the body's natural defence system to deal with disease. Healing quickens the body's natural healing processes on all levels.

The system of energy healing that we use acknowledges that all forms of life need spirit to provide the 'thought essence' or spark that motivates physical matter, infusing it with life. From our viewpoint, cancer is a living cell which is part of normal physical existence and which, if it comes out of balance, can proliferate indiscriminately in the human body, eventually taking over from the normal cells needed to maintain physical existence.

As healers, we endeavour to release and transmute the misplaced energy that stimulates the growth of the cancer cells, and then give appropriate healing to the physical body. Healing works within its own terms of reference. It is a non-manipulative therapy that works alongside any other form of therapy. It does not need the faith of the patient and does not conflict with any other therapy. It helps the patient to find that which he or she seeks on an inner level, for it can stir deeper levels of being that may unconsciously be blocking the flow of life.

It is encouraging that, today, healing is becoming accepted as a valid and credible therapy, offered in some medical centres as a complement to orthodox medical treatment (British Medical Association 1993).

The work of Denis Haviland, a retired senior civil servant, given in return for healing which had transformed his life, has played an important role in establishing healing as a recognized therapy (Booth 1994). As chairman of the CHO, he consulted both the medical establishment and the government on the degree of regulation required for a healing therapy that complemented the work of doctors. He headed a team that brought together a number of leading healing organizations under the banner of the CHO.

The CHO adopted a compulsory Code of Conduct to be administered by its members. This was written in consultation with the Royal Colleges, the British Medical Association, and the General Medical Council (British Medical Association 1986). A disciplinary procedure was established to enforce the code and the CHO introduced mandatory public liability and professional indemnity insurance for members, similar to that for GPs.

The CHO has also compiled a pilot scheme for a Competence Based Qualification (CBQ) with the idea of it becoming a National Vocational Qualification (NVQ) — the next step towards greater credibility.

College of Healing

Another big step forward took place in 1983, when a group of doctors and experienced healers founded the College of Healing. Together, they initiated a course designed to develop and maintain high standards for teaching healing. This has helped to bring healing to the forefront of complementary medicine, by providing a comprehensive, in-depth education in which both doctors and patients can have confidence.

The College of Healing now has a nationally accredited course in the theory and practice of healing (Booth 1994). In 1997, it was accepted by the Open College Network to Levels 2 and 3. This means that it can be available at any of 2500 Colleges of Further Education throughout the country.

The foundation course

This includes the following areas of study:

- Understanding how the mind, body, and spirit interact;
- Practising self-healing and visualization techniques;
- Developing and understanding the main energy centres (chakras) of the body;
- Nurturing a sensitivity to the human aura;
- Introduction to and practise of basic meditation techniques;
- Controlling breathing to induce a state of relaxation;
- Creating a safe environment for healing;
- Introduction to anatomy and physiology;
- Formulating your own personal development.

The professional diploma course

This includes:

- Integrating the physical, mental and spiritual systems;
- How colour and symbols affect the healing process;
- The role of the environment in health;
- How dreams affect our healing and well-being;
- The importance of nutrition;
- Using stress creatively;
- Starting a healing practice;
- Recognising the signs of emotional, mental and spiritual problems;
- Self-knowledge to avoid illusion and delusion;
- Developing sensitivity in chakric treatments;
- Giving healing to cancer patients.

The student has to prepare a portfolio on the course work, which includes six detailed case studies and also researches an aspect of healing. The curriculum includes plenty of practical healing and illustrates the study of healing for the modern-day healer.

In addition to the College of Healing, there are other members of the CHO, the foremost being the National Federation of Spiritual Healers which has a countrywide referral system. A full list of members is given at the end of the chapter.

Healing is regarded as a complementary rather than as an alternative therapy. In fact, it is a therapy that can support any other therapy because of its balancing, calming, and energizing qualities. Being non-invasive in a physical sense, it will not interfere with other therapies and all properly qualified healers will support conventional treatments.

Healing benefits

Healers regard cancer as a stress-related disease and recognize the emotional shock and trauma that can be brought about by the initial diagnosis. They are trained to channel universal energy not only to where it is needed, but to the person as a whole. Healers are trained to listen to what a patient is expressing and how they are expressing it, to help the patient to use breath more beneficially and to relax more deeply on all levels; to encourage the patient to use their mind to create realistic positive thoughts about their condition and hence to assist in their own healing process.

Healing is not about curing. We find the term 'curing' a misleading concept and have known so-called 'cured' patients who have been dismissed from hospital and have subsequently died through a weakened immune system. Healing helps to improve the quality of life, allowing the patient to play a part in the healing process. Conversely, if it becomes evident that the patient is approaching death, a healer can help support the patient in the dying process so that he or she is able to die with dignity and in peace.

Healers are drawn to the work because they are interested in the spiritual dimension of life and view human life as four-dimensional, comprising body, emotions, mind, and spirit. Indeed, healers draw upon the finer energy of the universe. So although some healers may follow a particular religion, others may embrace a spiritual understanding based on unconditional love — the love that motivates someone to become involved in a caring profession.

Healing is not an easy therapy to quantify as it is usually given as an addition to other forms of treatment. However, from anecdotal evidence, it supports other therapies, enhancing the healing process. The authors both work as healers and the energies they channel provide relief and improvement in patients' condition. Furthermore, all healing organizations have received countless testimonials to that effect.

Giving healing is not like giving a measured dose of a drug or adjusting a limb in a prescribed way. The healer subtly adjusts the energy to the energy of the patient. If patients are seriously ill, their energy level will be low and will need building gently. The healing energy will help relieve stress and may bring to the surface hidden or suppressed emotional issues. It can restore balance and harmony on an inner level, releasing barriers that may effect positively the success of other forms of treatment. It can also be helpful in relieving pain.

Above all, it can transform the attitude of the patient towards the illness, enabling them to accept it in a more positive and creative way. In this sense, it empowers the patient to take self-responsibility for helping his or her own condition. It is a totally supportive approach.

A healer should never give healing to a patient unless asked, as this could be invasive and possibly contrary to the patient's will. At this point, it might be interesting to describe four healing situations which bring in different aspects of healing:

◆ The patient asks for healing and this request is felt to be coming from his/her inner self. This is the most straightforward situation in which the healer will simply channel healing energy appropriate for the particular type of cancer;

◆ The patient requests healing, but the healer finds on 'tuning in', that the inner voice of the patient is rejecting it for whatever reason — usually because of unresolved issues that relate to an earlier situation in life. In this case, the healer would offer the healing mentally sending a thought to the patient, 'If it be your will,' so as to allow them to absorb or reject the healing in accordance with their deepest inner needs. In fact, it is always possible for the spirit or inner self to reject healing and override the patient's conscious wish. This can be felt intuitively by the healer, as if a brick wall were in place, or even physically, as a spark or slight shock;

◆ The healer is asked by a relative or friend of the patient to send healing, usually on a distant healing basis. The patient could be nearby or on the other side of the world. Distance does not seem to affect the efficacy of the healing process. However, because the patient's personal beliefs do not allow it, he/she would not ask for healing. Here again, the healer would 'tune in' and if it were felt that the inner voice was saying 'Yes please' would then proceed with the healing, very gently and again on an 'If it be your will' basis;

◆ The fourth example is where it is known that the patient would not ask for or wish to receive healing, but a close friend or relative is desperately seeking help. However, on 'tuning in', but not actually sending healing, the healer also feels that the inner voice is saying 'No'. In this instance, the healer would offer a prayer for that person.

In all instances, the healer respects the conscious freewill of the patient and, equally, the less conscious freewill of the spirit. These are very different criteria from those which face an orthodox practitioner, but it will help the reader to understand the different boundaries that the healer has to acknowledge.

Healing has now 'arrived' as a professional therapy and is being taught in a more structured and academic way, removing it from the irrational superstitions of the past. Nevertheless, healing must include an intuitive sensitivity which some healers may start out with naturally and others gradually develop. It is an aspect of all human beings used more or less unconsciously by most people, whether in business, science, the arts, or medicine, or simply in ordinary living. Many great scientists have been inspired through this intuitive faculty. Einstein is known to have said, 'Imagination is more important than knowledge.'

The following is a true story (Goldberg 1985):

> John is a philosopher — trained in mathematics. He is known for his orderly, systematic, impeccably logical arguments. Colleagues say that if John is on the other side of a disagreement you have your hands full. He was the last person I would have thought of as intuitive. Yet he told me, 'I've always been extremely intuitive. My mind is always making wild leaps that turn out right.' When I reminded him of his reputation as a quintessentially rational thinker, he said, 'I've learned to construct arguments. But they always come afterwards.'

Self-healing techniques

Visualization

As part of the healing process we give the patient visualization exercises. This supports the healing that is being given and helps them to take some responsibility for helping their condition. One such visualization which cancer patients really enjoy is the Sieving Exercise:

- Sit down, lie down, or stand up. Visualize a circular garden sieve in your hands, with a mesh that sieves out the cancer cells;

- Start at your feet and gradually bring the imaginary sieve up through your body, visualizing that you are sieving out all the cancer cells in your body;

- Bring the sieve right up through the body and over your head. As you do so, close an imaginary trap door just above your head so that the contents of the sieve cannot re-enter your body;

- After closing the trapdoor, empty the contents of the sieve into an imaginary bag, seal it, and send it off 'to its rightful place in the universe';

- Repeat the exercise three times, each time using a sieve with a finer mesh. The last time, it will be as fine as a coffee filter.

This enables the patient to feel that they are able to do something positive to help themselves. We also encourage them to find other visualization exercises of their own creation. This type of exercise gives an important psychological boost which the authors believe can also help boost the immune system.

Relaxation exercises

We encourage our patients to do simple relaxation exercises. This helps them let go of body tensions. Suggested simple exercises are listed here, although some of these would be discretionary according to the physical condition of the patient and the type of cancer involved:

- 10-minute relaxation. Lie down flat, knees up if you prefer. Take a few slow, deep breaths. Stomach out as you inhale, hold breath to the count of four, stomach in as you exhale. Out breath longer, relax and hold a moment. Tell your body to 'let go, let go'. Sink deeply and heavily into the bed or settee as you repeatedly remind every part of you to let go, again and again, until finally the whole body gives way. Do this at least once a day, two or three times if you get exhausted frequently;

- Yawn or sigh three times and have a good stretch;

- Imagine a punchball in front of you. Take a few powerful punches with each hand. Then focus on your natural breathing, allowing it to relax you;

- Massage the areas where tension is most felt. Use whatever movements feel best and most natural. These include stroking, rubbing, circular movements, kneading, squeezing, pressing and tapping. Self-massage is very effective for tension relief of head, neck, and shoulders;

- Choose a key relaxing word such as serenity, peace, tranquillity. Focus on a special place in the countryside and enjoy being there. Say the word 'relax' a number of times as you breath deeply, and then repeat your key relaxation word three times as you breathe slowly and deeply;

- Appreciate something good about yourself and smile inwardly. Feel good that you have taken time to take responsibility for your tension, smile kindly at yourself for having become so tense. Visualize how you would like to feel, and say to yourself, 'I am allowing myself to relax, to treat myself in a kind, respectful way, and to work through everything step by step';

- Reprogramming. Think of a recent stressful situation. What positive affirmation could you have given yourself to counter your tense reaction in that situation? Re-run the episode in your imagination, responding gently to it rather than reacting stressfully and repeat your affirmation.

Meditation

To enable the body, mind, and emotions to rest quietly, consciously letting go of fears and concerns must surely be a big plus for anyone with cancer. For this is when the parasympathetic system takes over, encouraging the healing forces on all levels to do their work. You can call it a self-healing meditation or simply, a relaxation.

In the following example, the mind is used to create a feeling of well-being and the important preparation and closing phases are included.

Preparation

Find a quiet place where you will not be disturbed and sit or lie down comfortably. …Starting at the feet, focus on each part of the body, giving it a moment's attention and consciously relax it, at the same time thanking it for the work it does for you. …Imagine your force field or auric field surrounding you and protecting you like a cocoon.

Meditation

Become aware of the very core centre of yourself, somewhere in the heart area … create a little space there, a place of stillness and serenity, of golden light and unconditional love. Hold it. …Allow this space to expand, radiating shafts of golden light that very gradually fill every cell in your body, energising you like a sun, your sun … sense the love you are radiating moving out beyond your body, filling your auric field with its glow … hold the sensation of radiating love and golden light for a few minutes … become aware of the healing energy of the universe within your sun, cleansing and balancing every cell in your body … enjoy the sense of well-being. …

Closing

Very gradually bring your attention back to your body, realigning yourself within it (you can think of two images on a screen coming into focus) … remain poised, still aware of the inner space of stillness and serenity in your heart area and your auric field surrounding you. …When you feel 'together', have a good stretch.

If you should ever feel unfocused at the end of a meditation, place your hands in cold water and have a cup of tea.

Lifestyle

We find it helpful for cancer patients to re-evaluate their lifestyle. In many cases this means looking at patterns of activity, recognizing that they need to plan their life more carefully rather than allowing their way of life to run them. We give below some ideas on adjusting one's life to changing circumstances:

- BE GENTLE WITH YOURSELF;
- Work no more than six hours per day;
- Have at least two days a week from normal work routine;
- Allow at least one hour for each meal;
- Eat slowly, chew well and, to assist the digestive process, avoid drinking water with your meals. But it is important to drink plenty of still mineral water between meals;
- Cultivate the habit of listening to relaxing music;
- Find a 'hermit' spot, use it daily and do not allow interruption;
- Take at least 10 minutes a day for physical exercise, preferably in the open air;

- Have a regular massage, float, or join yoga, or other exercise class;
- Cultivate a creative, non-competitive hobby, for example gardening, painting, making music. 'Sing your own song';
- Actively cultivate the habit of walking, talking, and moving at a slower pace;
- Smile and respond cheerfully whenever meeting anyone;
- Remind yourself that you can only change how **you** relate to people, you cannot change **them**;
- Give support to others and learn to accept support in return — to give is an indulgence, to receive is a gift;
- If emotional and/or sexual relationships are upsetting, seek advice;
- If you are unhappy at work or regularly get overtired — take stock and look at options, i.e. new areas of work, fewer hours, etc.;
- Avoid the tendency to dwell on the past — concentrate on the present;
- Avoid living in the future — always be in the 'now';
- Remember that fixed expectations can be a trap. Open expectancy is preferable;
- Express your feelings openly without antagonism or hostility;
- Do not accept or give yourself unrealistic deadlines. It can always be done tomorrow;
- Change your routine as often as possible;
- Before you go to sleep, remember 3 good things that have happened during the day;
- Say 'thank you' or 'well done' to yourself whenever you finish something that you feel satisfied with;
- Say 'I choose to', 'I need to', 'I want to', or 'I do not want to', rather than 'I should, could, ought or have to…';
- Avoid the 'Blame Game', you give away your power. Instead, take personal responsibility for your life and empower yourself;
- No-one, including yourself, need be a victim;
- Don't 'beat yourself up'. It's painful and you never win!
- IF YOU NEVER SAY **NO**, WHAT IS YOUR **YES** WORTH?

Counselling combined with healing

Most importantly, cancer patients need to be encouraged to find a creative activity through which they can truly express themselves. Everyone faces stresses in their lives. Some are straightforward and can be handled satisfactorily. Others relate to emotional traumas that we are unable to face or deal with. These seem to go right inside, disempowering us, building up some kind of emotional blockage that we are unable to resolve. It is this kind of blockage that can weaken the system and pave the way for susceptibility to some kind of illness such as cancer.

Often an unhappy childhood establishes repeat patterns in our lives from which there seems no escape. Unconsciously we choose a partner who already has or develops characteristics similar to those of one or both of our parents, resulting in a continuation of those unresolved challenges we faced in dealing with our parents. We may need to seek assistance and work with a counsellor or psychotherapist who will help us to let go of the need for those unwelcome repeat patterns.

When counselling is combined with healing, apart from the physical benefits, the changes that a person makes psychologically are speeded up, because the healing energy encourages submerged memories to surface. And the material that the psyche brings to consciousness is always just what is needed for the healing process at that moment. The healer/counsellor becomes the enabler.

How does one choose the right therapist for oneself? We are reminded of the words of that great cancer therapist, Dr Lawrence LeShan: 'It is rather like buying a new car. You go from garage to garage, trying out different models, until you find one that suits you!'

For anyone with cancer, counselling, in our opinion, is an essential part of the healing process. We see it as having five stages:

The problem

Recognizing that they have a problem, apart from the cancer. This is not always easy, for they may successfully sabotage this recognition. It can often feel safer to stay where we are than to stir up past and sometimes painful memories. We tend to subconsciously avoid those issues that lie in our past.

Finding the source

Having established that there is a problem, we need to help patients find the source of the blockage in their emotions. A good therapist will help discover where the past difficulty lies and how to confront it.

Dealing with it

Patients need to find a way of releasing the blockage. It may involve letting go of suppressed anger in a safe and contained way, re-establishing levels of self-worth and self-empowerment, finding independence from the past patterns of behaviour which can enable them to live in the present, freed from the past.

Moving beyond it

Moving beyond the need to be manipulated by those past patterns and the person or persons involved.

Stage of redemption

This is where patients now feel empowered and can look back and actually feel grateful for the lessons that those past difficulties may have taught them or enabled them to achieve; to realize that once anger is expressed in a safe way, it can provide the stimulus and motivation to step forward and tackle their own spiritual mission in this lifetime. It is a stage in which they can start to understand the true meaning of unconditional love. Interestingly, we consider that it is only at this stage that true forgiveness can be offered, for this too needs to be unconditional. It is a false trail to say, 'I forgive you, but …' and one that is ultimately damaging to both the patient and to the person they wish to forgive. Forgiveness needs to come from the heart.

Nutrition

We have dealt with healing, various forms of self-healing and what can be gained from counselling. But what about the body itself? A sensible nutritional regime can be highly beneficial, a de-tox approach, avoiding those foods which may contain suspected carcinogenic ingredients and are generally detrimental to good health.

However, in our experience, no diet will provide positive benefits if it creates emotional stress in the patient due to resistance. Indeed, some patients have said quite openly that they would sooner die from cancer than eat what they describe as 'rabbit food'.

Case study

Cancer patients come to us for a number of reasons. They are in a terminal state and have been told that orthodoxy has nothing more to offer them. They feel disempowered by the system. We remember the husband of a hospital Sister who had terminal cancer, telling us of his anger against the consultant who had told his wife quite bluntly that she was going to die and that there was nothing she could do about it. Thirdly, because they want to explore every possible avenue to find a way back to health.

The following case study illustrates how a change in attitude can be very powerful in the healing process:

> Denise is typical of many of our clients with cancer. She had felt a lump in her breast, was diagnosed and operated on three months later. She then went on to have a six-month course of chemotherapy, followed by a two-month course of radiotherapy. She first came to see Tony during this period and told him that she knew why she had cancer as three months before being diagnosed, she had been in a highly depressed state and had repeatedly said to herself, 'I want to die, I want to die'.
>
> However, she now felt that she wanted to live and enjoy a full life — she wanted to be of benefit to society and to feel she could do something worthwhile with her life. Her parents were not demonstrative people and consequently she had felt unloved as a child, which had created a feeling of insecurity and a need to please others in order that she would be appreciated.
>
> They worked together on a regular basis. Denise was given healing; they worked on unresolved issues from her childhood and she did various visualization exercises. She enthusiastically followed a diet and took nutritional supplements. Gradually she began to be less dependent on those issues that were pulling her down, she began to nurture herself and appreciate her self-worth.
>
> Eight years on, Denise, who is now in her late 40s, is living a full life with her husband and five children, having regained her self-confidence and self-empowerment. She supports and helps some of her friends who are facing similar challenges.

All cancer sufferers need to adhere to a golden rule: that they **never again** return to full-time, stressful employment. We have known cases in which that rule has been ignored because they have felt so well and perhaps have wanted or needed the money, with the result that the cancer has returned and usually been fatal. The body always needs that extra reserve to keep the immune system topped up and the general energy level well balanced. A slightly curtailed life, is after all, better than no life at all.

References

Booth, R. (1994). Keeping in touch. *Nursing Times*, 90, 29–31.

British Medical Association (1986). *Report on alternative medicine*. BMA, London.

British Medical Association (1993). *Complementary medicine — new approaches to good practice.* BMA, London.

Goldberg, P. (1985). *The intuitive edge.* Turnstone.

Jones, S. (edited by L. St Aubyn) (1983). *Healing: a short history.* Heinemann, London

Further reading

Angelo, J. (1998). *Your healing power.* Piatkus, London.

Dethlefson, T. and Dahlke, R. (1983). *The healing power of illness.* Element Books, Shaftesbury .

Furlong, D. (1995). *The healer within.* Piatkus, London .

Kubler-Ross, E. (1969). *On death and dying.* Tavistock/Routledge, London.

Krystal, P. (1982). *Cutting the ties that bind.* Samuel Weisher.

LeShan, L. (1989). *Cancer as a turning point.* Plume, New York.

LeShan, L. (1995). *How to meditate.* Thorsons (Harper Collins), London.

Levine, S. (1986). *Who dies?* Gateway Books, Bath.

Page, C. (1992). *Frontiers of health.* C W Daniel, Saffron Walden.

Organizations mentioned in text

College of Healing, Runnings Park, Croft Bank, West Malvern, Worcs, WR14 4DU, 01684 566450

Confederation of Healing Organizations (CHO), 113 High St., Berkhamsted, Herts., HP4 2DJ 01442 870660. A registered charity, it represents over 12,000 insured healers. CHO's objective is to establish healing as a standard therapy for the NHS as well as private medicine. Their 16 member associations (all charities) include:

Association for Therapeutic Healers,

Association of Professional Healers,

British Alliance of Healing Associates,

College of Healing,

College of Psychic Studies,

Fellowship of Erasmus,

Greater World Spiritual Healing Fellowship,

The Healing Foundation,

Maitreya School of Healing,

National Federation of Spiritual Healers,

Radionic Association (Distant Healing),

Rainbow Healing Association,

Spiritualist Association of Great Britain,

Sufi Healing Order of Great Britain,

White Eagle Lodge,

World Federation of Healing.

Chapter 12

Homoeopathy

George Lewith and Julian Kenyon

George Lewith is honorary senior research fellow at Southampton
University and honorary consultant physician at Southampton General
Hospital. His research interests include evaluating the effectiveness of
complementary medicine, particularly acupuncture and homoeopathy, in
a variety of clinical conditions.

Julian Kenyon is a partner in the Centre for the Study of Complementary
Medicine in Southampton and London. He is also Research Director of the
Dove Healing Trust, a medical research charity looking at the scientific
nature of subtle energies. He has a particular interest in cancer and its
treatment using an eclectic complementary approach.

The history and development of homoeopathy

Homoeopathy is the treatment of illness by giving very dilute medications derived from
plant, animal, and mineral sources. It was developed by Dr Samuel Hahnemann nearly
200 years ago. He became increasingly disillusioned by the cruel and ineffective medical
treatments of his time and took the courageous decision to give up his practice, concentrating instead on research. One of the main works that Hahnemann translated was William
Cullen's *A Treatise of Materia Medica*. Cullen (1710–90) was an Edinburgh teacher, physician, and chemist, and his book included an essay on Peruvian bark or cinchona (which
homoeopaths call 'china') from which quinine, a treatment for malaria, is derived. Cullen
attributed cinchona's ability to cure malaria, with its symptoms of periodic fever, sweating,
and palpitations, to its bitterness. Hahnemann was sceptical of this and tested small doses
on himself. He observed that cinchona produced in a healthy person the symptoms of
malaria, the very disease it was known to cure. This discovery was to be of great importance
in the development of homoeopathic theory and practice. By observing the symptoms
any substance produced when given to a healthy person, Hahnemann believed he could discover the healing properties of that substance. This procedure was called 'proving', a sort of
testing, which was then applied to a large number of remedies. Then the principle, medically, was to match the patient's symptoms to a homoeopathic drug picture, and give that

drug in a very dilute and 'potentized' (shaken after each dilution) form. The preparation of homoeopathic remedies using a plant such as cinchona involves the plant being macerated and dissolved in alcohol. One part of this so-called 'mother tincture' is mixed with nine parts (for a 'decimal one potency') or 99 parts (for a 'centesimal potency') of 90% alcohol. It is then shaken vigorously. This process can be repeated many times, resulting in very high dilutions indeed. Potencies of 24D, 12C, and higher, according to Avogadro's hypothesis, do not contain even a single molecule of the mother tincture.

Homoeopaths claim that the higher potencies (that is, the more dilute potencies) work more powerfully than the lower potencies. Using the 'similimum', which is the name given to the principle of fitting the disease symptoms to the substance which produces similar symptoms (homo = similar), then the unusual or uncommon symptoms which do not fit the condition as described by conventional medicine are often considered as pointers to the right remedy. Therefore homoeopathy is highly individual, resulting in different treatments for patients who, in conventional medicine, might receive identical treatment. This makes homoeopathy more difficult to evaluate from the point of view of clinical trials than conventional medical drugs. Homoeopathy can also involve mixtures with a combination of several homoeopathic substances, together with some herbal remedies. These are called 'complexes' and they are usually targeted either at specific organs or specific symptoms. A number of homoeopaths also use isopathic approaches in which the causative factor of the illness is diluted in the same way as homoeopathic medicines and is then given as a medication; for instance giving potentized pollens for the treatment of hayfever. Nosodes may also be used in homoeopathy. These are usually homoeopathic doses of the causative agents; for instance a homoeopathic dose of virus may be used to treat a viral illness and this is considered to be a nosode as the medication is made up from the original infecting organism.

Homoeopathy is an example of an anti-intuitive system — it would not be expected to work. This has led to much prejudice against homoeopathy, the main cause being that, 'it simply could not possibly work', that is the prejudice is based upon disbelief rather than on looking at the facts and appraising them in a reasonable way.

The evidence for homoeopathy

The evidence for the clinical effectiveness of homoeopathy is confusing. The first large meta-analysis in homoeopathy (Kleijnen *et al.* 1991) looked at the quality of the 107 published trials by scoring them on the following system:

- patient characteristics adequately described, 10 points;
- number of patients analysed, 100 or more patients, 30 points; and fewer patients, fewer points on a sliding scale;
- Randomization (if carried out correctly) was awarded 20 points;
- If the intervention was well described, then 5 points were awarded;
- A double-blind trial was scored at 20 points;
- If the effect measurement was relevant and well described, then 10 points were awarded. Lastly, the presentation of the results in such a manner that the analysis could be checked by the reader was given 5 points.

Therefore, a total of 100 points was possible for the best-possibly conducted trial. Out of 107 trials, 23 trials scored 55 points or more. Out of all the trials, 81 trials indicated positive results, whereas in the remainder no positive effects of homoeopathy were found. A similar analysis was published more recently in the *Lancet* (Linde *et al.* 1997). This came to substantially the same conclusions as Kleijnen *et al.*; homoeopathy did appear to be more effective than placebo, but it was not possible to be specific about the conditions that would benefit. Another meta-analysis (Linde *et al.* 1994) looked at the effects of homoeopathy in laboratory experimental systems; reaching the conclusion, from analysis of over 100 such studies, that homoeopathy does have a fundamental effect in a variety of carefully controlled and scientifically exacting experiments.

It therefore seems reasonable to suggest that there is some good basis for prescribing homoeopathy, but far more detailed clinical research is required. This must concentrate specifically on looking at new methods that help us to understand how the very individual process of homoeopathic prescribing can best be tested in a scientific context. Although it is possible to do double blind controlled trials to evaluate homoeopathy, the whole area of homoeopathic clinical practice does not lend itself easily to this scientific model.

The mechanism of homoeopathy

If it does work, and the evidence we have presented appears to suggest that it might, then we need to take a long, hard look at the mechanism, even though it may force us to challenge some of our basic scientific assumptions. Much of the scientific effort directed at understanding why homoeopathy works centres around the structure of water. Recent research would indicate that it may be possible for water to have a 'memory'. The nature of this effect, and the reason it may be so persistent, is very difficult to explain. A number of ways of looking at homoeopathic remedies have been tried, of which the most interesting is the use of nuclear magnetic resonance spectroscopy. Some work has been carried out with this using homoeopathic sulphur potencies. The spectra have been recorded with respect to the relevant intensities of the signals H_2O and OH^- between the homoeopathic remedy and the control using NMR. Interestingly, it was also found that homoeopathic dilutions gave higher NMR peaks than did ordinary dilutions which had not been potentized (Giudice *et al.* 1988). Other promising approaches to homoeopathy have come from new understandings of highly complex interactive systems such as chaos theory, but although there are interesting theories, as yet no definite answers have emerged.

The use of complementary and alternative medicine

There are several general reports on the use of complementary medicine by cancer patients, notably by Cassileth (Cassileth and Ernst 1998; Cassileth 1999). Cassileth suggests that complementary therapies for cancer are sought by the educated and relatively wealthy patient; the implication being that they are misguided in doing so. Furthermore, while Cassileth discusses unproven methods within complementary and alternative medicine (CAM), she ignores the confusion of papers supporting several well accepted conventional approaches to cancer; for example two multi-centre trials of Tamoxifen for the prevention of breast cancer, both rigorous, provide conflicting conclusions (Stat Bite 1998; Veronesi *et al.* 1998). Our impression is that patients seek complementary therapies for their cancer either because they feel that conventional medicine has no real answers for their particular tumour, or because they are desperate and 'at the end of the line'. There are also a substantial group of patients who seek to combine their conventional treatment with complementary medical approaches, in particular homoeopathy. Many patients have concerns about adverse reactions to chemotherapy and radiotherapy, another frequent reason for either seeking complementary medicine as the sole treatment or using it to complement and minimize the adverse reactions from their conventional intervention. In some surveys over 50% of patients attending oncology out-patients will seek some form of complementary medicine for their cancer (Cassileth 1999). The use of homoeopathy in cancer must be seen in this context.

At the Centre for the Study of Complementary Medicine in Southampton we use a range of different approaches of which homoeopathy is just one. When patients with cancer come to see us we attempt to define their needs, and exactly what they require from the service that we offer. In the context of managing cancer (as will be seen from the case studies), we usually then use a combination of homoeopathic, nutritional, herbal, and psychological techniques to help support the individual in the management of their illness, in conjunction with conventional medicine. This is very much the context of the approaches we use for the management of all chronic illnesses.

Homoeopathic treatments

Iscador

Iscador is the trade name of the European mistletoe extract (*Viscum album*). It has been used since the 1960s in Europe as an anticancer agent; it is claimed to possess both anti-tumour and immune stimulatory properties. Iscador is an anthroposophical medicine and, as such, is a homoeopathic medicine developed, grown, and manufactured in accordance with Rudolf Steiner's guidelines. Anthroposophical medicines are very much part of Steiner's philosophy which unite the body, mind, and spirit into a universal whole; as a consequence the plants that make up anthroposophical medical products are grown in a very specific manner, indeed with a recognition of the plant's and environment's own bio-rhythms. The medicines are potentized in a classical homoeopathic manner, but particular attention is paid to their integrative balance, both in the growth of the herbs and the manufacture of the product. Iscador is produced and registered in Germany and the appropriate booklets outline how the manufacturers feel it should be used in cancer. An excellent review of Iscador therapy for cancerous diseases has been produced by Helmut Kiene (1989).

To date, 46 studies on mistletoe therapy for cancerous diseases have been published. Of these, 6 collective studies and 30 controlled studies can be properly evaluated as part of a systematic review. The collective reports include the documentation of treatment histories and of individual tumour remissions during mistletoe therapy. Thirty-five reports involving controlled trials (11 historical studies, 12 retrospective studies, 10 prospective studies, and 2 randomized controlled trials) show an increase in the median or average survival time with Iscador therapy. The studies involve a wide range of cancers, including urinary cancer, prostatic cancer, cervical cancer, ovarian cancer, breast cancer, stomach and pancreatic cancer, colonic cancer, and lung cancer.

Unfortunately, the quality of many of these studies is unsatisfactory. Nevertheless, 9 of the 35 controlled trials show statistical significance in favour of mistletoe, and in general these studies form the better quality studies scientifically. The increase in survival time in the better studies, presumably as a consequence of mistletoe treatment, deserves some note and certainly further investigation. Some of these homoeopathic anticancer treatments may offer some real benefit to patients, beyond that of improvements in anxiety, depression, pain, and nausea.

Iscador represents one of the more promising areas for further, more detailed investigation and research. At the moment it is an approach that could be considered (both in terms of low cost and its low adverse reaction profile) for the treatment of cancer in situations where there is no clear evidence base for powerful chemotherapeutic or radiotherapeutic intervention.

Individualized classical homoeopathy

There are no controlled studies on the use of classical homoeopathy in cancer, but there are many case reports (Clover 1985; Kansak 1986; Panday 1987) and a few *in vitro* cell culture studies which are interesting but inconclusive in themselves (Karouby *et al.* 1987; Male *et al.* 1988). There are fewer reports on the use of complex homoeopathy in cancer (Ehring 1989). Many tracts describing the use of classical homoeopathy in cancer make unsubstantiated claims about 'cures' and these must be treated with a great deal of scepticism. Table 12.1 indicates the main classical remedies which are used, largely on an empirical basis, in cancer, by classical homoeopaths often in conjunction with conventional chemotherapy.

Ramakrishnan (1999), an Indian homoeopath who uses classical homoeopathy as his main therapeutic approach, reports his experience of treating over 4000 patients with this technique exclusively. He sees about 50 patients a day, which is untypical for classical homoeopathy in which a detailed constitutional consultation usually lasts for about 40 minutes. Such classical constitutional approaches are based on Kentian homoeopathy (Kent 1986). He found that the classical Kentian methods, which he practised for over 20 years, produced very poor results in cancer. He therefore developed his own treatment approaches in which he alternates the use of multiple remedies, frequent repetition of the dose and a particular formulaic method of homoeopathic prescription and medication

Table 12.1 Commonly used homoeopathic remedies and their indications in cancer

1. Baryta iodide	Any malignant problem involving lymph glands
2. Carcinosin	A well known carcinoma nosode
3. Sanguinaria	Lymphatic blockage
4. Conium	Stony hard glands similar to scirrhinum. It is used widely in breast, liver, prostate, and oesophageal cancer
5. Hydrastis	Cancer involving the abdominal organs
6. Opium (homoeopathic)	Pain relief
7. Plumbum	Malignancies of the nervous system
8. Sabal Serralata	For carcinoma of the prostate
9. Scirrhinum	A cancer nosode prepared from carcinoma of the liver
10. Cantharis	Bladder cancer
11. Thuja	Melanoma
12. Sulphur	Skin cancer

administration. He regularly uses nosodes which are homoeopathic dilutions of toxins relevant to the illness; in this case Carcinosin is frequently prescribed. Carcinosin is made from a potentized scirrhous carcinoma of the breast. Scirrhinum, prepared in potency from liver cancer, is another common remedy in his armamentarium. He divides his cases into four groups on presentation and describes grade 1 (first presentation of cancer), grade 2 (local progression), grade 3 (metastatic disease), and grade 4 (terminal disease). The exact clinical definition of how he divides patients into each of these grades is unclear from his publication. He has treated 330 cases in grade 1, 1040 in grades 2 and 3, and 2650 in grade 4. He claims a cure rate of 90% of patients who presented with grade 1 cancer.

Although this is a fascinating and interesting observation, it raises a large number of questions. First, follow up is often inadequate and certainly tends to occur only for a limited period of time and in a somewhat haphazard manner. It is difficult to be certain about the diagnosis and entry into this series of case reports; often no pathological or biopsy evidence seems to be available to substantiate the diagnosis of cancer. The use of the term 'cure' in cancer is very contentious: Ramakrishnan does not define what he means by 'cure'. Unfortunately, homoeopathy has many such unsubstantiated claims, but nevertheless Ramakrishnan's work is interesting and certainly worthy of further, more detailed investigation.

If homoeopathy works in cancer, it is possibly through a mechanism in which the homoeopathic consultation provides a healing environment in which spontaneous remissions can take place. Spontaneous remission of cancer has been widely reported, and well documented (Clover *et al.* 1995; Boyd 1966; Everson and Cole 1966; Papac 1990).

Classical homoeopathy has been used empirically as a method of symptom relief in cancer. Again, such work is uncontrolled and empirical, but it is commonly used by classical homoeopaths in the United Kingdom in conjunction with conventional chemotherapy. Table 12.2 indicates six important palliative homoeopathic remedies used in cancer.

Homoeopathy can also be used to help anxiety, depression, and a number of other emotional problems that may be associated with cancer. The use of homoeopathy in this way is again empirical and requires a detailed homoeopathic consultation in which usually a constitutional remedy will be prescribed. The Royal London Homoeopathic Hospital reports a study of complementary cancer care looking primarily at quality of life and symptom relief (Clover *et al.* 1995) for patients attending a complementary cancer therapy clinic. The treatments offered were homoeopathy, Iscador, relaxation, diet, and acupuncture. Health-related quality of life was measured using the Hospital Anxiety and Depression Scale and the Rotterdam Symptom Check List. Patients attended with many different primary cancers but predominantly the breast (36%). The mean delay between diagnosis and attendance at the clinic was 2 years; 74% of patients had confirmed metastases when first seen. There were significant improvements in psychological distress (P < 0.005 on the Rotterdam Symptom Check List) and anxiety (P < 0.01 on the Hospital Anxiety and Depression Scale) after 3 visits. Physical symptoms remained stable. It was concluded that complementary cancer therapy appears to have a positive effect on psychological distress and anxiety, and offers clinically useful improvement in quality of life. This study supports the idea that classical homoeopathy has value in palliative care, but it is also interesting to note that many of the patients entering this study remained far more stable clinically than one would have expected from the staging of their particular illness. It would certainly be worthwhile investigating the use of this 'package of care', not only to measure improvement in distress and symptoms, but also to investigate its value in the long-term survival of such patients.

Table 12.2 Six remedies in cancer care

Any indicated homoeopathic remedy could be helpful in cancer, provided it is appropriate to symptoms of the case. Because the polychrest remedies have such large materia medicas, they fit more cases than smaller remedies with less proving data to their credit. The patient's constitutional remedy needs to be sought, so that it can be prescribed in alternation with more specific organ or tissue remedies. The latter are a number of remedies with a specific field of action in certain types of cancer. These are beyond the scope of this chapter, as are the homoeopathic nosodes, made from cancer tissue itself. The six remedies selected below are illustrative of the use of homoeopathy in general in palliation of the symptoms common in cancer.

1. Nux vomica

This remedy has pathology mostly related to the gastrointestinal tract and therefore used to treat gut symptoms. The alkaloid strychnine is a major component, and so abdominal cramps are a common feature of the remedy. The principal use in cancer patients is for nausea and vomiting when intestinal spasm is a prominent feature. Often there is pyloric spasm with a sensation of weight in the epigastrium. There is frequently queasiness after breakfast, followed by nausea with much ineffectual retching. This can progress to vomiting of food as soon as it is swallowed, and although this is distressing for the patient, the vomiting brings some relief. Often the patient feels chilly, and there may be a desire for the very things that are likely to exacerbate the nausea, such as fatty and tasty foods and even coffee or other stimulants. The nauseated patient may become very irritated with the slowness or perceived inefficiency of his nurses, which symptoms alone could lead to this remedy.

2. Cocculus

This remedy is mostly used where there is on overstimulation of the central nervous system, leading to vertigo, often accompanied by restlessness and agitation. It suits patients who have become weak and confused as a result of their illness. It can be used for motion sickness, and can be of help when the patient's medication mimics this set of symptoms. The main use of the remedy, however, is not in the cancer patient, but in his relatives. The well-known keynote 'aggravation from night watching' makes the remedy eminently suitable for the relatives of the cancer patient, who through lack of sleep, have been overcome by their own worry.

3. Opium

The materia medica of opium is well known to everyone, and it is likely that the cancer patient will be taking opiates or similar analgesics at one time or another for pain relief. Opium is particularly useful when there is paralytic ileus, or sufficient paralysis of the intestines as to lead to a total absence of the urge to stool. Sometimes there are bouts of overflow diarrhoea associated with this type of constipation. Extreme drowsiness accompanies the constipation, which can progress to loss of sphincter control of both bladder and rectum. Faecal impaction often occurs at the late stages of the opium state. Occasionally opium can help in cases where there is urinary retention, particularly when the sphincter is in spasm.

4. Terebinthina

This remedy is very specific, as it can be extremely effective in the symptoms of cancer of the bladder. Whenever there are burning pains in the mucus membranes, with strangury and haematuria, this remedy offers relief. It can be helpful in severe urinary tract infections, with marked burning on urination. It is particularly useful when bladder cancers lead to recurrent infection, when it can be given in low potency to provide symptomatic relief.

Table 12.2 Six remedies in cancer care (*continued*)

5. Carbo vegetabilis

This remedy has two main uses in cancer patients. Firstly, it is of special help in patients who are desperately ill from their tumours. When there is low vitality as a result of a long and debilitating illness, with persistent ill health resulting from the cancer, this remedy can literally revive the spirits. Although the remedy is more appropriate for lack of physical vitality, it can help when the problems are also mental. When the head feels heavy as lead, and the picture is one of collapse, it has the reputation of helping to overcome the deepest indifference and apathy. The second use is for weak digestion causing bloating and flatulence or eructation. As a potency of medicinal charcoal, it shares the ability of the crude form to deal with intestinal gas. The lack of tone, or collapse, of the muscle wall of the gut leads to the flatulence, and so homoeopathically the two uses depend on the same properties of carbo vegetabilis.

6. Podophyllum

This remedy is a specific in acute diarrhoea, and so is useful when there is profuse loss mixed with gas and sputtering. Such explosive diarrhoeas soil the entire toilet bowel. The remedy is so useful in loose stools, that it is used in cases of inflammatory bowel disease. When these have led to cancer, the remedy is the first choice in controlling symptoms. Whenever the stool is watery and profuse, or horribly offensive, podophyllum can relieve. In its provings, the remedy has all the expected abdominal pains and cramps, together with the interesting symptom of the prover being unsure of whether he is about to vomit or pass stool.

Complex homoeopathy

Complex homoeopathy is a method of formulating medications which was initially developed by one of Hahnemann's pupils. It involves the use of mixtures of mother tinctures and low potency homoeopathic preparations (usually between 6C and 12C). These mixtures have been formulated so as to minimize any aggravation that might be caused by the homoeopathic preparations and to maximize the effect of that preparation on a particular organ, or for a particular symptom complex. They combine the best features of homoeopathy and herbal medicine. Classical homoeopathy fails to address the naturopathic principles of drainage via the colon, urinary tract, and skin; complex homoeopathy combines these approaches with the idea of classical homoeopathy.

The most commonly used complex homoeopathic remedies are mixtures of herbal and homoeopathic preparations targeted on particular organs. In cancer treatment the main organ-based remedy used would be liver targeted. Complex homoeopathic mixtures have been developed empirically over the last 150 years, largely in France and Germany. From a clinical point of view, a complex preparation has a wider range of action than a single remedy, which may make it more likely to produce a useful clinical result.

An eclectic approach to cancer

Although homoeopathy is certainly an important part of our approach to cancer, we almost invariably use it in conjunction with dietary and nutritional strategies. We are not the only group to have come to such practical conclusions; the approach used by the cancer group at the Royal London Homoeopathic Hospital also involves a 'package' of treatment which combines dietary advice, nutritional advice and supplementation, classical homoeopathy, Iscador, and a variety of different psychological support techniques as well as massage and aromatherapy (Clover *et al.* 1995). Cancer is regarded as a complex disease in which a number of biochemical systems within the body begin to interact in a negative and destructive manner; an interrelated process which is probably best described by systems theory (Heraway *et al.* 1976). It is therefore important to have a multisystem approach to therapy. The following case reports illustrate that approach.

Case reports

Mr D. R. — a seventy-five-year-old semi-retired surveyor

This gentleman's history began in 1991 when he had an apparently benign pleural effusion; subsequently, he became ill in early 1997 and in September of that year a very advanced left sided mesothelioma was diagnosed. From 1944–46 he had served in the naval reserve and at that time had exposure to asbestos. His clinical state when he came to see us was of a very ill-looking man with much restricted movement on the left side of his chest. He was manifestly breathless and could only manage short walks; he was also losing weight.

He consulted a Centre doctor in October 1997, and we pursued a number of unconventional investigative approaches. An electrical test which measures micro-amperage readings using a fast circuit over terminal points of acupuncture meridians on the fingers and toes was employed. This is known as an acupuncture measurement instrument (AMI); in clinical practice we have found it to be a reliable and consistent investigation that indicates organ function in a traditional Chinese context (Jessel-Kenyon *et al.* 1998). There was a marked liver dysfunction on his AMI, as well as deficiencies in the kidney and stomach meridians. Blood tests demonstrated that there were tissue deficiencies in magnesium, selenium, zinc, and B vitamins.

Treatment was then designed around a nutritional, dietary, and homoeopathic approach. He was prescribed six intravenous drips containing vitamin C, B group vitamins, zinc, magnesium, selenium, and chromium. His vitamin and mineral levels were checked a month after these infusions and were found to be normal. There are many papers in the literature indicating that nutritional deficiencies, both mineral and vitamin, are contributory towards the development of cancer. There is a dearth of literature indicating that supplementing these deficiencies, which in my clinical experience are found in most cases of cancer, has a curative effect in the cancer process. Our anecdotal impression is that parenteral supplementation of nutritional deficiencies is clinically useful, and that oral supplementation is very much less effective. Patients who decided not to avail themselves of the opportunity of parenteral supplementation, on subsequent remeasuring of their mineral and vitamin levels following on average 6 months of oral supplementation, often revealed little to no improvement of their nutritional parameters (Blott *et al.* 1993; Li *et al.* 1993; Potera *et al.* 1977; Cameron *et al.* 1979).

Mr D. R. was also tested on computerized electrodermal equipment which looks at the electrical measurements (impedence) over acupuncture points. The aim of this technique is to define the medications required by a patient through a 'bio-resonant response'. These medications are then given to the patient. Treatment usually consists of a mixture of complex homoeopathic preparations (mixtures of herbs and homoeopathy which are organ targeted) and nosodes, which are homoeopathic potencies of toxic substances that are thought to have triggered the illness. Mr D.R. also began a course of

Iscador injections which were injected subcutaneously over the left side of the chest. He received a diet based on large amounts of raw organic vegetables, with a low sugar and low fat content and alcohol avoidance.

By the end of 1997 he was beginning to feel much better and was significantly less breathless, and the weight loss had stopped. He was seen approximately monthly, and remeasured each time with the computerized electrodermal testing equipment, and each time the medication was changed depending on the 'bioresonant response'. The course of Iscador was completed in March 1998. He had an X-ray in March 1998 which showed that the mesothelioma was static. He was then started on a course of pleomorphic bacteria vaccine, a vaccine made from a cell wall deficient bacterium known as *Progenitor cryptocides*. The prescription of this particular medication is based on the hypothesis that the bacterium is pathological and may be responsible for encouraging tumour growth (Macomber 1990; Cantwell *et al.* 1979). The vaccine is injected subcutaneously, near to the site of the tumour, and may lead to the disappearance of the bacterium within the tumour. It is also suggested that this organism releases a human chorionic gonadotrophin (HCG) like substance (Bacus and Affronti 1981), and that the effect of treatment can be monitored by measuring serum and urine levels of HCG. He had a course of 30 pleomorphic bacteria vaccine injections which were self-administered. During the treatment he began to improve substantially, to the extent that a chest X-ray carried out in September 1998 showed only a little pleural shadowing of the left base. His tumour was then rechecked and repeat histology carried out in October 1998 confirmed the original diagnosis of mesothelioma. In spring 1999 (at the time of writing) he continued to feel well and could manage long walks with his dog. He was no longer short of breath, and we hope his mesothelioma will remain in remission.

Case 2 — Mrs C. J. B.

A 52-year-old patient with a Dukes C carcinoma of the colon (confirmed histologically) and resected in September 1998, presented to us with metastatic abdominal disease in late 1998. She had recently been prescribed chemotherapy and had four doses. She had found the side-effects intolerable and discontinued chemotherapy. An AMI suggested deficiencies in the large intestine and gallbladder and blood tests demonstrated a low red cell magnesium, red cell selenium, white cell zinc, and a generally low tissue vitamin B level. As a consequence, she received six intravenous infusions with appropriate nutritional supplements (Blott *et al.* 1993; Li *et al.* 1993; Potera *et al.* 1977; Cameron *et al.* 1979). During December 1998, as a result of further MRI scans, she was found to have two distinct deposits in her liver. On a further consultation in late December 1998, electrodermal testing was used to define an appropriate complex homoeopathic prescription, principally directed at the liver. She also began a course of pleomorphic bacterial vaccine at this time; she received 30 doses (a dose on alternate days) and self-injected subcutaneously over the liver area. In February 1999 she had her two discrete liver metastases resected with the result that on histology there were no malignant cells in either of the deposits; an unusual finding. Furthermore, at the operation in February 1999 there was no evidence of any recurrence of the carcinoma in the colon, or indeed any evidence of lymphatic spread which had been reported in the previous operation notes and confirmed histologically. At the moment the patient appears to be in remission and treatment is continuing.

These two anecdotal case reports involve providing cancer patients with a package of treatment. While every attempt has been made to use each particular therapeutic intervention in a rational and considered manner, it is difficult to be sure whether a particular approach will work on its own or whether it only has efficacy in combination with other approaches. Furthermore, the use of complementary and alternative medicine in cancer may simply be to provide an environment in which spontaneous remission can occur.

Conclusion

There is some evidence that specific homoeopathic preparations may have some benefit for cancer patients; perhaps the only area where we can be even tentative, because some controlled studies exist, is the use of Iscador. Classical homoeopathy is used on an empirical basis with little sound controlled trial evidence with which to substantiate its use as the primary treatment for cancer. Both the Centre for the Study of Complementary Medicine in Southampton and the Royal London Homoeopathic Hospital in London have devised packages of treatment in which a homoeopathic approach forms part of a broader therapeutic approach to cancer. From the evidence that we have, the clinical effects of homoeopathy in cancer cannot be dismissed, and this particular therapy may hold some real clinical value for patients with malignancy. Further research is desperately needed if we are to understand the place of homoeopathy in the management and treatment of cancer.

References

Bacus, B. T. and Affronti, L. F. (1981). Tumour associated bacteria capable of producing a human choriogonadotrophin-like substance. *Infection and Immunity*, **81**, 1211–15.

Blott, W. J., and Li, J. Y. (1993). Nutrition intervention trials in Linxian (Supplementation. This specific vitamin/mineral combinations, cancer incidence and disease specific mortality in the general population). *Journal of the NationalCancer Institute*, **85**, 1483–92.

Boyd, W. (1966). *Spontaneous regression of cancer*. Charles C. Thomas, Springfield, Illinois.

Cameron, E., Pauling, L., and Leibovitz, B. (1979). Ascorbic acid and cancer: a review. *Cancer Research*, **39**, 663–81.

Cantwell, A. R., Kelso, D. W., and Rowe, L. (1979). Hypo-dermatitis Sclerodermiformis; an unusual acid fast bacteria. *Arch. Dermatol.*, **115**, 449–52.

Cassileth, B. R. (1999). 'Complementary' or 'Alternative'? It makes a difference in cancer care. *Complementary Therapies in Medicine*, **7**, 35–7.

Cassileth, B. R. and Ernst, E. (1998). The prevalence of complementary-alternative medicine in cancer. *Cancer*, **83**, 777–82.

Clover, A. (1985). Some experiences in the treatment of cancer by homoeopathy. *British Homoeopathic Journal*, **74**, 96–9.

Clover, A., Last, P., Fisher, P., *et al.* (1995). Complementary cancer therapy: a pilot study of patients, therapies and quality of life. *Complementary Therapies in Medicine*, **3**, 129–33.

Ehring, F. (1989). Regression von uber 150 Haugmetastasen eines malignen melanoms bei homoophehischer komplextherapie. *Hautarzt*, **40**, 23–7.

Everson, T. C. and Cole, W. H. (1966). *Spontaneous remission of cancer*. W. B. Saunders, Philadelphia PA.

Giudice, E. D., Preparata, G., Vibiello, G. (1988). Water as a free electric dipole laser. *Physical Review Letters*, **61**, 1085–88.

Heraway, D. J. (1976). *Crystals, fabrics and fields: Metaphors of organicism in twentieth century developmental biology.* Yale University Press, Newhaven.

Jessel-Kenyon, J., Pfeiffer, L., and Brenton, M. (1998). A statistical comparison of repeatability in three commonly used bio-electronic devices: Kirlian photography, the segmental electrogram, and the AMI Motayama. *Acupuncture in Medicine,* 16, 40–2.

Kansak, K. (1986). Role of homoeopathy in malignant diseases. *Hahnemann Homoeoopath. Sand.* 10, 138–45.

Karouby, Y., Dorfman, P., Bastide, M., *et al.* (1987). A pharmacological study of Thuja in mice; and anti-tumoural and immuno-modulating effects of very low doses. *Cancer Detection and Prevention,* 11, 100–5.

Kent, J. T. (1986). *Repertory of the homoeopathic materia medica and a word index.* Homoeopathic Book Service, 45 Museum Street, London, WC1A 1LR.

Kiene, H. (1989). Clinical studies on mistletoe therapy for cancerous diseases. A review. Personal Communication.

Kleijnen, J., Knipschild, P., and ter Riet, G. (1991). Clinical trials in homoeopathy. *British Medical Journal,* 302, 316–23.

Li, J.Y., and Blott, W. J. (1993). Nutritional trials in Linxian (multi-mode vitamin/mineral supplementation, cancer incidence, and disease specific mortality among adults with oesophageal dysplasia). *Journal of the National Cancer Institute,* 85, 1492–8.

Linde, K., Jonas, W. B., Melchart, D., *et al.* (1994). Critical review and meta-analysis of serial agitated dilutions in experimental toxicology. *Human and Experimental Toxicology,* 13, 481–92.

Linde, K., Clausius, N., Ramirez, G., *et al.* (1997). Are the clinical effects of homoeopathy placebo effects? A meta-analysis of placebo-controlled trials. *Lancet,* 350, 834–3.

Macomber, P. B. (1990). Cancer and cell wall deficient bacteria. *Medical Hypotheses,* 32, 1–9.

Male, R. R., Rodgers, T., and Male, A. G. R. (1988). Homoeopathic cancer considerations. *British Homoeopathic Journal,* 177, 30–3.

Panday, P. (1987). Rectal carcinoma cured by homoeopathy. *Journal of the American Institute of Homoeopathy,* 80, 101–3.

Papac, R. J. (1990). Spontaneous regression of cancer. *Conn. M. Med.,* 54, 179–82.

Potera, C., *et al.* (1977). Vitamin B6 deficiency in cancer patients. *Am J Clin Nutr.,* 30, 1677–9.

Ramakrishnan, K. (1999). *Homoeopathic treatment of cancer.* Conference. Brighton, England. 20–21 February.

Stat Bite. (1998). Breast cancer incidence in the breast cancer prevention trial. *Journal of the National Cancer Institute,* 90, 648.

Veronesi, U., Maisonneuve, P., Costa, A., *et al.* (1998). Prevention of breast cancer with Tamoxifen: Preliminary findings from the Italian randomized trial amongst hysterectomised women. *Lancet,* 352, 92–9.

Chapter 13

Music therapy

Colin Lee

Colin Lee is Head of Music Therapy at Wilfrid Laurier University, Canada. His research interests include the analysis of clinical improvization and his developing theory of Aesthetic Music Therapy.

Introduction

The use of music therapy can be crucial for many patients living with cancer. When diagnosed with a life-threatening illness many people feel the need to re-evaluate their lives; to find that creative part that has been suppressed by the realities of day-to-day living. Music therapy, as a co-creative process between patient and therapist, can empower people to find their artistic selves and use their musical expression as a means for exploration and health. Music provides the opportunity to communicate that which cannot be spoken. It can facilitate powerful experiences of reminiscence and distract from the realities of physical pain. It is the portend of this chapter that music should not be used casually or prescriptively. Often in healthcare settings music is abused; the constant use of background sounds from radios, televisions, and hi-fi systems can become aggravating and potentially stressful. Silence is preferable to the use of uninformed music. Music chosen with and for the patient can, however, be intensely therapeutic. Music therapy as an intricate therapeutic phenomena, should only be practised by qualified and experienced individuals. Music should, however, be embraced and used by all healthcare professionals and is an ideal therapeutic tool that can be used in conjunction with more formal treatment procedures. The empathic use of music, and its potential to inspire the spirit, can enrich all our lives.

A brief history

Music therapy in North America began in the 1940s with the inception of training programmes at academic institutions across the United States (Boxberger 1962). The first professional organization, the National Association for Music Therapy (NAMT), concentrated on validating standards of clinical practice and curriculum, promoting research and establishing professional publications that included the introduction of the *Journal of Music Therapy* (JMT) (Davis *et al.* 1999). In 1971 a second professional organization, the American Association of Music Therapy (AAMT) was established, culminating in the recent merger of both associations to form the American Music Therapy Association (AMTA) in 1998.

In Britain music therapy began in the 1950s with the pioneering work of Nordoff and Robbins (1971) and Alvin (1965). The British Society for Music Therapy (BSMT) was formed in 1958 as a charitable organization dedicated to promoting and publicizing music therapy. In 1976 the Association of Professional Music Therapists (APMT) was formed to provide professional warranty and trade union status (Gilroy and Lee 1995). In 1987 the *British Journal of Music Therapy* began as the official publication of both organizations. Recent changes have included the expansion of training courses and the State Registration of music therapy under the Council of Professions Supplementary to Medicine.

Other countries' organizations include the Australian Music Therapy Association, Austrian Association of Professional Music Therapists, Canadian Association for Music Therapy, New Zealand Society for Music Therapy, Swedish Association for Music Therapy, Uruguayan Association for Music Therapy, and the World Federation for Music Therapy (Bruscia 1998). As music therapy increases internationally, as more research is undertaken, and as more journals develop, so the credibility of music therapy and its place within the field of complementary medicine is secured.

Definitions

Music therapy has many definitions that come from diverse international beliefs and individual practitioners therein. The definition as proposed by the World Federation of Music Therapy states:

> Music therapy is the use of music and/or its musical elements (sound, rhythm, melody, and harmony) by a music therapist, and client or group, in a process designed to facilitate and promote communication, relationship, learning, mobilization, expression and organization (physical, emotional, mental, social, and cognitive) in order to develop potentials and develop or restore functions of the individual so that he or she can achieve better intra- and interpersonal integration and, consequently a better quality of life (Ruud 1998, p. 52–3).

In attempting to define music therapy one is caught between the 'art' and 'science' of its practice. Music is as elusive to empirical scrutiny, as medicine is in its clinical meticulousness. That is not to say that music is not a precise discipline. Music has mathematical elements that indeed could be linked to the precision of medicine. However, it is the creative expression of music, its ability to transcend and highlight emotional states, that clearly separates it from scientific outcome studies. Music therapy as an evolving and comparatively recent discipline is diverse in its beliefs and boundaries of what constitutes clinical practice. Music therapy in essence is fundamentally both 'art' and 'science'. It draws its beliefs and rigour in varying degrees from a continuum that encompasses the exactness of *Behavioural Music Therapy* (Madsen 1981) to the spontaneous freedom and clinical precision of *Creative Music Therapy* (Nordoff and Robbins 1977).

The music therapy process

Music therapy is precise in design and takes its structure from assessment and ongoing evaluation. Music therapy is held individually and with groups. Sessions, although geared to the immediate needs of the client, should have determined long-term and short-term objectives. These objectives come from an understanding of the client, evaluation of previous work, and a perception of potential clinical directions. Descriptions and interpretations enable the therapist to provide a music therapy pathway that best suits the needs of each client. Many techniques and clinical philosophies are available to the music therapist. The relationship between therapist and patient lays the foundation for clinical clarity and is essential for the ongoing process. It is the relationship and clinical purpose that separates music therapy from the recent forms of music healing.

The architecture of music therapy exists on many levels; from the immediacy of the moment to the overall design of a complete course of treatment. As the patient discovers their place within the presenting musical surroundings, so assessment and interpretation should reflect this co-creative process. Music therapy has a clear focus that guides the efficacy of its process and outcome. As it continues to find its place within medical and artistic settings, so the accuracy of assessment, evaluation and documentation is crucial for its professional future.

Music therapy in cancer and palliative care

The developing literature and growing number of therapists working in cancer and palliative care has placed the work as an important contemporary specialization of music therapy practice. Qualified music therapists now work with patients in medical, palliative, and hospice settings. In 1989 the first international symposium of music therapists in palliative care was held in New York (Martin 1989), followed by a similar gathering in Oxford in 1994 (Lee 1995). A third international conference was held in 2000, in conjunction with the international congress on care of the terminally ill in Montreal.

Susan Munro (1984, Porchet-Munro 1993; Munro and Mount 1977) laid the theoretical foundations that have been developed and enhanced by such pioneering figures as Aldridge (1993,1998,1999), Bailey (1986), Bruscia (1991,1992), Lane (1993, 1996), Lee (1995, 1996), Martin (1989, 1991), O'Callaghan (1996a, 1996b, 1997), Salmon (1989, 1993), and Whitall (1989, 1991). Aldridge's recently edited book (1999) introduces us to music therapists newer to the field. Their voices combine to present a literature base that establishes this discipline as unique, not only in the field of music therapy, but in its contribution to the field of palliative medicine.

Music therapy is defined here as the clinical use of both active and receptive music to assist persons diagnosed with a life-threatening illness encountering physiological, psychological, emotional, and spiritual distress. Music therapy is a primary intervention, working alongside conventional treatment approaches. It offers aesthetic fulfilment and creative expression as well as diversion in managing pain and anxiety. Music therapy can positively affect a patient's physical and/or emotional well-being. The qualities of the musical relationship enable a patient to face and transcend the realities of their living and dying.

There are many music therapy techniques available, each having its own quality and characteristic. The patient is empowered to choose approaches that are relevant to their needs, the therapist helping and guiding from an understanding of the developing therapeutic relationship. Techniques can be combined to provide sessions that are rich in diversity. Some are best suited to groups whereas others need the intimacy of an individual relationship. Due to the intense nature of their expression, several techniques should be used independently, for example guided imagery and music (GIM). Music therapy as an adjunct to conventional treatment practices is also effective. Many of the techniques and outcomes described here can be used in conjunction with other disciplines.

Active music making either individually (Hartley 1999) or in groups (Salmon 1989) can provide the opportunity for creative expression and non-verbal communication. It can be physically releasing and help promote mobility. Improvization (Lee 1996), the playing and singing of songs (Bailey 1984), musical performance, and song writing (O'Callaghan 1996a, 1997) can help as distraction from perceptions of pain and facilitate communication between family members. Creative music making can additionally be used as an opportunity for life review (Beggs 1991) and as a means to explore immediate emotional needs. Music making can take place on many levels; from songs that invite simple dialogue, for example guitar and percussion, to using patients' past musical history, such as playing classical music on orchestral instruments. Some patients will never have experienced music making while others may be musicians, requiring a more sophisticated musical palette. Performing in organized concerts (Jackson 1995) can be a life-affirming experience for both patients and their families. Inviting a patient to enter a musical dialogue should be approached with care. Music has the potential to elicit responses that can be distressing as well as exhilarating. The music therapist should be experienced in using these opposing forms of musical expressions, as an affirming part of the therapeutic process.

Verbal reflections may allow patients an opening for therapeutic and personal growth. The therapist should have the necessary verbal skills to allow patients the opportunity to discuss all the complexities of their illness. From the lyric analysis of song writing (O'Callaghan 1999), the psychotherapeutic interpretations of improvizations, to the discussion of patients' musical history, verbal communication can be influential in securing and enhancing the therapeutic relationship. Some patients may never make music, the relationship developing from a musical core that does not necessitate the actual physical act of making or listening to music.

The receptive use of taped and live music can have specific effects on symptom management and the general well-being of the patient. Music relaxation can be used as a support and distraction during medical and nursing interventions (Porchet-Munro 1993), to promote sleep and as a form of physical and emotional release. Auditory stimulation has proven effects in controlling pain (Zimmerman et. al. 1989) with cancer patients. The emotional impact of pain can also be affected by music. Tapes of live or pre-recorded music compiled with the guidance of the music therapist can aid the patient with their individual pain control. Taped music can also serve as a diversion and relaxant, relieving nausea and vomiting before, during, and after chemotherapy (Standley 1992). Music can help lower heart and respiratory rates (Clynes 1982), as well as decreasing dyspnoea and insomnia (Munro 1984). Improvized music can be used to help comatose patients' breathing patterns as well as providing non-verbal human contact (Dun 1999). Guided imagery and music (Bonny 1978) is a method that uses specifically designed tapes of classical music to elicit subconscious mental images. These images are explored and illuminated with a trained guide (Bruscia 1998). GIM is now being used as a powerful intervention for patients with cancer (Erdonmez 1995; Wylie and Blom 1986).

Experimental research studies in cancer and palliative care are small. Whitall (1989) noted a lowering of heart and respiration rates when using guided imagery, deep breathing, and progressive relaxation exercises. Bailey (1983) discovered that listening to live versus recorded songs had a more positive effect on patients, and Curtis (1986) concluded that music can benefit relaxation and pain relief. O'Callaghan (1998, 1999) has pioneered recent practical studies by using a modified grounded theory design to investigate the lyrical themes in songs written by palliative care patients. The results indicate that the writing of songs can help patients and families to explore life experiences during their time of illness. Forinash (1990) balanced quantitative research developments with an illuminating phenomenological study, contemporary qualitative research designs concentrating on the analysis of the expressive qualities in music (G. Aldridge 1999; Lee 1996), and their impact on the music therapy process in patients with cancer and AIDS. The use of music therapy with pediatric cancer patients has also been researched and documented. Brodsky (1989) found that music could help children in medical isolation feel less anxious and Magill *et al.* (1997) used music to soothe and relax children in cancer pain management. More descriptive explorations of work with children (Ibberson 1996; Dun 1999) has added to the growing literature in this field.

Clinical philosophy

During my years as a music therapist working with cancer patients, I came closer to understanding the immediacy of music and its power to heal. We live in a world of paradoxes that lurch us from experience to experience and decision to decision. Our cluttered striving for life and future often prevents us from staying still and being silent. 'Why work with the dying?' (Delmonte 1995) is a fundamental question all people working with cancer patients must face. Exploring one's sense of impermanence, living with the unknown, and travelling with patients' struggles in the face of death, can be both painful and enlightening. The ultimate enigma is that music fundamentally expresses life. Music can mirror a myriad of expressions that will encompass the spectrum from birth to death. It is music that defines the music therapist's role and music that facilitates the many vagaries of living and dying.

Offering music for people who are facing loss is a delicately balanced process. If the music therapy relationship has already been created, or if the relationship is in its inception, the boundaries of professionalism and the individual responses of the therapist may become unclear. This may be seen to negate the potency of the therapeutic process and even adulterate the efficacy of the work. However, in my experience providing music when a patient is facing decline and/or death, must be flexible in terms of the relationship and the personal exposure both parties will offer (Lee 1996). A patient with little time left to live, will not have the energies to proceed with the normal stages of a developing relationship. The music therapy process must therefore be immediate and vital, if any sense of growth and meaning is to occur.

Music therapy techniques range from listening, through the use of songs and songwriting to in-depth clinical improvisations. Once the relationship is established, ongoing sessions may be transferred from the music therapy room to the ward. The therapist will then dispense with the structure of ongoing sessions and move toward a time that is more flexible. This can develop naturally from the preceding work and the immediate needs of the patient. Working from the onset at the bedside is a critical dynamic that is different from the normal beginnings of the therapeutic relationship encompassing the boundaries of a music therapy room. The clinical options are more limited, but may be more liberating as the relationship develops. Clinical solutions find a balance that reveal the strength of the process.

Working with patients who are near death demands that the therapist stays true to their clinical philosophy. Moving into the unknown territory of the patient's feelings, while keeping a professional distance, is a balance that is constantly shifting. Attempting to understand the enigmas of the developing music therapy relationship within the therapeutic context perhaps will, and should, remain a mystery. It is this sense of mystery for music, the relationship, and the final human passage, that makes the use of music therapy with cancer patients so compelling.

Moving from music to silence

One of the most powerful elements of music therapy is silence. The silence immediately following musical dialogue often holds the most potent therapeutic outcome. Time that is caught and frozen from the preceding musical dialogue can translate the compelling nature of the process and future direction of the work. We should never underestimate the power silence has to contain music. Silence that comes before, during, and after music, transcends the human condition and provides the fracture for patients to assimilate and make sense of the experience. There are many textures and tones of silence and many emotional responses. Just as music is a multicomplex phenomena, so silence in music therapy demands sensitivity and understanding.

The silence that moves from sound when a person is dying is potentially a highly charged and spiritual experience for both patient and therapist. Clinical evaluations and interpretations during this, the most challenging human test, are touched with that which is not spoken, played, or sung. In moving from life and sound there is a movement toward the membrane between life and death. It is this metaphoric use of the word membrane that best describes the living sense of this experience — a voice that is tangible yet fluctuating and unshackled. Holding silence and allowing it to be part of the patient, the therapist, and the therapeutic relationship is one of the most challenging aspects of working with cancer patients.

These expressions of moving from sound to silence are manifestations of the patient's certainty at being in the transition between life and death, and the therapist's struggles in holding this experience while ultimately standing apart and returning to life. Silence here knows no bounds; can fly, be still, and at once complete. Relinquishing oneself to this intense silence, while remaining in the present is a clinical technique that takes many years of experience to understand and interpret. This reality is tangible, metaphysical yet free, and has presented me with many questions in attempting to validate music therapy and the paradox of therapeutic growth within the face of uncertainty and loss. Silence speaks and completes; in silence we are equal and it is in silence that true strengthening occurs.

Case-study — David

This case study explores work with David, a twenty-one-year-old man dying of cancer. My work as a music therapist in the Hospice was carried out in conjunction with Gill, the physiotherapist. The linking of disciplines came directly from David's physical and emotional needs. After David died Gill and I met to reflect on our work. The session was recorded and transcribed, her comments coming directly from that meeting.

The sessions took place during the last two weeks of David's life. He was admitted to the Hospice because his tumour was developing rapidly. David also had secondary complications of spinal cord compression. When David arrived he was frightened and in great pain. David was initially referred to music therapy because he played guitar and was known to be musical. During our first meeting he was eager to discuss music and the group he had formed with his girlfriend. We discussed his favourite bands and the growing importance of music since his illness. Although not able to move freely he could sit up in bed. There was a sense of life and urgency about him. We agreed to hold our first session in his room and that I would bring a guitar.

In between this meeting and our next David was admitted to the pain clinic as his condition rapidly deteriorated. On his return to the ward, I took a guitar to the session as promised. As I entered his room, however, I realized that it would be impossible to entertain any notions of music-making. He lay on his back. The pain appeared to be so intense that he moved his head only slightly to acknowledge my presence. We sat in silence, the suspension of time holding us both. There seemed to be no words to describe the enormity of his situation. I eventually dared to speak: 'It must be hard with so much time to think?' Time was again suspended as David considered my words: 'Yes, it certainly is.' I felt foolish at my words. After a lifetime of silence I stood up to leave. At this moment Gill entered the room. She too saw the desperate physical and emotional pain of David's presence. Gill immediately and insightfully suggested that we might try relaxation work with touch and music. David nodded in agreement.

I began the reflective meeting with Gill after David's death by trying to describe the awkwardness I felt during the first session. The suggestion of our working together was liberating for me. Up until now I was sitting in silence with David. At first the silence was comfortable, but after a time I thought 'What can I say?' 'What should I say?' 'How can I begin to acknowledge the death and dying of such a young man?' When I finally spoke I knew the enormity of my words would be awkward. I trusted the silence between us, but on another level it seemed so strong as to be crushing me. Gill replied, 'David was a frightened young man. He was on his back constantly. He couldn't sit up and face his situation.' She paused as if considering the depth of our work, 'We enabled him to let go.'

The format of sessions consisted of relaxation and touch along with improvized music on a sounding bowl (a stringed instrument of contemporary origin) [1]. The music balanced the movements of Gill's hands, as well as trying to capture David's disposition and the ensuing tripartite relationship. The physical and musical responses were clinically graded to provide David with the opportunity to relax and release tension, as well as being able to enter a non-verbal relationship that was hopefully representative of his fears and emotions.

Gill commented on the therapeutic process, 'When the music started, and after I touched him, you could feel the tension coming out. The three of us became one. It was like following the dream lines.' We offered David two sessions each day; one in the morning and the other in late afternoon. The intensity of our relationships deepened at every

---

[1] The sounding bowl is an instrument created by an English wood craftsman, Tobias Kaye (1995). Turned bowls of various sizes are strung with strings. They are now becoming standard instruments for music therapists working in palliative care, in the UK.

meeting. There were few words spoken. During our third session however David opened his eyes and spoke in spite of himself, 'It's all so avant-garde. So enlightened.' We can offer no explanation for these words. We accepted them as a statement deep from inside. Gill spoke at length about our quickening relationship and these moments of opening, 'There were many occasions when he moved his lips, as if he were saying things. It seemed as if from this time each session continued as one. There were no preliminaries. His face became remarkably beautiful. He lost all his lines of tension and pain. It was almost as if he decided to move away, but then came back. After he spoke these words he was, I'm sure, ready to let go completely.'

Gill further articulates the efficacy of our work from her perspective, 'What we did with David was clear and not in any way a vague undefined process. We had clear aims; we knew what we were doing and why we were doing it. I was aware that when the music started my approach to touching him changed. In the early sessions he would come back, more vigorous, and then ease away. I was fascinated how your music matched that experience. The music seemed related to his strength. Spiritually the music was aware. It was like being in a beautiful bubble. Yet we still had to remain in control, to be in the present. During these moments we glimpsed a union. We were terribly privileged. It wasn't uncomfortable, it was magical.' I respond, 'To reach out and touch the layer between life and death?' Gill acknowledged my thoughts, 'A communion that produced a whole that was greater than the parts. We were able to allow our intellect and emotions to come together. It was something more than communication, it was a joining, a oneness of minds. It's you being allowed into someone else's space, but allowing other people into your space as well. I felt that our work was something he needed. It was a release for him. He could move away, move from his bed. David was tied to the pain and his bed. This experience allowed him to move away and fly. For me this was one of the most profound experiences I have had in my work at the Hospice. It was a tremendous honour to be there. It was giving and taking. The satisfaction that you were able to make a difference, a totally generous sharing and giving. It became a special bubble and he would always say, 'I've been waiting for you.' We both knew at the final session that we wouldn't see him again. We didn't want him to die. We wanted the experience to continue.'

These insightful and reflective comments by Gill helped us both to place the immensity of the experience. As the sessions progressed so David's physical and spiritual presence became evermore distant. Perhaps we may never fully know the impact of our work with David. However we do know the influence David left on both our lives. His gift to us was that he allowed us into his life at this time of transition. The intensity of our relationship has not diminished with the passing of time. I remember our beautiful bubble with continued clarity; it enriches my living and keeps David's spirit alive in me professionally and personally.

Conclusion

Reflecting on music therapy in cancer and palliative care, through assessment, research, and writing is essential for the development of the work. Music therapy is on the brink of enormous change. Music is of-itself and in-itself, one of the most enigmatic and creative practices known to humanity. Perhaps it is impossible to understand fully the science and mechanics of its process, because that would ultimately invalidate the power of music itself. However, music can act as a clear clinical tool in the therapeutic arena. Gradually the outcome of music therapy is beginning to be understood (Wheeler 1995). How the inspiration of music influences the presence of people's lives, however, is still an enigma. What are the musical qualities that may influence profound change for a person faced with cancer, what musical ingredients help relax and divert patients from pain and why are music and spirituality so intertwined? The answer to these and other questions, now stand before music therapy in cancer and palliative care, demanding new and innovative thought.

Acknowledgments

With thanks to the staff at Sir Michael Sobell House Hospice for their constant belief in music therapy. To Gill McEvedy, physiotherapist, for her openness in combining our disciplines and Dr Rosemary Fischer for constantly challenging my clinical and artistic arguments.

Organizations dedicated to the promotion of music therapy in cancer/palliative care

1. The Towersey Foundation, St. Pauls House, Devon Square, Newton Abbot. Devon TQ12 2HH, UK.
2. Jessie's Fund, 10, Bootham Terrace, York YD3 7DH, UK.
3. Music Therapy Programme, Hospice of Palm Beach County Inc. 5300 East Avenue, West Palm Beach, Florida 33407, USA.

References

Aldridge, D. (1993). Hope, meaning and the creative art therapies in the treatment of AIDS. *The Arts in Psychotherapy*, **20**, 285–97.

Aldridge, D. (1998). Life as jazz: hope, meaning, and music therapy in the treatment of life-threatening illness. *Advances in Mind-Body Medicine*, **14**, 271–82

Aldridge, D. (ed.) (1999). *Music therapy in palliative care*. Jessica Kingsley Publishers, London.

Aldridge, G. (1999). The implications of melodic expression for music therapy with a breast cancer patient. In. Aldridge, D. (ed.) Music therapy in palliative care. Jessica Kingsley Publishers, London.

Alvin, J. (1965, revised 1975) *Music therapy*. John Clare Books, London.

Bailey, L. (1983) The effects of live music versus tape-recorded music on hospitalized cancer patients. *Music Therapy*, **3**, 17–28.

Bailey, L. (1984). The use of songs with cancer patients and their families. *Music Therapy*, **4**, 5–17.

Bailey, L. (1986). Music therapy in pain management. *Journal of Pain Symptom Management*, **1**, 25–8.

Beggs, C. (1991). Life review with a palliative care patient. In K. Bruscia (ed.) *Case studies in music therapy*. Barcelona Publishers, Gilsum NH.

Bonny, H. (1978). GIM Monograph #2. *The role of taped music in the GIM process*. Baltimore: ICM Press.

Boxberger, R. (1961). Historical bases for the use of music in therapy. In *Music therapy* (ed. E. H. Schneider), pp. 125–66. Lawrence, KS: National Association for Music Therapy, Inc.

Brodsky W. (1989). Music therapy as an intervention for children with cancer in isolation rooms. *Music Therapy*, **8**. 17–34.

Bruscia, K. (1991). Embracing life with AIDS: psychotherapy through imagery and music (GIM). In *Case studies in music therapy* (ed. K. Bruscia), pp. 581–602. Barcelona Publishers, Gilsum NH.

Bruscia, K. (1992.) Visits from the other side: healing persons with AIDS through guided imagery and music. In *Music and miracles* (ed. D. Campbell), pp. 195–207. Quest Books, Wheaton IL.

Bruscia, K (1998). Defining music therapy. 2nd edn. Barcelona Publishers, Gilsum NH.

Curtis, S. (1986). The effect of music on pain relief and relaxation of the terminally ill. *Journal of Music Therapy*, **23**, 10–24.

Clynes, M. (ed.) (1982). *Music, mind and brain: the neuropsychology of music.* Plenum Press, London.

Davis, B., Geffler, K., and Thaut, M. (1999). *An introduction to music therapy. Theory and practice.* 2nd edn. Mc Graw-Hill, Boston.

Delmonte, H. (1995). 'Why work with the dying.' In *Lonely waters* (ed. C. Lee), pp. 109–18. Sobell House, Oxford.

Dun, B. (1999). Creativity and communication. Aspects of music therapy in a children's hospital. In *Music therapy in palliative care* (ed. D. Aldridge), pp. 59–67. Jessica Kingsley Publishers, London.

Erdonmez, D. (1995). A journey of transition with guided imagery and music. In *Lonely waters* (ed. C. Lee). Proceedings of the International Conference, 'Music therapy in palliative care.' Sobell Publications, Oxford.

Forinash, M. (1990). The phenomenology of music therapy with the terminally ill. University Microfilms, 91–02617, Ann Arbor.

Gilroy, A. and Lee, C (1995). Introduction: juxtapositions in art therapy and music therapy research. In *Art and music: therapy and research*, (ed. A. Gilroy and C. Lee). Routledge, London.

Hartley, N. (1999). Music therapists' personal reflections on working with those who are living with HIV/AIDS. In. *Music therapy in palliative care* (ed. D. Aldridge), pp. 105–125. Jessica Kingsley Publishers, London.

Ibberson, C. (1996). A natural end: one story about Catherine. *British Journal of Music Therapy*, **10**, 24–31.

Jackson, M. (1995). Music therapy for living: a case study on a woman with breast cancer. *Canadian Journal of Music Therapy*, **111**, 19–33.

Kaye, T. (1995). The voice of the sounding bowl. In *Lonely waters* (ed. C. Lee). Proceedings of the International Conference, 'Music therapy in palliative care'. Sobell Publications, Oxford.

Lane, D. (1993). Music therapy: gaining an edge in oncology management. *Journal of Oncology Management*, Jan/Feb, 42–6.

Lane, D. (1996). Songs of love: music therapy can make a difference in the care of dying children. *Hospice*, 7, 6–7.

Lee, C. (1995), *Lonely Waters*. Proceedings of the International Conference 'Music Therapy in Palliative Care'. Sobell House, Oxford.

Lee, C. (1996). *Music at the edge. The music therapy experiences of a musician with AIDS.* Routledge, London.

Magill, L., Nessa, C., Handzo, G., and Loscalzo, M. (1997). Cancer and pain: a creative multidisciplinary approach in working with patients and families. In *Music therapy and pediatric pain* (ed. Loewy), pp. 000–00. Jeffrey Books, Cherry Hill, NJ.

Madsen, C. (1981). *Music therapy: a behavioural guide for the mentally retarded.* National Association for Music Therapy, Washington, DC.

Martin, J. (1989). Music therapy in palliative care. In *The next step forward: music therapy with the terminally ill* (ed. J. Martin), pp. iii–viii. Calvary Hospital, New York.

Martin, J. (1991). Music therapy at the end of life. In *Case studies in music therapy* (ed. K. Bruscia), pp. 617–632. Barcelona Publishers, Gilsum NH.

Munro, S. (1984). *Music therapy in palliative/hospice care.* Magna Music Baton, St. Louis, MO.

Munro, S. and Mount, B. (1977). Music therapy in palliative care. *Canadian Medical Association Journal*, **119**, 1029–34.

Nordoff, P. and Robbins, C. (1971). *Music in therapy for handicapped children.* Victor Gollancz Ltd, London.

Nordoff, P. and Robbins, C. (1977). *Creative music therapy.* John Day, New York.

O'Callaghan, C. (1996*a*). Lyrical themes in songs written by palliative care patients. *Journal of Music Therapy*, **33**, 74–92.

O'Callaghan, C. (1996*b*). Pain, music creativity and music therapy in palliative care. *American Journal of Hospice Palliative Care*, **13**, 43–9.

O'Callaghan, C. (1997). Therapeutic opportunities associated with the music when using song writing in palliative care. *Music Therapy Perspectives*, **15**, 32–8.

O'Callaghan, C. (1998). Effect of the music therapy intorduction when engaging hospitalized cancer patients. *Music Therapy Perspectives*, **16**, 67–74.

O'Callaghan, C. (1999). Lyrical themes in songs written by palliative care patients. In Music therapy in palliative care (ed. D. Aldridge), pp. 43–58. Jessica Kingsley Publishers, London.

Porchet-Munro, S. (1993). Music therapy. In *Oxford textbook of palliative medicine* (ed. D. Doyle), pp. 555–9. Oxford University Press, Oxford.

Ruud, E. (1998). *Music therapy: improvisation communication and culture,* pp 52–3. Barcelona Publishers, Gilsum NH.

Salmon, D. (1989). Partage: group work in palliative care. In *The next step forward: music therapy with the terminally ill.* (ed. J. Martin). Calvary Hospital, New York.

Salmon, D. (1993). Music and emotion in palliative care. *Journal of Palliative Care*, **9**, 48–52.

Standley, J. (1992). Clinical applications of music therapy and chemotherapy: The effects on nausea and emesis. *Music Therapy Perspectives*, **9**, 91–6.

Wheeler, B. (1995). Music therapy research: quantative and qualitative perspectives. Barcelona Publishers, Gilsum NH.

Whitall, J. (1989). The impact of music therapy in palliative care. In *The next step forward: music therapy with the terminally ill* (ed. J. Martin), pp. 69–72. Calvary Hospital, New York.

Whitall, J. (1991). Songs in palliative care: a spouse's last gift. In *Case studies in music therapy* (ed. K. Bruscia), pp. 603–610. Barcelona Publishers, Gilsum NH.

Wylie, M. and Blom, R. (1986). Guided imagery and music with hospice patients. *Music Therapy Perspectives*, **3**, 25–8.

Zimmerman, L., Pozehl, B., Duncan, K., and Schmitz, R. (1989). Effects of music in patients who had chronic cancer pain. *Western Journal of Nursing Research*, **11**, 298–309.

Chapter 14

The focused mind: hypnosis, relaxation, guided imagery, and meditation

Claire Edmonds, Catherine Phillips, and
Alastair Cunningham

The authors are based in Toronto, Canada. Claire Edmonds is a research
associate at the Ontario Cancer Institute, where she studies the effects of
psychosocial interventions on both the quality of life and survival of
cancer patients. She is also a psychotherapist, leading groups that focus
on support, coping, and the spiritual concerns of cancer patients.
Catherine Phillips is a researcher and therapist with the Healing Journey
Program at Princess Margaret Hospital. Alastair Cunningham is a senior
scientist and psychologist at the Ontario Cancer Institute. His research
interests include mind-body theory, and investigating the effects of
adjunctive psychological therapy on quality and length of life in cancer
patients.

Introduction

Cancer patients are increasingly interested in participating in their healing by using self-
help strategies and complementary care techniques. Of the supportive care services offered
in the National Cancer Institute's designated cancer centres, some of the most popular are
relaxation/meditation, guided imagery, and hypnotherapy (Coluzzi et al. 1995). Healthcare
practitioners have some awareness of these techniques but are relatively unlikely to recommend them to patients coping with cancer (Zaza et al. 1999). Although none of these techniques are replacements for good medical care, we believe that there is ample evidence of
their efficacy as adjuncts to help cancer patients cope with anxiety, distress and physical
pain as well as the treatments and their side-effects.

Hypnosis, relaxation, guided imagery, and meditation can be viewed as part of the broader
category of cognitive behavioural interventions which focus on changing specific thoughts or

behaviours (Meyer and Mark 1995). These terms are often poorly defined in the literature and used interchangeably to describe any coping technique that involves the intentional relaxation of the body or thought stream. The following definitions will clarify some of the differences between these techniques and demonstrate how they can be used in various combinations.

Definitions

Hypnosis

Hypnosis has been described as a class of induction procedures (rather than a single technique) in which the patient becomes very attentive and absorbed in a relaxation-inducing activity prescribed by a therapist (Carey and Burish 1988). The practitioner guides the patient to become aware of internal sensations of heaviness and warmth, encouraging her to relax consciously while ignoring external stimuli and any cognitive judgement that may interfere with the process. After the induction, feelings of relaxation are often deepened by the use of guided imagery, for example visualizing scenes of a safe and peaceful beach. Patients may become deeply absorbed in the process and have various experiences such as time distortions, alterations in physical perceptions (tingling, heaviness in extremities), a suspension of critical thought, and enhanced suggestibility (Spiegel 1985; Levitan 1992; Pattison 1997). With practice, patients can perform self-hypnosis thereby producing this state of deep relaxation for themselves.

Relaxation

Relaxation training can refer to a variety of mental and physical techniques that produce feelings of relaxation and reduce physiological arousal, for example progressive muscle relaxation, abdominal breathing, and autogenic training (Jacobsen 1997; Benson 1989). All of these techniques draw the patient's attention away from feelings of tension and distress towards feelings of comfort and calmness. Progressive relaxation training was first developed by Jacobsen in the 1930s (see Carey and Burish 1988 for a brief history). The patient is guided through his body to tighten and then relax muscle groups in order to identify muscle tension and replace it with feelings of relaxation. Redd (1994) refers to this procedure as 'active' relaxation because of the muscle tensing component. By contrast hypnosis is more passive. Often progressive relaxation is used as a first step in helping patients learn self-hypnotic techniques. Autogenic training is a passive technique directing the patient to focus on sensations of warmth in the limbs and abdomen and the rhythm of the breath (Benson 1989). Abdominal breathing is similarly passive, the patient intentionally focusing on deep and slow breathing which has a calming effect.

Guided imagery

Guided imagery is another cognitive tool in which purposeful mental images are used to achieve a desired therapeutic goal such as relaxation, emotional calm, or feelings of being in control (Achterberg 1985). It may begin with a relaxation technique (passive or active as above) after which patients are given or encouraged to develop an image suggesting relaxation and safety, often from the repertoire of their own personal experience, for example a safe beach or forest. This technique can also be used for cognitive activities, such as the mental rehearsal of stressful events like medical interventions or treatments (Stephens 1993). Simonton and his colleagues (Achterberg and Lawlis 1978; Simonton *et al.* 1980) developed a technique in which cancer patients image their immune systems defeating their cancer. Although there is no evidence that imagery of this kind can influence the immune system to fight cancer, cognitive behavioural stress management programs have been associated with improvements in immune outcomes (Ironside *et al.* 1995). Guided imagery can also be used in psychotherapy to help patients identify deeper feelings and fears, to define goals for themselves, deal more effectively with death issues (Levitan 1992) or spiritual issues (Brown-Saltzman 1997).

Meditation

Meditation is both a process and a state: it might be described as focused attention in the relative absence of thoughts. As with the previous techniques, meditation begins by instilling a physical sense of relaxation. However, rather than being led in a cognitive activity like guided imagery, the mind is stilled more deeply, often by focusing on the breath or some other neutral material like counting. Through this quietening process, there are qualitative changes in awareness in which the attention is extended beyond the usual somatic and cognitive levels of experience. Patients can experience profound feelings of peace, calm ,and tranquillity during and after meditation (Kutz *et al.* 1985a; Kutz *et al.* 1985b; Walsh 1996).

All of these techniques are similar in that they encourage the relaxation response, defined by Benson as a state characterized by physiological changes associated with decreased arousal of the sympathethic nervous system (lowered heart rate, blood pressure, breathing rate etc) as well as psychological calm (Benson *et al.* 1974; Benson 1989). As a learned behaviour, the patient's ability to invoke the relaxation response improves with practice and in time can be produced at will. Techniques evoking the relaxation response have been used to treat a wide range of medical and psychological disorders including hypertension, cardiac arrhythmias, addictive behaviours, post traumatic stress disorder, phobias, and anxiety (Everly and Benson 1989). Fundamental to all of these techniques is the intentional focus on internal sensations that lead to relaxation and quietening. Spiegel (1985) has used the metaphor of the camera lens to describe this; in hypnosis the aperture is tightly focused on specific details of experience while sacrificing details from the surrounding environment. This metaphor can be broadened to describe other techniques. In progressive relaxation, the aperture of attention is slightly expanded beyond the specific focus of hypnosis to include the whole body, as the patient learns to identify sensations of tension and replace them with relaxation. Mental imagery widens the aperture again, to include cognitive and emotional material such as memories and images. Finally, meditation has the widest aperture because the body is stilled, the mind is quietened and the consciousness is expanded even more to allow for the disengaged observation of the body, thoughts, emotions and the existential context of life.

What do these techniques have to offer cancer patients?

There are at least three areas of application for these techniques in the treatment of cancer patients; two widely agreed upon, and the third controversial:

• Physical symptom control, e.g. nausea associated with medical treatments for cancer, and coping with pain and distressing medical interventions;

- Relieving emotional distress and promoting adjustment;

- Possibly life extension: this is an unproven concept, as yet. If there is an effect, it presumably occurs by improving the body's defences against the disease.

This chapter will briefly review the literature assessing the effectiveness of these techniques for cancer patients. Hypnosis, relaxation, guided imagery, and meditation are often used in various combinations, and it has proven almost impossible to separate them. Therefore, the studies will be organized by the three sets of dependent variables they measure. We will then illustrate some of these benefits for patients using qualitative data from our own program. The chapter concludes with recommendations for healthcare practitioners.

Physical symptom control

A substantial body of literature suggests that behavioural interventions have an important role to play in alleviating physical symptoms and the emotional distress they cause (Redd and Hendler 1982; Walker 1992; Carey and Burish 1988; Trijsberg *et al.* 1992; Redd 1994; Meyer and Mark 1995; Wallace 1997).

Interventions for nausea and vomiting

Chemotherapuetic interventions are highly cytotoxic causing nausea, vomiting, anorexia, hair loss, fatigue, vulnerability to infections, anxiety, and depression. Over time, patients can also develop a conditioned response of anticipatory nausea up to 24 hours prior to their chemotherapy. Antiemetic drugs are available, but behavioural interventions can augment their effects and ameliorate some of the psychological distress associated with treatment.

In an early study, Lyles *et al.* (1982) found that progressive relaxation and guided imagery reduced nausea and negative affect in chemotherapy patients, both in the clinic and at home following the chemotherapy, compared to a control condition of meeting with a supportive therapist. Intervention patients also reported feeling more in control of their lives and disease. Contanch and Strum (1987) compared the effects of listening to an audiotape of progressive muscle relaxation and guided imagery to a placebo condition of relaxing music as well as a no treatment control. They found that the intervention group experienced significantly less vomiting and anxiety than either control group, as well as improved caloric intake in the two days following their chemotherapy.

Walker (1992) assessed two interventions (progressive relaxation training versus hypnosis) in combination with antiemetic medication. While the antiemetic medication was effective in reducing nausea in all groups, the hypnotherapy group reported less anxiety, and those receiving progressive relaxation reported less late onset nausea, suggesting these techniques added benefits over the drug alone. Troesch *et al.* (1996) also assessed the effects of guided imagery in combination with antiemetic medication. Patients randomized into the intervention group received an audiotape that encouraged patients to visualize a positive chemotherapy experience with no side-effects. There were no statistical differences between the groups in nausea or vomiting; however, those in the intervention group reported feeling more in control and relaxed than the control group.

In summary, behavioural techniques can ameliorate the unpleasant and distressing side-effects of chemotherapy when compared to randomized no-treatment controls. While newer antiemetic medication may be more effective in decreasing physical symptoms, behavioural techniques still have a role in decreasing emotional distress.

Interventions for pain

Behavioural interventions have also been used to alleviate pain in cancer patients. Pain and discomfort can be caused both by the treatments used for the disease and the disease itself, particularly in advanced cancer (Redd *et al.* 1991). Pain is also associated with disturbances in sleep, appetite, energy, and mood (Ferrell *et al.* 1994; Ferrell *et al.* 1993). While pharmacological treatments for pain are available, they are not without harmful or unpleasant side-effects. Combining behavioural interventions with medication can enhance the effectiveness of the analgesics in addition to helping to instil a sense of control and self-efficacy in patients.

Fleming (1985) examined the effects of an intervention using a breathing-based relaxation technique and positive thinking in combination with analgesics on 58 patients with advanced cancer. In total, 62% of subjects noted an improvement in pain and reported feeling calmer and less anxious. Spiegel and Bloom (1982) found that hypnosis was effective in reducing pain in metastatic breast cancer patients randomized to a supportive-expressive group therapy compared to controls. Ferrell *et al.* (1994) developed a comprehensive pain program for elderly cancer patients. The program had a large educational component but also used audiotapes for progressive muscle relaxation and guided imagery. Compared to randomized controls, the intervention was effective in decreasing pain and anxiety and improving sleep.

Relieving distress and promoting adjustment

A diagnosis of cancer can cause tremendous emotional distress. Supportive interventions, both professional and peer-led, can assist patients by providing information, emotional catharsis, role modelling, problem solving, and mutual support (Taylor *et al.* 1986). Cognitive behavioural interventions, however, help patients control emotional distress directly. The behavioural components may include hypnosis, progressive relaxation, and guided imagery as well as other cognitive strategies such as reframing, thought stopping, and positive affirmations to help patients with recurring negative thoughts and anxieties. Again, there are numerous reviews concluding that such psychological interventions can help reduce the emotional distress experienced by patients (Cunningham and Edmonds 1996; Devine and Westlake1995; Fawzy *et al.* 1995; Greer 1989; Meyer and Marks 1995) and that training in coping skills or stress reduction techniques added to support programs confers additional benefits (Anderson 1992; Trijsburg *et al.* 1992).

There are relatively few randomized trials on these interventions and studies are often small and limited in terms of standardized measurement and follow-up (Meyer and Mark 1995). However, some good controlled studies have been performed. This section reviews interventions that include coping skills such as relaxation, guided imagery, or meditative techniques.

Some coping skills interventions have been offered in an individual rather than a group format. Weisman and Worden (1976) found that distressed cancer patients improved in mood after four sessions of an individual psychological intervention compared with historical controls. Moorey *et al.* (1994) also found that patients randomized into an 8 hour individualized cognitive behavioural intervention had less anxiety and distress at a 12 month follow-up compared to controls. Cain *et al.* (1986) compared 8 weeks of thematic counselling (including relaxation) given either individually or in a group format and found that both were equally effective in producing mood and coping improvements up to 6 months later in randomized cancer patients.

Two randomized studies directly compare the effects of coping skills training with the effects of a support group. Telch and Telch (1986) randomized psychologically distressed cancer patients into a 6-week coping skills group, an unstructured support group, or a standard care control group. The coping skills instruction produced large and highly significant improvements in mood, coping, and self-efficacy, while the support group showed small but generally non-significant improvements, and the control group deteriorated.

Cunningham and Tocco (1989) found that subjects in a 6-week coping skills program improved in mood and quality of life two-fold compared to subjects randomized into a professionally led supportive discussion group. A further analysis of over 400 patients taking the same coping skills course (Cunningham *et al.* 1993) showed that it provided similar benefits to patients with a wide range of disease types and stages, marital status, gender, educational level, and religious orientation.

Two more recent studies have also found coping skills training effective in improving distress. Bindemann *et al.* (1991) randomized patients either into a 12-week relaxation program or a no-treatment control group, after which the intervention subjects demonstrated less anxiety, depression, and less psychiatric morbidity than controls. In a non-randomized study, Baider *et al.* (1994) reported on 123 highly distressed cancer patients who chose to take a 6-week program of progressive relaxation and guided imagery. Psychological distress improved after the intervention and was maintained over the 6 month follow-up.

Research suggests that coping skills improve mood and quality of life because patients develop more resources to help themselves. In fact, one study found a strong association between perceived self efficacy and improved mood (Cunningham *et al.* 1991*a*), suggesting that at least some of the additional benefits from coping skills are derived from the sense of control they impart.

Studies on long term (more than 3 months) interventions for cancer patients are relatively rare in the literature, possibly due to the expense of such trials. Farber and Wienerman (1981) and Ilnyckyj *et al.* (1994) found no significant improvements in psychometric measures in cancer patients with various diagnoses who were randomized into a 6 month intervention, despite 75% of the patients reporting that the intervention had been helpful. Spiegel *et al.* (1981) also reported only modest improvements in the mood of metastatic breast cancer patients after 9 months of supportive-expressive therapy compared to controls, who deteriorated in mood over the same period. In our own long term randomized trial, metastatic breast cancer patients showed no significant psychometric improvements in mood after an 8 month support and coping skills program; however, these same patients experienced a significant improvement in mood after an intensive weekend coping skills course (Edmonds *et al.* 1999). We have concluded that there are different effects from long-term and short-term groups; clinical improvements were observed in these patients that did not show on standardized instruments. We are now using qualitative techniques to better understand how long-term groups help patients.

Life extension

In the 1970s, researchers began exploring whether these behavioural techniques could extend survival in cancer patients. The early work of the Simontons and their colleagues introduced the idea of mental imaging of the immune system overcoming cancer cells as an adjunctive technique for cancer patients (Achterberg and Lawlis 1978). Simonton *et al.* (1980) reported on 130 patients enrolled in their program and found that the median survival of their participants was twice that of national norms. Critics have noted that these results may be biased by the highly selected nature of their sample (educated, motivated, and likely wealthy) and they have been criticised for advancing claims of efficacy based on insufficient evidence (American Cancer Society 1982). Two other researchers have also reported improved survival in non-randomized research. Meares (1980), an Australian psychiatrist, assessed the effects of meditation on advanced cancer patients. Of the 73 patients who underwent at least 20 sessions of intensive meditation, several eventually experienced unexpected remissions and longevity. Newton (1982) also found that patients who had undergone over 10 weeks of hypnosis and visualization did well physically, as the median survival of the lung, breast, and bowel patients he treated was longer than national norms.

Two randomized studies have found survival advantages in post-hoc tests. Fawzy *et al.* (1990) demonstrated that distress was alleviated and active coping styles enhanced by a 6-week structured intervention (cognitive problem solving) in patients with malignant melanoma. Six years later there were significantly fewer deaths among these people than in the controls who did not attend a group (Fawzy *et al.* 1993). Furthermore, a good medical outcome (lack of recurrence or survival) was correlated to active coping with high levels of initial distress. It appeared that 'mobilization, not minimization', was predictive of survival. Spiegel *et al.* (1989) reported the results of a randomized trial of supportive expressive therapy (with a hypnosis component for pain control) and found that the intervention patients survived longer than the control group. Several other studies have not found a survival effect (Ilnyckyj *et al.* 1994; Morganstern *et al.* 1984) as well as our own which was specifically designed to assess survival (Cunningham *et al.* 1998). More controlled studies are forthcoming which may clarify this relationship.

Self-help and guilt

Although it is not clear whether guided imagery changes immune parameters significantly in ways that would influence cancer, many therapists still find the technique clinically helpful (LeShan 1989; Cunningham *et al.* 1991*b*; Levitan 1992). Spiegel and Moore (1997), however, have questioned whether these techniques, particularly guided imagery, used expressly for life extension or immune system enhancement, can harm patients who face terminal illness. In our own experience (illustrated in the next section), these techniques do not create 'false hope' but rather offer concrete skills for coping in the face of progression. Patients understand that their self-help efforts, like medical interventions, offer no guarantees of success, but to most patients they are worth the investment of time, especially because they offer other benefits such as symptom control and mood improvements.

The Healing Journey Program

For twenty years we have conducted a progressive program in a large metropolitan hospital that incorporates a variety of coping skills including relaxation, guided imagery, and meditation. Patients are able to move through three levels, from basic training in coping skills, to a second level introducing meditation, and more advanced coping skills, then, to the third level, writing a life history and sharing it with a small support group (Cunningham and Edmonds 1996). Some patients with metastatic cancer join a fourth level group consisting of long-term psychotherapy with a strong spiritual component as well as coping skills (see Chapter 15 on Psychospiritual therapy). The following excerpts are taken from patients' written homework in the fourth level and were selected to illustrate the benefits attained from the techniques, and other issues highlighted by the research.

Physical symptom control

Tension reduction and sleep

Training in relaxation requires time and practice to develop proficiency. Patients usually begin by becoming aware of where they hold tension in their bodies and attempting to release it. With repeated practice at home, often with the aid of audio tapes, they become more adept at recognizing their tension and releasing it. Such techniques help patients feel more relaxed and sleep better.

> When I first used a (relaxation/imagery) tape in February, I found I frequently lost my concentration and the tape would end with me feeling frustrated that I had not achieved any sense of relaxation. However, it is definitely getting easier with practice. In the afternoon, I find by the end of the tape, I relax so profoundly that I am able to drift off into my afternoon nap quite effortlessly. BM

> I do a mental check-list of my muscles frequently during the day, particularly my neck and shoulders, jaws, and my lower back and I'm finding that they are less likely to be tense than they were several months ago. I also don't clench my fists together which has been a long-time habit … Sometimes, if I don't sleep well, I go through the relaxation exercises and I find them very helpful. I do have some times where my mind is so busy that I can't make it quiet, but I think that's happening to me less often, now. I've really noticed the improvement lately, as I seem to be able to handle what is, for me, the busiest time of the year at work, when I usually get very stressed. BA

> I can let my body relax by thinking about the relaxing and letting go. I do this when I think of it — it makes my mind think about itself and I try to slow things down. If I do this often enough and long enough I generally feel quieter — I sleep better at night. IM

> The best time for me to do relaxation is usually late afternoon, as I begin to feel fatigued at this time and often have a sense that I need to slow down. I do relaxation exercises at other times though, if I feel I need it, e.g. if I wake up in the morning feeling anxious, or if I feel like I need to calm down in the evening before going to bed. BL

Some patients are empowered by imagining their immune systems defeating their cancer, however, others find this process anxiety provoking. For example, they may fear the emotional engagement required to image their cancer or worry their immune system imagery will be inadequate. The clinician must be sensitive to how the patient feels about this process, helping her to understand that these images reflect deeper feelings that can be worked with and do not necessarily reflect biological events.

Excellent results [from guided imagery] that enables me to be transported to my favourite spot on a beach in Naples, Florida; there I can smell and feel the sea, hear the birds, and visualize my powerful white cells eradicating the weak cancer cells aided by the bright light of the sun's powerful rays. I achieve complete relaxation and am then able to drift off to sleep by counting backwards from 1000. BM

Once I was able to master imagery, I had a tremendous feeling of accomplishment. When I could not fix my mind on a healing process, I was worried as to what message this was sending me. Once I was able to easily picture myself being healed, I had a higher level of comfort as to my ability to be healed. KC

Coping with pain and medical procedures

Patients frequently comment on how helpful these techniques are in coping with physical pain.

During relaxation/meditation, I feel a quieting effect. My mind tends to focus on fewer things and sometimes only on one. My body feels more relaxed and tends to slow down. If I have pain, I can often breathe into the pain and relieve it for the time being. IST

The other thing that is important about this past weekend is that when I had extreme pain there were a few times I allowed myself into that realm and everything seemed to get worse. However, when I went into a relaxed state and tried my various visualizations the pain seemed to diminish … Thoughts and feelings definitely impact our physical experience. Having become far too familiar with the operating room and stages of recovery I know my thoughts, passive and visual meditations impacted my need for pain relief. There is no comparison between my initial surgery to my most recent one. The only difference being the last surgery was significantly more serious and anticipated recovery time much longer, yet I required almost no pain medication and rebounded more quickly than most. My surgeon wanted to know what exactly I was doing to facilitate all of the above. MC

In some cases pain might interfere with patients' ability to practise the techniques. In these instances a patient must work with his doctors to find an analgesic that helps. Care must be taken to ensure that the patient does not feel as though he has failed in helping himself when pain medication is required.

The obstacles that interfere during the meditation sessions are related to nagging pain in my shoulder or chest area making concentration and complete relaxation difficult. SM

Nausea and vomiting

Nausea and vomiting can also be ameliorated with these techniques.

My chemo worked well and I had very few side-effects. I think the meditation and imaging helped this. IS

In the following passage, notice how physical symptoms cause great emotional distress and how meditation helped the patient feel more in control.

> It was also interesting this past weekend as the impact of this high level of chemo kicked in and kicked me. At moments I felt so totally helpless, ill, and discouraged. The helpless feeling came from the fact that I just was not able to do anything, most importantly looking after my youngsters. As well, my body was functioning in a way I had never seen before — no energy, nausea, unable to eat, and a sense of total weakness. With all of this came a feeling of bleakness and being totally discouraged. I understand that the emotions had much to do with the physical reaction to the chemo as well as the news about the CEA (a tumour marker). However, I was able to relate to my meditations and call on the calm I receive from them to help me through. MC

In patients who become very skilled in these techniques, great peace of mind can be achieved. Suffering, both physical and emotional, can be ameliorated, as the attention is drawn away from the physical-emotional realm, into a transcendent level. In a sense this transcendence, the widest aperture of experience, dilutes suffering in a broader spiritual context.

> From the time I got home from chemo at 4:00 till I take sleeping pills at 10:00 is quite difficult. The physical discomfort is very bad (nausea, headache). I'm awake, but have to lie down very still. This time I tried something different and it really affected my mental outlook, even though my physical discomfort remained the same. I tried out some of the techniques that I've learned from the tapes … I did a body scan and tried to describe the specific physical sensations in each part of my body. The nausea was hardest to describe but I tried. I notice that the pain fluctuated as I went from one area of the body to another, and that some areas (hands and feet) felt OK. I noticed the negative thoughts I'd been having ('I can't wait for this to be over, this feels awful, I wish I could make it go away, etc'.) and replace those with positive thoughts. I remembered things I had seen during the day that made me feel hope or compassion (several things had happened at the hospital). I then thought about how lucky I was to have so much love in my life, and it helped me to 'get out' of my body. I had a real sense that everyone experiences suffering, that I am not alone — that the people who love me are suffering as they imagine me going through these procedures, and facing the unknown future. Through feeling compassion for them I felt closer to a Divine presence, and a belief that there is a lesson here for me to learn — that my impulse to try to direct this path when it is uncomfortable for me will only interfere with my freedom and ability to connect with the Divine. This was a challenge to think about in that physical state, and I felt hopeful that I could at least try. BL

Relieving distress and promoting adjustment

With practice, patients can use these techniques to cope with specific worries or concerns such as upcoming appointments and procedures.

It is amazing how important meditation, imagery, relaxation etc. can become to you in a time of stress. The events of this week threw me into meditation frenzy. I was more focused this week than ever before. I suspect it was the fear induced on Thursday by being pointed at [i.e. given a pessimistic prognosis] and the inability of my efforts to remove that fear because I could not get the results of my test ... I meditate here (in her 'special place') at least twice each day. I take long walks into the woods and my special healer meets me. Sometimes the shadow in the pathway is gone when I get there, and other times he is there waiting to take me to my inner healer. Still other times, he is my inner healer. This has been a wonderful new experience for me ... It is following these walks in the woods that I have completed my imagery exercises. It has allowed me to be in an environment where the cancer cannot grow. It has helped me to remove some of my fears and think more positive about what the future has to offer. For the first time, I am not feeling anxious about my upcoming doctor's visit. KC

There can be great ongoing anxiety and stress in living with metastatic disease, and facing the likelihood of premature death. These techniques help patients remove themselves from their anxiety and be 'in the moment' rather than anticipating the future.

One of the biggest obstacles I have faced to healing has been the stress I have experienced from fear, since I was diagnosed with metastatic cancer. I found that this fear manifested in a number of physical symptoms: tightening in my chest, abdominal discomfort, headache, sleeplessness. I believe that prolonged anxiety affects the ability of my immune system to function, and that the more relaxed and peaceful I feel, the easier it is for my body to heal. I also found that this fear affects my emotional state. It sometimes leads to feelings of sadness, disappointment, anger, resistance, helplessness, etc. The spiritual work I do helps me in both the physical and in the emotional realm. It has helped me to focus outside of my body and physical state, on something bigger than myself. It has given me hope that my life can have purpose, even if my physical abilities are diminished. It has helped me to reach a still, tranquil state of mind, which is useful in dealing with fear. I have learned to accept the range of emotions that come up, and to let them come and go, rather than getting 'stuck' in the emotional and related physical states. I think that this is probably better for healing, as the physical effects of stress are reduced. BL

Some patients describe how their general quality of life has improved in areas beyond their illness. They notice enhanced emotional expression and concentration, a deeper appreciation of the people around them and a shift in their priorities.

Either the mind or the body have to be ready to relax before you actually can relax. If one is busy, the other can relax it. Once I realized this, I found that it was easier to relax. As I slow down in general, I am finding that I am gaining more opportunities for relaxation. Also I am finding that few things bother me, and I am learning how to express my feelings more quickly and forgetting about the situation. This gives me less worrying time and more relaxing time.... I find that the effects of relaxation/meditation is to learn to focus on one thing at a time. I have not been able to do that in the past, because I moved a lot of activities forward simultaneously. This change is now beginning to penetrate other activities in my life. My ability to concentrate as well as my enjoyment of the things that I do have increased. I can now spot the time-wasters and work at getting rid of them too. DL

Often as patients become calmer and more peaceful, they relate better with those around them and feel deep gratitude for their family and friends. They also find that they can connect with and express their feelings more effectively.

> When I wake up in the morning feeling well and the sun is shining and Jack is beside me, I feel this overwhelming sense of love and security. Also when I'm in the kitchen or living room and he comes up and puts his arms around me, I feel that I could live forever. When I look at the photos of my children and the smiling face of my grandson on the wall, I feel a warm glow in my heart which makes me smile back every time. I go into the garden and smell the roses, see the butterflies, hear the birds and I know that I want to live for a very long time. BA

> When I did my relaxation this afternoon, I felt so good. My body and mind were relaxed. I thought about the wonderful friendships I have and the many blessings that I enjoy. KC

> I am working on heightening my awareness of what happens between myself and others — particularly when I experience anxiety or tension. As soon as it happens I try to be quiet for a while and be aware of what is really happening between us. I like myself better as a consequence. ZJ

> I have had some symptom anxiety, I think triggered by some reading. I also feel some anxiety about wanting to share some of my feelings with my parents, but not knowing how. I first tried to calm my anxiety, and to observe what my fearful thoughts actually were. I listened to a tape, practised some new meditation techniques, and cried a little — after this some of my sadness and anxiety were relieved. BL

Survival

Many patients express the hope or belief that these techniques may help them live longer and some may credit their self-help work with periods of disease stability or remission. Although this belief can be very motivating and confer a sense of control to the patient, it does not necessarily mean that there is a causal relationship between self-help practice and longer survival. This is one of the caveats that pertain to retrospective case studies and self-reports of remarkable survivors (e.g. Hirschberg and Barasch 1995; Berland 1995; Huebescher 1992); just because a patient believes that psychological attitude or self-help has increased their life span does not necessarily make it so. The therapist needs to be aware of the patient's beliefs and goals with regards to his self-help practice. The following excerpts illustrate the beliefs that some patients have in the effectiveness of these techniques to lengthen their lives.

> I truly believe that my own efforts can make a difference. I suppose that it is a question of having faith in God and myself and standing steadfast when anxiety and doubt rear their ugly heads. I believe that if other 'incurable' people have healed themselves there is no reason why I cannot do the same. I believe that if I can get past this hurdle, I can lead a long, productive, active life … I feel that being unable to locate the cancer, the cells are still floating around and haven't collected in one place yet. So if I can work hard enough I may be able to destroy them. MS

Since I had radiation in January ... and minor surgery..., my main efforts to control my cancer have been related to using self-help techniques such as meditation/relaxation and exercise. My tumour has not progressed since then. I believe my ability to help my mind/body to help itself is related to self-help....I am definitely excited about learning self-help techniques. The benefits will serve me well to live with my cancer and to enhance the quality of my life beyond the illness. DM

My body is a miracle — I really believe that. I am happy to tell people that I am a miracle. It's not my doing.... But I would get teed off if I did get sick again. IST

I feel that my body must be trying to get me to learn more. I need to pay attention and figure where it wants me to go. I believe that my body has a wisdom that I am only partially reading. I give it lots of relaxation and visualizations to communicate to it that I want it to help me get healthy — that I want to work together to figure out what I need to do from here on. ZJ

I believe that through my self-help I will be able to:
1. Keep my cancer under control. My quarterly scans indicate that nodes seem to appear and disappear. I am convinced that it is through my efforts that these disappearances occur — seems to follow logically since I am on no medication — and I am convinced that through my own efforts I will eventually be able to control the appearance of new nodes ...
2. Add a degree of serenity to my existence. I feel that I have made respectable progress in this area. My relaxation and meditation exercises have helped me a great deal. Our group work has been an enlightenment....The group has helped me to disentangle a number of matters in this area that I otherwise would have overlooked ... self-help will lead me to a better understanding of the self which, in my opinion, is a necessary step in my search [for serenity]. OK

Failure and guilt in the event of progression

Inevitably, for most patients with metastatic disease, progression and ultimately death do occur. Do these techniques, and the possibility of influencing the disease, create feelings of failure in the event of progression? As patients sicken and die in the groups, this issue needs to be raised by the therapist and addressed. We have found that patients are able to see that often the disease is too difficult to overcome, even with a combination of medical and self-help techniques. Group members often conclude that their self-help practices have made significant improvements in the quality of their lives and were worth learning. In the following excerpts, patients describe how they are able to use the techniques to help them cope and to gain some emotional control in the face of bad news. Some patients develop a spiritual perspective and an existential stance in the face of death (see Chapter 15 on Psychospiritual therapy).

When I feel discouraged I sometimes question how much effect I can have on this cancer. But each day I do my prayers, meditation, and visualization, and it restores my hope.... I saw my oncologist briefly on Wed. last week and found out that my pelvic ultrasound shows a slight increase in the size of my ovarian tumours. Although I was disappointed by this news and experienced some initial fear, I think that I accepted the news more calmly than I might have in the past. I think that my daily relaxation has helped me to gain more of a feeling of trust that everything will be OK. I find it helpful to sit more than once in the day and am finding I'm motivated to do this. Yesterday I experienced some anxiety about my back pain, so I sat quietly and focused on feelings of love, compassion. I experience this in a very physical way, a kind of warmth and opening in the chest area. It was very calming, and shifted my focus away from my worries. BL

I find it much easier to go right into my meditation and can actually use the calming impact of the meditation instantly if I need it during my every day activities. My example of this was when I received my CEA results last week, only to find the levels elevated 50%, which indicates that the cancer has developed a resistance to the chemo we are currently using. My immediate response was that 'cold' feeling running throughout my entire body. However, within a matter of a couple of minutes I was totally calm and relaxed and ready to investigate the next step of the medical process. I was able to leave behind the fear and sense of being discouraged, and replaced it with the calmness. MC

Symptomatic or asymptomatic, I truly believe that my [self-help work] has already given me fantastic returns. It would not be fitting for me to question whether my self-help efforts could bring about changes in my life since they have, in my opinion, already paid off in spades ... replaced stress with harmony, anger with peace, despair with hope, mental paralysis with possibility, and isolation with community. OK

Patients often respond with great disappointment, fear, and anger in the face of advancing disease. The following excerpt was taken from a patient who experienced serious disease progression early in her practice of self-help strategies:

After discovery of spread to lungs ... 6 months after surgery, in preparation for adjuvant radiation, ... I was sitting in the adjacent room calmly beside my husband, my inner self was screaming 'NO, NO, NO!' to the diagnosis that I knew would be given to me. I considered this ... rotten and unfair ... I felt betrayed, angry and fearful.... I felt that I had read extensively and followed ALL the rules and guidelines religiously, including ... relaxation, visualization and meditation.... I felt in shock immediately after in the hallway, with many ambivalent feelings ... I lost my composure and started to cry... IM

After her diagnosis of metastatic disease she entered long term therapy with our groups and was encouraged to work through her feelings of anger and develop a broader understanding of what self-help might offer her. While she recognized the risk that cancer would spread, she ultimately found that her self-help practice enhanced her daily life, enabling her to focus on the pleasures of the present, not fears of the future.

I don't perceive that I have 'doubts' rather a strong sense of 'reality' that the cancer might continue to spread. However, my self-help efforts have changed most definitely my moment-to-moment living in a new awareness, a new dimension that I otherwise would not have had. My efforts can and are making a difference ... I am truly living every minute of life now. IM

Conclusions

The research literature describes the benefits from these cognitive behavioural techniques in terms of psychometric scores and statistical significance. Qualitative data, however, flesh out the literature and richly illustrate the nature of the improvements patients can experience. The patients quoted in this section are unusual in that they have chosen to enter a program that is long term, intensive, and includes a large spiritual component. Future qualitative research might focus on patients' processes in learning and acquiring these skills and to compare and contrast the techniques with each other. It would also be helpful to examine patients' reactions to disease progression, comparing their feelings and ability to cope with patients who do not choose to learn self-help strategies. However, we believe that value of these techniques in helping patients cope with cancer and its treatment has been amply demonstrated, especially when the disease is metastatic.

Recommendations for practitioners

Cancer patients experience both physical and emotional distress and there are techniques that they can learn to help them feel more in control. The research demonstrates that hypnosis, progressive relaxation, guided imagery, and meditation can produce reliable improvements in physical symptoms (pain, nausea, and vomiting), mood (anxiety and depression) and quality of life and while these techniques, and psychological interventions generally, have not yet been shown to have a reliable effect on survival, this must not be discounted.

These techniques are cost effective and easily taught to individuals or groups. They are not designed to replace medical interventions but to assist patients in coping with both the physical and emotional effects of living with cancer. They can be helpful to patients at any point along the disease trajectory: in coping with the diagnosis and treatment, after treatment is over when the patient must live with regular medical monitoring and fears of recurrence, and when the disease is metastatic. In our experience, any feelings of guilt associated with recurrence must be recognized and processed with the patient on a continuing basis. The techniques need to be presented as ways of trying to feel better and even fighting the disease, but it should be pointed out that some cancers may be too difficult to overcome with any combination of techniques, medical or psychological. We believe that these techniques should be made available in all hospitals that treat cancer patients and that practitioners should be aware of their usefulness as a valuable complementary therapy.

References

Achterberg, J. (1985). *Imagery in healing: Shamanism and modern science.* Boston: New Science Library.

Achterberg, J. and Lawlis, G. F. (1978). *Imagery of cancer.* Institute of Personality and Ability Test, Chicago.

American Cancer Society (1982). Unproven methods of cancer management: O. C. Simonton. CA-A *Cancer Journal for Clinicians*, 32, 58–61.

Anderson, B. L. (1992). Psychological interventions for cancer patients to enhance the quality of life. *J. Consult. Clin. Psychol.*, 60, 552–68.

Baider, L., Uziely, B., and Kaplan De-Noir, A. (1994). Progressive muscle relaxation and guided mental imagery in cancer patients. *General Hospital Psychiatry*, 16, 340–47.

Benson, H. (1989). Hypnosis and the relaxation response. *Gastroenterology*, 96, 1609–11.

Benson, H., Beary, J. F., and Carol, M. P. (1974). The relaxation response. *Psychiatry*, 37, 37–46.

Berland, W. (1995). Unexpected cancer recovery: why patients believe they survive. *Advances J. of Mind-Body Health*, 11, 5–19.

Bindemann, S., Soukop, M., and Kaye, S. B. (1991). Randomised controlled study of relaxation training. *European Journal of Cancer*, 27, 170–4.

Brown-Saltzman, K. (1997). Replenishing the spirit by meditative prayer and guided imagery. *Seminars in Oncology Nursing*, 13, 255–9.

Cain, E. N., Kohorn, E. I., Quinlan, D. M., *et al.* (1986). Psychosocial benefits of a cancer support group. *Cancer*, 57, 183–9.

Carey, M. P. and Burish, T. G. (1988). Etiology and treatment of the psychological side-effects associated with cancer chemotherapy: a critical review and discussion. *Psychological Bulletin*, 104, 307–25.

Coluzzi, P. H., Grant, M., Doroshow, J. H., *et al.* (1995). Survey of the provision of supportive care services at the National Cancer Institute-designated cancer centres. *Journal of Clinical Oncology*, 13, 756–64.

Contanch, P. H. and Strum, S. (1987) Progressive muscle relaxation as antiemetic therapy for cancer patients. *Oncology Nursing Forum*, 14, 33–7.

Cunningham, A. J. and Tocco, E. K. (1989). A randomized trial of group psychoeducational therapy for cancer patients. *Pat. Ed. and Counsel*, 14, 101–14.

Cunningham, A. J. and Edmonds C. V. I. (1996). Group psychological therapy for cancer patients: a point of view, and discussion of the hierarchy of options. *International Journal of Psychiatry in Medicine*, 26, 51–82.

Cunningham, A. J., Lockwood, G. A., and Cunningham, J. A. (1991a). A relationship between perceived self-efficacy and quality of life in cancer patients. *Patient Education and Counselling*, 17, 71–8.

Cunningham, A. J., Edmonds, C. V. I., Hampson, A. W., *et al.* (1991b). Helping cancer patients cope with, and combat, their disease: report on a group psychoeducational program. Advances, *Journal of the Institute for Advancement of Health*, 7, 41–56.

Cunningham, A. J., Lockwood, G. A., and Edmonds, C. V. I. (1993). Which cancer patients benefit most from a brief, group, coping skills program? *Internat. J. Psychiat. in Med.*, 23, 383–98.

Cunningham, A. J., Edmonds, C. V. I., Jenkins, G. P., *et al.* (1998). A randomized controlled trial of the effects of group psychological therapy on survival in women with metastatic breast cancer. *Psycho-Oncology*, 7, 508–17.

Devine, E. C. and Westlake, S. K. (1995). The effect of psychoeducational care provided to adults with cancer: meta-analysis of 116 studies. *Oncology Nursing Forum*, 22, 1369–81.

Edmonds, C. V. I., Cunningham, A. J., and Lockwood, G. A. (1999). Psychological response to long term group therapy: A randomized trial with metastatic breast cancer patients. *Psycho-Oncology*, 8, 74–91.

Everly, G. S. and Benson, H. (1989). Disorders of arousal and the relaxation response: speculations on the nature and treatment of stress related diseases. *International Journal of Psychosomatics*, 36, 15–21.

Farber, J. and Weinerman B. (1981). A comparison of different support group formats in aiding cancer patients in coping with their disease and treatment. *Proceedings of American Social Clinical Oncology*, April, C-422.

Fawzy, F. I., Cousins, N., Fawzy, N. W., *et al.* (1990). A structured psychiatric intervention for cancer patients, I. Changes over time in methods of coping and affective disturbances. *Archives of General Psychiatry*, 47, 720–25.

Fawzy, F. I., Fawzy, N. W., Hyun, C. S., *et al.* (1993). Malignant melanoma. Effects of an early structured psychiatric intervention, coping and affective state on recurrence and survival 6 years later. *Archives of General Psychiatry*, 50, 681–9.

Fawzy, F. I., Fawzy, N. W., Arndt, L. A., *et al.* (1995). Critical review of psychosocial interventions in cancer care. *Arch. Gen. Psychiatry*, 52, 100–13.

Ferrell, B. R., Rhiner, M., and Ferrell, B. A. (1993). Development and implementation of a pain education program. *Cancer*, 72, 3426–32.

Ferrell, B. R., Ferrell, B. A., Ahn, C., *et al.* (1994). Pain management for elderly patients with cancer at home. *Cancer*, 74, 2139–46.

Fleming, U. (1985). Relaxation therapy for far-advanced cancer. *The Practitioner*, 229, 471–5.

Greer, S. (1989). Can psychological therapy improve the quality of life of patients with cancer? *British Journal of Cancer*, 59, 149–51.

Hirshberg, C. and Barasch, M. I. (1995). *Remarkable recovery*. Riverhead Books, New York.

Huebscher, R. R. (1992). Spontaneous remission of cancer: an example of health promotion. *Nurse Practitioner Forum*, 3, 228–35.

Ilnyckyj, A., Farber, J., Cheang, M. C., and Weinerman, B. H. (1994). A randomized controlled trial of psychotherapeutic intervention in cancer patients. *Annals Royal College of Physicians and Surgeons of Canada*, 27, 93–6.

Ironside, G., Antoni, M., and Letendorf, S. (1995). Can psychological interventions affect immunity and survival? Present findings and suggested targets with a focus on cancer and human immunodeficiency virus. *Mind/Body Medicine*, 1, 85–110.

Jacobsen, P. B. (1997). The Spiegel/Moore article revisited. *Oncology*, 11, 1179–89.

Kutz, I., Leserman, J., Dorrington, C., *et al.* (1985a). Meditaion as an adjunct to psychotherapy. *Psychotherapy and Psychosomatics*, 43, 209–18.

Kutz, I., Borysenko, J. Z., and Benson, H. (1985b). Meditation and psychotherapy:a rationale for the integration of dynamic psychotherapy, the relaxation response and mindfulness meditation. *American Journal of Psychiatry*, 142, 1–8.

LeShan, L. (1989). *Cancer as a turning point*. Dutton, New York.

Levitan, A. A. (1992).The use of hypnosis with cancer patients. *Psychiatric Medicine*, 10, 119–31.

Lyles, J. N., Burish, T. G., Krozely, M. G., *et al.* (1982). Efficacy of relaxation training and guided imagery in reducing the aversiveness of cancer chemeotherapy. *Journal of Consulting and Clinical Psychology*, 50, 509–24.

Meares, A. (1980). What can the patient expect from intensive meditation? *Australian Family Physician*, 9, 322–5.

Meyer, T. J. and Mark, M. M. (1995). Effects of psychosocial intervention with adult cancer patients: A meta-analysis of randomized experiments. *Health Psychology*, 14, 101–8.

Moorey, S., Greer, S., Watson, M., *et al.* (1994). Adjuvant psychological therapy for patients with cancer outcome at one year. *Psycho-Oncology*, 3, 39–76.

Morganstern, H., Gellert, G. A., Walter, S. D., *et al.* (1984). The impact of a psychosocial support program on survival with breast cancer: the importance of selection bias in program evaluation. *Journal of Chronic Disease*, 37, 273–82.

Newton, B. W. (1982). The use of hypnosis in the treatment of cancer patients. *American Journal of Clinical Hypnosis*, **25**, 104–13.

Pattison, J. (1997). Hypnotherapy: complementary support in cancer care. *Nursing Standard*, **11**, 44–6.

Redd, W. H. (1994). Advances in behavioral intervention in comprehensive cancer treatment. *Supportive Care in Cancer*, **2**, 111–15.

Redd, W. H. and Hendler, C. S. (1982). Behavioral medicine in comprehensive cancer treatment. *Journal of Psychosocial Oncology*, **1**, 3–17.

Redd, W. L., Silberfarb, P. M., Anderson, *et al.* (1991). Physiologic and psychobehavioral research in oncology. *Cancer*, **67**, 813–22.

Simonton, O. C., Mathews-Simonton, S., and Sparks, T. F. (1980). Psychological intervention in the treatment of cancer. *Psychosomatics*, **21**, 226–33.

Spiegel, D. (1985). The use of hypnosis in controlling cancer pain. Ca-A *Cancer Journal for Clinicians*, **35**, 221–31

Spiegel, D. and Bloom, J. R. (1982). Pain in metastatic breast cancer. *Cancer*, **52**, 341–5.

Spiegel D. and Moore, R. (1997). Imagery and hypnosis in the the treatment of cancer patients. *Oncology*, **11**, 1179–89.

Spiegel, D., Bloom, J. R., and Yalom, I. D. (1981). Group support for patients with metastatic breast cancer. *Archives of General Psychiatry*, **38**, 527.

Spiegel, D., Bloom, J. R., Kraemer, H. C., *et al.* (1989). Effect of psychosocial treatment on survival of patients with metastatic breast cancer. *Lancet*, Oct. 14, 888–91.

Stephens, R. (1993). Imagery: A strategic intervention to empower patients Part 1 — Review of the Literature. *Clinical Nurse Specialist*, **7**, 170–4.

Taylor, S. E., Falke, R. L., Shoptaw, S. J. and Lichtman, R. R. (1986). Social support, support groups, and the cancer patient. *Journal of Clinical and Consulting Psychology*, **54**, 608–15.

Telch, T. F. and Telch, M. J. (1986). Group coping skills instruction and supportive group therapy for cancer patients: A comparison of strategies. *Journal of Consulting and Clinical Psychology*, **54**, 802–8.

Trijsberg, R. W., van Knippenberg, F. C. E., and Rijpma, S. E. (1992). Effects of psychological treatment on cancer patients,: a critical review. *Psychosomatic Medicine*, **54**, 489–517.

Troesch, L. M., Rodehaver, C. B., Delaney, E. A., and Yanes, B. (1996). The influence of guided imagery on chemotherapy-related nausea and vomiting. *Oncology Nursing Forum*, **20**, 1179–85.

Walker, L. G. (1992). Hypnosis with cancer patients. *American Journal of Preventive Psychiatry and Neurology*, **3**, 42–8

Wallace, K. G. (1997). Analysis of recent literature concerning relaxation and imagery interventions for cancer patients. *Cancer Nursing*, **20**, 79–87.

Walsh, R. (1996). Meditation research: State of the art. In *Textbook of Transpersonal Psychiatry and Psychology* (ed. B. W. Scotton, A. B. Chinen, and J. R. Battista), pp. 167–75. New York: Basic Books.

Weisman, A. D. and Worden, J. W. (1976). Psychosocial analysis of cancer deaths. *Omega*, **6**, 61.

Zaza, C., Sellick, S. M., Willan, A., Reyno, L., and Browman, G. P. (1999). Health care professionals' familiarity with non-pharmocological strategies for managing cancer pain. *Psycho-Oncology*, **8**, 99–111.

Chapter 15

Psychospiritual therapy

Alastair Cunningham, Joanne Stephen, Catherine Phillips, and Kimberley Watson

The authors are based in Toronto, Canada. Alastair Cunningham is a senior scientist and psychologist at the Ontario Cancer Institute. His research interests include mind-body theory, and investigating the effects of adjunctive psychological therapy on quality and length of life in cancer patients. Catherine Phillips is a researcher and therapist with the Healing Journey Program at Princess Margaret Hospital. Joanne Stephen and Kimberley Watson are doctoral candidates and researchers with the Healing Journey Program.

Introduction and definitions

'Psychospiritual' is a new and barely recognized term, and because there is confusion about what 'spiritual' means, we need to begin with definitions. The problem with definitions of spirituality, as Walsh and Vaughn (1993) noted, is that they tend to draw on assumptions about the nature of 'reality'. Thus we offer one that is historical, and based on the world's spiritual traditions, and one that is 'popular', and reflects contemporary trends. They are not incompatible, but differ in the assumptions required.

The traditional definition of 'spiritual' is based on a common core of insight or wisdom, sometimes called the 'Perennial Philosophy' (following Spinoza), that has been held by many cultures, and for thousands of years. Happold (1970) describes the main ideas of this philosophy in his book *Mysticism*: the world of matter is held to be a manifestation of a different (non-material) reality, that can be known by direct intuition or apprehension, but not solely by logical reasoning. It is claimed that beneath man's ego or phenomenal self lies an eternal inner self, sometimes called spirit, with which we can identify, and that this realization is the chief end of earthly existence. In the words of a modern sage (Easwaran 1989), when we do realize this goal we discover that the spirit or divinity within ourselves is one and the same as that in all individuals and all life.

A contemporary scholar, Krippner (1995) provides a simple definition that follows from this understanding. Spirituality, he says 'can be used to describe aspects of human behaviour and experience that reflect an alleged transcendent intelligence or process'. He goes on to point out that 'spiritual' is not synonymous with 'religious', a religion being an institutionalized body of beliefs, practices, and rituals, based on an assumed underlying spiritual reality. People can be spiritual without being religious, and vice versa. Our discussion then is not about the value of religious beliefs or social practices such as attending church, although these appear to have a healthful influence (Levin and Schiller 1987). Our discussion is about spiritual experience.

Many people may be uncomfortable with the idea of a spiritual dimension underlying material reality, yet nevertheless have a sense of 'something' powerful and mysterious that is transcendent, beyond the usual concerns and preoccupations of the personal self. Depending on our beliefs, we may prefer more limited definitions of 'transcendence'. Aldridge (1993), for instance, defines spirituality as 'a relationship to a higher authority (God or life force for example) as defined by an individual to identify meaning and purpose in life, and to transcend a given moment'. Coward (1990) offers another definition that 'humanizes' the transcendent even further: 'the capacity to reach out beyond oneself, to extend oneself beyond personal concerns and to take on broader life perspectives, activities and purposes'. Aldridge (1993) investigated many definitions of spirituality and two components were common: a relationship to a higher power, and finding meaning and purpose in life. We have likewise found that patients who become deeply involved in psychospiritual therapy may or may not have theories about spirituality, but nevertheless describe experiences of connecting with some form of a 'higher power', and as a consequence, discover greater meaningfulness and peacefulness in their daily lives.

Our present purposes are not, of course, theological but psychological. We aim to contribute to a discussion that is at an early stage, that is, how to bring such a transcendent dimension, however it is conceived, into the healthcare of interested individuals who have cancer or other diseases. We would, however, insist that spirituality implies some attempt to go beyond material goals and ego needs. Many philosophies of life do not advocate this. We also acknowledge the vagueness of much of the terminology surrounding spirituality, and the need to use metaphors like 'dimension' or 'level' to refer to events that cannot be measured in concrete ways, although they may have profound effects on individuals.

'Psychospiritual' is a curious term that has emerged recently as the idea of incorporating spiritual issues into psychotherapy has become more common. Strictly speaking, the linking of these two words is redundant; the route to spiritual awareness is necessarily through the mind. However, it may usefully be compared with 'psychosomatic', which refers to the connections between body and mind. In a similar way, 'psychospiritual' acknowledges the connections of mind and spirit, or the conscious awareness of a spiritual dimension. We define 'psychospiritual therapy' as psychologically-based therapy designed to assist patients in bringing a sense of the transcendent into their daily lives, that is to have spiritual experience. Psychospiritual therapy is not a single technique, or even a single therapeutic approach, but rather a broad orientation towards assisting people with techniques that have been used for many centuries. Some of the techniques taught or advocated to patients are: meditation, guided imagery, prayer, reading works from the world's great spiritual tra-

Table 15.1 Types of psychological intervention for cancer patients, arranged in order of increasing requirement for change on the part of the patient

Nature of group	Hierarchy of Group Programs[a]	
	Therapeutic aims	Main activity required of patients
1. Providing information	To inform	Listening
2. Support	Acknowledgement of problems and expressions of emotion	Sharing accessible feelings
3. Coping skills training	Acquisition of new cognitive skills	Cognitive and behavioral change; taking some control
4. Psychotherapy	Increased self-understanding	Retrieval of repressed ideas and affect, with resulting change
5. Spiritual/existential therapy	Discovery of meaning; experience of transcendent order	Meditation, study, reflection; some relaxation of ego control

[a] Each program includes most of the elements of programs lower on the hierarchy.
Reprinted from *International Journal of Psychiatry in Medicine* (1996), **26**, p. 56, with permission.

ditions, breath work, expressive artwork, body awareness techniques such as yoga and tai chi, and dream analysis. The emphasis, perhaps even more than in conventional psychotherapy, is on helping clients have their own experience. As in psychotherapy, however, the therapist needs a base of relevant personal experience to be an effective guide.

One way of positioning psychospiritual therapy relative to other kinds of psychological help offered to cancer patients is shown in Table 15.1. This describes a hierarchy of interventions, arranged in order of the extent of the contribution required from the patient (Cunningham and Edmonds 1996). Thus receiving information, at the 'low' end, needs no effort; attending a support group or counselling session requires willingness to risk the expression of emotion; and learning coping skills needs the further investment of time to acquire skills. Psychospiritual therapy is placed at the top of the hierarchy because it asks a great deal from the patient; an initial awareness of one's own thought processes, a willingness and ability to control basic psychological functions such as the flow of ideas, an interest and openness to exploring spiritual concepts, and the application of techniques, notably meditation in its various forms.

As the term 'spiritual' becomes more widely accepted in the popular culture, and used to embrace everything from sensuality to goal setting, it is important to list what psychospiritual therapy is not. Traditional religious observance is not necessarily effective in causing spiritual connection or experience. Likewise, when unconscious or repressed material is tapped through dream analysis or psychoanalytic interpretation or mental imaging, this is usually not spiritual, although, as for prayer, these methods may be used to facilitate spiritual experience. Distant healing, 'energy work' and 'spiritualism' are not psychospiritual therapy, although they may somehow access spiritual mechanisms (if such a term can be used to describe non-material events). And humanistic/existential therapies do not typically have an explicit intention to connect clients with the spiritual, although individual practitioners may well include this as part of their therapeutic plan.

The neglect of the spiritual dimension in the health field

Modern western healthcare is highly materialistic; the psychological attributes of patients are usually accorded little prognostic significance, and their spiritual beliefs even less. Historically this reflects the philosophical split between mind and body, and between science and religion. Yet the consumers of this healthcare may have different priorities. Most Americans, for example, identify themselves as religious in some way (Hoge 1996; Kosmin and Lachman 1993). Spirituality tends not to be differentiated from religion in discussions of the role of both in health and disease, and most of the research literature exploring the relationship of these human qualities to disease have used such simple measures as attendance at church to assess the religious dimension (Dein and Stygall 1997; Larson *et al.* 1998). Part of the resistance to integrating spirituality into healthcare may derive from this confusion, leading to a view that religion and spirituality are the business of professions other than medicine or psychology. Lukoff *et al.* (1999, p. 64) believe that although religious and spiritual issues are integral to all aspects of healthcare, 'health professionals report minimal or no training in dealing with them'. Likewise in psychology: 'religion and religious beliefs are basically neglected in psychology text books' (Jones 1996, p. 113). Psychology and psychiatry, since Freud, have tended to ignore or pathologize religion and spirituality, although there are, of course, many individual psychologists, physicians, and counsellors from other disciplines to whom religion and/or spiritual experience are of great importance, and many who bring this background into their practice. The neglect of this vital aspect of the life of patients occurs at the institutional level. This is most unfortunate, since as we will see later in this chapter, spirituality may be or become the prime concern of many people dealing with life-threatening cancer. To ignore this part of their experience is to miss an important avenue for providing help.

Frameworks for understanding psychospiritual therapies

If spirituality is to become a regular part of psychological counselling we need some theoretical framework in which to place it in relation to physical, cognitive, and emotional issues. Such a framework should obviously not depend on any particular metaphysical beliefs, and should guide the use of spirituality in practice. This conceptual task is barely begun; it will take time and effort from many interested people. Here we offer some ideas that we have found helpful in our own practice.

As has often been the case in psychology, to conceptualize patterns of experience we need to draw on metaphor. We have found two models useful: the 'levels' model and the concept of personal growth as evolution towards spiritual understanding. The first of these is shown in Fig. 15.1. There is a relatively old understanding that humans are made up of a hierarchy of levels of increasing complexity, from atoms to molecules to cells to organs, and so on. To this we can add a second idea, much less commonly stated, that there are two aspects of this organization; the materials or substance out of which the different levels are constructed, and the complexity or patterns of information embodied in these structures (Cunningham 1995). 'Mind', on this view, is an informational idea rather than a thing, a pattern of functioning, the 'software' of the brain, to use a computer analogy. Figure 15.1 shows a series of material levels of increasing complexity, and it also shows examples of informational or pattern terms that correspond to some of these material levels. 'Spirit' seems more of an informational concept than a material entity, almost like a greatly expanded form of mind.

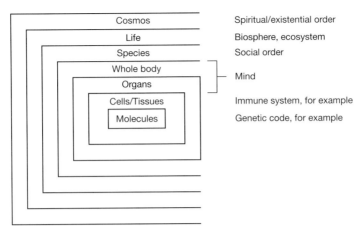

Fig. 15.1 Principal structures of the human being, with some informational correlates. Reprinted from Advances, *Journal of Mind–Body Health*. (1995), **11**, 7, with permission.

This description certainly does not capture all that 'mind' and 'spirit' are, but it can be an aid to thinking. For example, we are familiar with helping clients to 'get in touch' with what is going on in their minds, their stream of thoughts, and it can equally be helpful to think of contacting the spiritual dimension as similarly tapping into a kind of 'giant mind'. Further, laying out a 'map' of the human as a series of levels like this, or in even more simplified form (Cunningham 1986), becomes a useful guide for patients and therapists. The psychological work can be seen as an attempt to become aware of what is happening at each level, changing where necessary. The spiritual work is a natural part of this, contacting that level of oneself, becoming more aware of it, and making adjustments in lifestyle and thought-style to be in harmony with the spiritual part of the self (Cunningham *et al.* 1991).

A second kind of orienting model is the view that human psychological development is an evolutionary process, with spiritual connection at its apex. Incorporating transcendent experiences into one's life, and having an expanded sense of self and greater feeling of connectedness, are seen from this perspective as natural outcomes of psychological growth. Most western psychological models of personal development (e.g. Erikson 1963; Kohlberg 1976; Loevinger 1976; Piaget 1969) have viewed the development of a strong ego as the ultimate human attainment, although Abraham Maslow (1971) and Carl Jung (1959) have argued that man has a 'higher' or transcendent dimension. Maslow (1971), for example, documented the experiences of self-actualizing persons: loving feelings, joyousness, acceptance, feelings of awe and wonder were some of the experiences regularly reported. On the other hand, traditional spiritual disciplines, like Buddhism, Sufism, and Yoga, take it for granted that the higher reaches of personal growth are largely concerned with increasing spiritual understanding and connection, which paradoxically entails relinquishing exclusive identification with the ego. Some modern western scholars (e.g. Wilber 1995; Shafii 1985) have begun to map these 'higher' stages.

The value of the developmental model, as with the 'levels' idea, is that it can guide practice; it suggests that spiritual practices such as meditation are more appropriate for people who have already undergone some basic psychological development, and who are interested in exploring questions of ultimate meaning in their lives. Psychospiritual therapy, bringing spiritual development, may lead to a much greater awareness of how the individual fits in to a larger scheme, an enhanced sense of meaning in one's life, increasing tolerance of others, and a readier acceptance of personal death. Some examples are given below of these benefits to patients with life-threatening disease.

There are strong similarities between psychospiritual therapy, as defined here, and transpersonal psychotherapy. The latter is the practical, therapeutic arm of the emerging (but unconventional) field of 'transpersonal psychology', which attempts to bring together the traditions of modern, western psychology and the world's spiritual traditions. Transpersonal psychotherapy 'views all psychological processes against the backdrop of spiritual unfolding' (Cortwright 1997). It is thus broader than, and includes, psychospiritual therapy. For the present, it seems wise to retain the more conservative term, since transpersonal therapy makes assumptions that most healthcare professionals would currently not accept. 'Existential therapy' (Spira 1997) is another psychological approach that shares some of the aspirations of spiritual work, but is concerned with helping patients create meaning in an apparently meaningless world, without invoking a transcendent order.

The relevance of psychospiritual therapy

Why use psychospiritual therapy for cancer patients? The criterion must be, 'does it help them?' and the clinical observation is that, as with most approaches, it helps some people a lot, some a little, and others not at all. Although this is perhaps best illustrated with concrete examples (see below), we can suggest three main ways in which cancer patients may be helped by psychological assistance intended to promote spiritual connection or spiritual growth:

1) *Quality of life may be enhanced.* There is evidence that in patients who are confronting their own mortality, spiritual awareness is associated with less distress and an ability to maintain a sense of well-being (Reed 1987; Coward 1990, 1991). Women with advanced breast cancer, for instance, described their spiritual experiences as leading to a relief of pain and the sense of burden, of feeling mentally uplifted, feeling a greater closeness with others and their environment, an increased valuing of self and a 'savoring of the small moments in life' (Coward 1990). Kaczorowski (1989) and Smith *et al.* (1993) reported an association between spirituality and reduced distress in cancer patients, and argued that an intervention able to increase a patient's level of spiritual awareness would be highly beneficial, given the erosion of well-being that typically accompanies cancer, especially advanced cancer.

2) *A sense of greater meaning and purpose may emerge.* A diagnosis of cancer often comes to dominate a person's experience and identity. Connecting spiritually may counter this disabling effect, so that psychological and spiritual growth, rather than cancer, becomes the primary focus. This often leads to increased sense of meaning in daily life. Coward (1990) found that women who had self-transcending experiences reported a sense of purposefulness in helping others, and a greater meaningfulness in everyday activities. We have witnessed this also. 'Meaning' is a slippery term, but we intend here to signify an awareness of being part of a larger order. This is often accompanied by a sense that all will be well, even if one dies, and by feeling loved and cared for by God or some higher

power, as in the examples cited later. Such impressions are hard to explain rationally — the point is not whether they do or do not contact a transcendent reality, but that they are the patient's experience and such experiences can greatly ease the emotional pain of facing premature death.

3) *Life may be longer, as well as better.* There has been considerable speculation in the trade literature, especially in relation to cancer, that spiritual growth may prolong life. Scientific evidence is, of course, lacking, and hard to obtain. There is evidence that religious observance is associated with longer life (Levin and Schiller 1987), although this may be attributable to good lifestyle habits and social support rather than directly to spirituality. Not the least of the technical problems in assessing the efficacy of psychospiritual therapy is to disentangle the spiritual work from the many other strategies (e.g. regular psychotherapy, relaxation practice, visualization) used by patients who become involved in self-healing efforts. From our own research, in a prospective longitudinal study on a small sample of such people who had metastatic cancer, there was a strong correlation between dedicated use of a psychospiritual therapy program, including a lot of meditation and spiritual reading, and longer survival (Cunningham *et al.*, 2000). We are not aware of any other systematic attempts to test the efficacy of psychospiritual therapy in prolonging the life of cancer patients.

The Healing Journey Program

Our program, operating in a Canadian cancer hospital, has four levels each requiring greater involvement from the participant. The first is a series of classroom-style presentations and experiential practice introducing mind-body approaches to healing. Three to four hundred patients attend this level annually. The second focuses more intensely on specific coping techniques and includes small group participation. Approximately one hundred and fifty patients attend level two annually. A small proportion attend a third level, which involves writing a life story. The fourth level, open only to selected patients with metastatic illness, consists of long-term (nine months) small group psychotherapy. This level requires significant involvement from the participants in the form of weekly homework assignments and self-help practice at home.

Thus patients in our program choose the extent of their involvement by opting to proceed or drop out at the end of each level. The topic of spirituality is introduced, with instruction on meditation, at the second level. At the fourth level, participants actively engage in systematic, spiritual practice through the process of homework assignments, reading spiritual material, and initiating regular meditation and/or prayer. The work in the spiritual area is done in conjunction with work in other areas. These include: the body — paying attention to diet, exercise, and developing awareness of where tension is held in the body; conscious mind — watching the mind and learning to manage negative thoughts and emotions; 'deeper mind' — using imagery to explore thoughts and feelings more intensively, and a social level — developing greater awareness and harmony in close relationships. Thus the program promotes an integrated and extensive self-help effort; for the purpose of the current discussion, the descriptions here will pertain only to spiritual development.

The following excerpts are from recent participants in our fourth level program, taken from homework assignments or from personal interviews.

Getting started

Participants come into the program with different levels of spiritual experience and aware-ness. Most are open to exploring spirituality and believe that such exploration may be beneficial to themselves (initials are not those of the patients):

> It's [spirituality] another whole area that I want to make sense of. I believe it can work. IS.

Some already have a developed understanding, an established practice of meditation and can describe significant experiences that confirm the meaningfulness of this kind of work for them. Their goal is to heighten their awareness and to continue their work in a commu-nity of like-minded fellow explorers.

> I have this feeling of being part of something interconnected and greater than myself. I have been trying to articulate this in my thoughts and writings lately and it is something that I would like to discuss with others. BL.

Blocks to exploration

A few participants are reluctant to explore spirituality because of previous experience with religion. Issues related to their religious upbringing may need to be dealt with before they can be open to the idea of spiritual meaning.

> I continue to smart from my first experiences with religion. It's very tender and I shy away from things like acts of faith. It has to be demonstrated to me somehow. AM

Some participants are blocked by their sense that it would be 'hypocritical' to explore spirituality now that they are unwell. They see it as turning to God simply because they are in need of healing and are deterred by the apparent expediency of such motivation.

> It feels hypocritical to pray to God only when I am in trouble. BA.

Such blocks are often overcome after raising them in the group and hearing how others worked through them, by witnessing the benefits of spiritual experience in others, and most importantly, by starting their own practice of meditation. A few remain resistant to the idea that spiritual exploration could be beneficial to them and choose to avoid the area although they usually remain in the group for other reasons, such as emotional support.

Deepening spiritual exploration

Homework assignments encourage participants to initiate or deepen meditation practice, read spiritual texts, and attend activities or gatherings that have a spiritual purpose. Through such activities, participants begin to develop a sense of connection with some-thing larger than themselves. They start to have experiences that 'feel right'. These experi-ences and their growing spiritual awareness motivate them to further exploration.

I think spirituality means a connection with something bigger than ourselves. I feel like I've taken baby steps along the spiritual path and that would be the best way I could describe it. Because I haven't found words that I'm comfortable with describing how I feel. But I do feel a very powerful or very strong connection to something bigger than myself.

The interesting thing is I had always pictured or thought of that entity as being outside myself, whereas what has developed has been very much something I'm finding within myself. When I thought of prayer, I always pictured it as being on your hands and knees praying to something outside yourself whereas it is very much an inner voice that I'm connecting to. But that voice, although it's within, it also seems to be something bigger than myself and also it's the connection that we all have with each other and the universe — the oneness that I have read about and thought about and still have some trouble grasping.

I have started the practice of praying each evening. I'm not sure how conventional it is, but it is very much a review of the day and the practice of letting go of any resentments or any negative feelings that have built up over the course of the day and praying for guidance or help with letting [them] go. An example from last week is meeting with that insurance person [about disability benefits]. I built up a lot of anxiety and worrying.

I've done that in a number of situations and it worked just beautifully. I guess through reading and talking to different people [in the group] I've started different [spiritual] practices that have developed meaning for me. So they really have — I'm looking for a word — blossomed or continued to build experience by experience. AD.

I am finding that the most helpful part of my spiritual practice at this moment is to continually imagine the presence of God around me. It's difficult to describe how I experience this — first I have to remember to do this and focus on feeling a Divine presence. The more often I think to do this during the day, the easier it is for me to remain calm. Sometimes when I do this I feel a rush of energy through my body, sometimes I can imagine a warm light surrounding me, and sometimes it's more a thought. When I'm doing this it feels like I am building a feeling of trust in Divine support or guidance. My main goal right now is to bring this feeling more into my life. BL.

Experiencing benefits

As sense of spirituality deepens, participants feel differently. They describe a greater sense of comfort, often expressed as a new lightness or easiness in relation with one's self and with others. New meaning and purpose in life emerge, as well as a greater sense of connectedness with something larger than oneself.

I think fundamentally I feel happier about myself. That is a gift, I think, in and of itself. Nothing really fantastic or wonderful, but it's sufficient to make me feel like I'm a happier person. I feel more contented. I'm able to deal with some things a little bit better, stresses are a little bit easier to deal with. I feel there is some direction to my journey, whereas before there didn't seem to be a lot of clear purpose. I was spinning in circles more or less. I feel now there is a way I'm following or being led. AM.

Perhaps the most common description of the benefits of spiritual exploration is the achievement of greater peace.

> I think that I have developed a stronger trust in God in the past year. One way I measure this is by the extent and degree of anxiety I feel. When I was first diagnosed last summer I experienced weeks of intense anxiety — difficulty sleeping, fearful thoughts, etc. I still have those thoughts, but they come and go more quickly. I've found that when I am able to bring my attention back to God I feel relief. A few days ago I found out that I have bone metastases in my lower spine and pelvis. Initially I felt overwhelmed when I heard this news — that evening I had many catastrophic thoughts, and had a feeling of panic like I had lost all control. By the time I was ready to go to bed I was able to calm down, and I did this by reminding myself that I could accept whatever happened, that it is God's will, and I could pray for strength and peace of mind. As I've intensified my daily prayer, I have felt relief from these initial feelings of panic. BL.

> The times when I have a deep meditation or a very good Qi Gong session I sense that all is well in my world and that sense of peace and ease takes over above everything else and allows calm to prevail. I just feel at these times that everything will be OK. This is a new feeling and although I was initially cautious, I am becoming more relaxed and familiar with this state and starting to enjoy this way of being. I know during those times when fear takes over I am able to more readily handle it now, as I focus on the universal power to keep me safe and guide me. MC.

Specific issues for cancer patients: why me?

Having cancer often raises specific issues related to spiritual exploration. Some participants struggle with the question, 'If there's a God, why would He let this happen to me?'

> I think a cancer diagnosis, or other life crisis, challenges most people's spiritual faith, no matter how strong it is. Suddenly facing my own mortality helped me to examine my spirituality and find ways to discover and develop it. In a very meaningful way, it put my beliefs to a test.
>
> When I was first diagnosed, I think that I had very little understanding of my own spirituality. I saw God as something separate from me and outside of myself. This allowed me to blame him and accuse him of punishing me. It also allowed me to question the existence of a God. If there were a God, why would he let this happen to me?
>
> Because I was not sure about my beliefs, I was able to use this time as an opportunity to discover what I believe. In the process of exploring my faith I have been able to identify with my spiritual self and give thought to what the meaning of my life is. I think that the inner resources I have discovered have played a major impact on my healing and enabled me to find a peace in my life that I never felt before. KC.

Physical cure versus personal meaningfulness

Initially, many participants embrace spiritual exploration in the hope that it will cure their cancer. As they develop spiritually, some describe a shift away from focusing solely on physical cure to an expanded view of emotional and spiritual healing. Spiritual work becomes meaningful for itself, not just as a means to promoting physical health.

I think one of the most positive effects of my spiritual work is that it has broadened my view of what healing means, to one that goes beyond physical healing. Because the course my illness will take is quite uncertain, I find that having a goal of physical recovery isn't enough. Certainly I hope for physical recovery, but realize that the extent and time span of this recovery are unknown, and may be less than I would ideally like. Although I understand this intellectually, it has been difficult for me to accept at a deeper level. There are times when I feel deep sadness at the possibility that I will die before I reach the old age I had previously assumed I would reach. At times I feel a burning desire to be alive, and to have years stretching ahead of me when I can do all of the things I still want to do in my life. I find I am beginning to be able to let go of my sadness and anger about the uncertainty of my future when I am able to think of healing in a broader sense, which includes emotional and spiritual healing. BL

I think if physical healing continues to be the only reason for doing this, it would somehow be empty of its real meaning. I've had to accept the uncertainty of whether or not I'm going to achieve physical healing. I do look at it in more of a broader sense and I guess the ultimate healing is having peace of mind. AD.

Fighting spirit versus spiritual acceptance

As spiritual development progresses and participants become more accepting of whatever may happen to them, this acceptance in turn raises new concerns. Does this mean they are losing their 'fighting spirit' and 'giving in to their illness'?

What I've wrestled with sometimes is the question of whether or not that means giving into the illness. How can you have peace of mind when you're facing this?

But I don't see it as giving into the illness at all. And that's why now what I feel really expresses it and what I feel comfortable saying is that I've accepted the uncertainty. I haven't accepted that because I have metastatic breast cancer that I'm going to die, but I have accepted that I don't have total control and no matter what I do, it is uncertain what the outcome will be. AD.

A thought that I found helpful today is 'We mistakenly believe that if we accept our death, we will begin to die. Curiously, the reverse is true: when we accept we are already dying, we are set free to live.' This spoke to me because I often focus on my fears of dying (in my random thoughts, not purposely) and wonder if I could shift this focus to a desire to be set free? I have been concerned that if I focus too much on accepting death that it might be a form of giving up, when I need a 'fighting spirit'. I'm not sure how to 'surrender' without giving up. Joseph Goldstein makes a distinction between 'letting go' and 'letting it be'. I certainly try hard to 'let go' and will try letting it be instead. BL

Integrating spiritual awareness and experience into everyday life

For many of the patients in our 'advanced' groups (level 4) spiritual exploration becomes the focal point of their healing process. They see their spiritual work as an integral part of their lives. It is no longer a belief or practice separate from themselves, but rather the core of their being. As one participant said 'I'm feeling it, personalizing it, living it.'

> My spiritual development has become a primary focus in my life. I don't see it as a separate category, but something integral to my life and part of everything I do. The more deeply I've become involved in spiritual practice, the more effortless it seems to lead a spiritual life. I don't mean 'effortless' in the sense that it isn't hard work, but rather that a spiritual focus or outlook comes to me more naturally now than in the past. My spiritual development is the most important thing now in my life, because it affects so strongly how I am living each day, and also because it prepares me to accept my own death when the time comes. BL.

New perspectives on death

As we have noted, spiritual development brings a greater acceptance of whatever may happen and a sense of connectedness with a larger order. Many participants describe a trust that 'no matter what happens, I will be OK'. Developing this trust helps them face the emotional pain and fears associated with confronting their death and the prospect of leaving loved ones behind. It also helps them find meaning in their present life and to place emphasis on living fully and enjoying each day.

> I think that one of the greatest gifts I have received from my spiritual journey is the realization that my spirituality can encompass all of my life. It is not something that belongs in a special compartment, separate from the rest of life. It has to do with a basic sense of what life is all about.
>
> Life has to be about more than an exercise that leads to death and decay in a grave. Life begins with breath and ends with breath. With the beginning of the first breath, spirit and body are connected. When our physical self dies, our spirit moves on. It is this faith and belief that helps me to have an inner sense of wholeness and peace, even if my body is not perfect. Developing, growing and maturing in my spirituality helps me to understand that the death of my physical body is not the end of my spiritual self. A healed person is not necessarily a person without any physical disease. KC.

Final comments

Over the years of observing participants in our program develop spiritually we have noted the substantial benefits they have experienced, such as greater acceptance of themselves and others, greater comfort and meaning in their illness, and a more profound sense of peacefulness. Unfortunately, only a small proportion of the participants reach this level of development. This is partly explained by the hard work involved which relatively few choose to do, and partly by limited resources which restrict participation in advanced level programs. We believe there is a need for institutionalized training and support for psychospiritual therapy in cancer care settings. Given such support, the great benefits of this work would be made available to a much larger proportion of patients than is currently the case.

References

Aldridge, D. (1993). Is there evidence for spiritual healing? *Advances: Journal of Mind-Body Health*, **9**, 4–21.

Cortwright, B. (1997). *Psychotherapy and spirit: Theory and practice in transpersonal psychotherapy.* State University of New York Press, New York.

Coward, D. (1990). The lived experience of self-transcendence in women with advanced breast cancer. *Nursing Science Quarterly*, **3**, 162–9.

Coward, D. (1991). Self-transcendence and emotional well-being in women with advanced breast cancer. *Oncology Nursing Forum*, **18**, 857–63.

Cunningham, A. J. (1986). Information and health in the many levels of man: towards a more comprehensive theory of health and disease. *Advances: Journal of Mind-Body Health*, **3**, 32–45.

Cunningham, A. J. (1995). Pies, levels and languages: Why the contribution of mind to health and disease has been underestimated. *Advances: Journal of Mind-Body Health*, **11**, 4–30.

Cunningham, A. J., and Edmonds, C. V. I. (1996). Group psychological therapy for cancer patients: A point of view, and discussion of the hierarchy of options. *International Journal of Psychiatry in Medicine*, **26**, 51–82.

Cunningham, A. J., Edmonds, C. V. I., Hampson, A. W., Hanson, H., Hovanec, M., Jenkins, G., and Tocco, E. K. (1991). Helping cancer patients cope with and combat their disease: A group psychoeducational program. *Advances: Journal of Mind-Body Health*, **7**, 41–56.

Cunningham, A. J., Edmonds, C. V. I., Phillips, C., Soots, K. I., Hedley, D., and Lockwood, G. A. (2000). A prospective, longitudinal study of the relationship of psychological work and change to duration of survival in patients with metastatic cancer. *Psycho-oncology*, **9**, 323–339.

Dein, S. and Stygall, J. (1997). Does being religious help or hinder coping with chronic illness? A critical literature review. *Palliative Medicine*, **11**, 291–8.

Easwaran, E. (1989). *Original goodness*. Nilgiri Press, Tamales, CA.

Erickson, E. (1963). *Childhood and society*. Norton, New York.

Happold, F. C. (1970). *Mysticism: A study and an anthropology*. Penguin, New York.

Hoge, D. R. (1996). Religion in America: The demographics of belief and affiliation. In *Religion and the clinical practice of psychology* (ed. E. P. Shafranske). American Psychological Association, Washington, DC.

Jones, S. L. (1996). A constructive relationship for religion with the science and profession of psychology: Perhaps the boldest model yet. In *Religion and the clinical practice of psychology* (ed. E.P. Shafranske). American Psychological Association, Washington, DC.

Jung, C. (1959). *The basic writings of C. G. Jung*. (ed. Violet De laszlo). Random House, New York.

Kaczorowski, J. M. (1989). Spiritual well-being and anxiety in adults diagnosed with cancer. *The Hospice Journal*, **5**, 105–16.

Kohlberg, L. (1976). The collected papers on moral development and moral education. Center for moral education, Cambridge, Mass.

Kosmin, B. A. and Lachman, S. (1993). *One nation under God: Religion in contemporary American society*. Crown Trade Publications, New York.

Krippner, S. (1995). A cross-cultural comparison of four healing models. *Alternative Therapies*, **1**, 21–9.

Larson, D., Swyers, J., and McCullough, M. (1998). *Scientific research on spirituality and health*. National Institute of Healthcare Research, Rockville, MD.

Levin, J. S. andSchiller, P. L. (1987). Is there a religious factor in health?. *Journal of Religion and Health*, **26**, 9–36.

Loevinger, J. (1976). *Ego development*. Jossey Bass Publishers, San Francisco.

Lukoff, D., Provenzano, R., Lu, F., and Turner, R. (1999). Religious and spiritual case reports on Medline: a systematic analysis of records from 1980 to 1996. *Alternative Therapies*, **5**, 64–70.

Malsow, A. H. (1971). *The farther reaches of human nature*. New York: Viking.

Piaget, J. (1969). *The psychology of the child*. Harper Torchbooks, New York.

Reed, P. (1987). Spirituality and well-being in terminally ill hospitalized adults. *Research in Nursing and Health*, **10**, 335–44.

Smith, E. D., Stefanek, M. E., Joseph, M. V., Verdieck, M. J., Zabora, J. R., and Fetting, J. H. (1993). Spiritual awareness, personal perspective on death, and psychosocial distress among cancer patients: An initial investigation. *Journal of Psychosocial Oncology*, 11, 89–103.

Shafii, M. (1985). *Freedom from the self: Sufism, meditation and psychotherapy.* Human Sciences Press, New York.

Spira, J. L. (1997). Existential group psychotherapy for advanced breast cancer and other life-threatening illnesses. In *Group psychotherapy for medically ill patients* (ed. J. L. Spira). The Guilford Press, New York.

Walsh, R., and Vaughn, F. (1993). On transpersonal definitions. *Journal of Transpersonal Psychology*, 25, 199–207.

Wilber, K. (1995). *Sex, ecology and spirituality.* Shambala Publications, Boston.

Part III

Professional settings and personal experience

Chapter 16

Patient heal thyself

Heather Goodare

Formerly an academic editor, Heather Goodare was treated for breast cancer in 1986/7 and subsequently trained as a counsellor. She is particularly interested in consumer issues, complementary medicine, and psycho-oncology.

When I was diagnosed with breast cancer in 1986 I knew almost nothing about complementary medicine, except that my husband had been greatly helped by an osteopath to overcome a recalcitrant back problem. Coincidentally I had had lower back pain only two months before my cancer diagnosis, and in view of my husband's experience decided to go straight to an osteopath rather than my GP — and the problem was solved in three sessions. I was also given exercises to do, which have kept my back relatively trouble-free ever since.

I had suffered from clinical depression for some years, only just escaping hospitalization, and my GP, though very supportive, did not offer psychotherapy beyond the visits of the community psychiatric nurse, who was kind but ineffective. The main treatment was antidepressants, with the dose doubled when I was referred to a psychiatrist (which only made me constipated and even more depressed). My recovery from depression was achieved through the visit of my brother from Australia: he listened to me for a whole week, and supported me while I came off all my medication. But the long years of 'mental misery' (Walshe 1846) had taken their toll on my body (no doubt the prescribed drugs including HRT didn't help either), and three months later I noticed a lump in my breast. It was 5 cm in diameter, Grade III, and two lymph nodes were involved — as I later learned.

Contact with survivors

The first thing I needed to do on receiving the bad news was to talk to another woman who had had breast cancer and survived. This person was an old publishing colleague living in London. We talked on the phone. 'You must go to Bristol', she said. What was 'Bristol'? It turned out to be the Bristol Cancer Help Centre, and I rang them straight away to book a one-day visit between my surgery and the start of radiotherapy. I can honestly say that since that day I have never looked back, and so far I have remained disease-free.

In those days the one-day visit included an hour with a holistic doctor, another hour with a counsellor, and various group meetings for relaxation and visualization, discussion, and sharing of experiences. Healing, art therapy, and biofeedback were also available, and during that first year I made several return visits to sample everything on offer, though I did not actually stay there as a resident. Dietary advice was an important element, and the doctor there also wrote to my GP suggesting vitamin and mineral supplements, which he duly prescribed on the NHS. This must have been a lot cheaper than the previous antidepressants, tranquillizers, and sleeping pills, and I greatly regret that they are no longer available on NHS prescription.

Cancer and the mind

For me the most important element of the Bristol programme was the counselling. The sessions there helped me to turn around, to free myself from the crippling weight of my previous emotional history, especially the break-up of my first marriage. Since many of my deep-rooted problems were linked with my religious background, I felt I needed to sort them out with a member of the clergy. First I had weekly sessions with my vicar, who though not trained as a psychotherapist had a natural talent for listening, and when necessary, challenging. When he felt he could not help further, I found a Jungian analyst who was also a priest. Later I moved on to therapists using other models, mainly humanistic, for by now I had started to train as a counsellor myself. The book that helped me greatly during this time was *Cancer as a Turning Point* (LeShan 1989). I saw myself in the case histories quoted, and in the end was able to be my own therapist.

Something I found magical about the Bristol Centre was that the staff were not afraid to touch, even to hug. This obviously has its dangers, and is eschewed by traditional psychotherapy, but I am convinced that touch has an important part to play in work with cancer patients (de Hennezel 1997), even those who are are not nearing the end of life. People with cancer often feel isolated, stigmatized, untouchable, and I have even been asked if cancer is 'catching'. To have a totally loving welcome on arrival at Bristol was something quite unexpected and life-enhancing, which contrasted with the cold, impersonal reception later in the hospital oncology centre, with its railway-carriage rows of chairs in the waiting room.

Mind and body

Exercise became important too. During my depression I had been inactive: now I made a deliberate effort to get fit. My right breast and armpit were damaged by surgery, and later by radiotherapy, but I was determined to minimize this by appropriate exercise. I managed to avoid lymphoedema by religiously doing rehabilitation exercises every morning (these are still necessary 14 years later), and after a year, took up yoga. This I found to be a wonderful combination of the physical and the spiritual, and since it is not competitive, it is entirely suitable for people with disabilities. I played my violin in the local orchestra throughout my radiotherapy, and I am sure that this helped too, both emotionally and physically (my right arm being the one affected, which I had to keep up for bowing, thus helping to drain the lymph).

Meditation was also taught at Bristol, and this I found the hardest of all. I used to practise visualization under the radiotherapy machine: each bout of one and a half minutes was about as long as I could keep it up for initially. Then halfway through the radiotherapy I had a firm conviction that every cancer cell in my body had gone (washed out by the cool waterfall that was my favourite image). I nearly refused further treatment, but since I still possessed that submissive, compliant personality theoretically characteristic of cancer patients, and didn't want to offend my oncologist, I persevered, and used the time for meditation, following the technique taught by John Main OSB (Main 1985). Strangely, some of my religious acquaintances thought this meditation was very weird, almost smacking of dabbling in the occult. The fact that meditation is found at the core of all the great religions didn't seem to have dawned on them. I returned to some of the mystical writers I had studied previously as literature — the anonymous medieval *Cloud of Unknowing*, Mother Julian of Norwich, and the seventeenth-century metaphysical poets.

Nutrition

During my radiotherapy I followed the diet recommended by the Bristol Centre, which was almost entirely vegan. This I found refreshing and excellent, and since it excluded all fried and fatty foods, there was nothing in it to incline one to nausea during the treatment. I was grateful however to be allowed a glass of wine each evening. My young son, aged 15 at the time, went his own carnivorous way and became an excellent chef, while my husband made the best of both worlds. I was lucky not to have to cook meals for a large family. I stuck to the vegan diet for the prescribed three months of 'detoxification', and then slowly introduced some dairy foods and occasional fish and free-range chicken. Fourteen years later I am still following this regime, which is now a great deal easier to manage since even the supermarkets have introduced organic fruit and vegetables: we also grow our own in our back garden. Moreover, vegetarian menus are now widely available when eating out.

Healing

In the early days after my first visits to Bristol I had regular healing from a lovely, serene ex-nurse who attended my local church, where services of healing were also held. I am sure it helped. When I first felt a hard pea-sized lump in my right breast that turned out to be radiotherapy-induced fibrosis, healing seemed to be able to reverse the process. But it started up again, and when the lump slowly grew into a huge banana-shaped crescent on the inside of my breast, with new lumps elsewhere including the back of my shoulder, where the rays had made their exit, I finally had to come to terms with the fact that this fibrosis was irreversible. I tried acupuncture, which certainly seemed to soften it for a while, but when the treatment (which was pretty expensive) had to stop, the fibrosis hardened once more. I now know that if I had had a radiotherapy regime of daily treatment with smaller fractions (instead of larger fractions five times a fortnight) I might have escaped these problems. In those days we were warned not to use any creams or lotions whatever, only baby powder: now patients are 'allowed' to use certain vegetable-based creams to prevent burning, and I still use aloe vera lotion to nourish the skin, which though not burnt became very thin, dry, and papery.

A European perspective

In 1989 my husband and I went on a cycling holiday in Brittany, and in a bookshop in Rennes I discovered a book by Patrice Guex, a Swiss psychiatrist, called *Psychologie et cancer* (Guex 1989). I started reading it, then bought it, and decided to try and translate it. Negotiations were set in train, and Routledge agreed to commission a translation. The book contained an interesting chapter on complementary medicine (*médecines parallèles*) which was however somewhat slight, and Routledge's adviser, Professor Karol Sikora, suggested it should be revised and expanded. I thought a good person to do this would be Dr Michael Wetzler at the Bristol Centre, and he agreed: but in September 1990 the troubles resulting from the publication of the flawed and erroneous study of women with breast cancer attending the Centre (in which I myself was a 'subject') caused such an upheaval that many of the staff left, including Michael, who emigrated to South Africa. So I decided to tackle the job myself, since it did not require medical training. In researching the subject, besides finding the best published papers that I could to provide reference material, I personally experienced each therapy myself, from Alexander technique to T'ai Chi. Re-reading this chapter (Guex 1994) I am delighted to find the following sentence under the heading 'Towards integration':

> It is important to respect the patient's autonomy and to encourage his desire to explore therapies that may help him to feel better (Cosh and Sikora 1989), even if they have no impact on his prognosis. If we condemn complementary therapies, the patient will simply have recourse to them without telling us (Eisenberg *et al.* 1993).

Seven years later this remains as true as ever. The BMA book *Complementary Medicine: new approaches to good practice* (BMA 1993) was published just as my translation of Guex was going to press: unfortunately the reference to it which I added at proof stage was missed in error from the final pages. This publication represented a *volte-face* from the earlier BMA position on 'alternative therapy', which was very dismissive (BMA 1986). Fleur Fisher's compilation, under the auspices of the impressive Board of Education of the BMA, was, by contrast, a beacon of clarity and common sense.

How the doctor can help

So what do I require of my cancer doctor in relation to complementary therapy? First of all, 'the recognition that I have a mind' (Dennison 1990). I too can read books and medical journals, explore different therapies, and make my own judgements. Yes, it is true that there are some queer people about in the complementary medicine field, as there are also in orthodox medicine. I had a very odd experience with one therapist who claimed to be an acupuncturist: let the buyer beware. An important difference between complementary and orthodox medicine, however, is that it is much easier to change your complementary practitioner than it is to change doctors, especially oncologists, since there are so few of them anyway in the UK.

A person with cancer (as with many other diseases) is suddenly thrust into a strange country, not knowing the language, with no map, guidebook, or dictionary. The gatekeeper to this foreign country is the doctor. He plans the route. He chooses the guides — referring people on to the surgeon and the oncologist, for example. But as in a totalitarian state, these guides don't often deviate from the prescribed text, nor do they encourage the tourist to go off the beaten track: if they did, their jobs would be at risk. Much less (with a few honourable exceptions) do they encourage fraternisation with the natives — other patients who have survived the disease and the treatments and might have a few useful tips to offer.

But this is exactly what the tourist wants to do. He wants to learn the language, even if only on a phrase-book level. He wants to talk to the inhabitants of this country directly, without an interpreter. He wants to meet people who have trodden this way before him. He wants to hear at first hand what are the best paths up the mountain, where are the picturesque byways and backstreets, where are the good views, the interesting bistros. Yes, it may be more difficult than following the guided tour, more risky even, but it may be more interesting.

The doctor as facilitator

The patient requires the doctor to provide a glossary, map, phrasebook, and take care to maintain the signposts in good repair. The traveller will be confused if some vandal comes and switches round the arms of the signposts so that they point in the wrong direction. Equally, if roadblocks are set up he will become very frustrated. A friendly guide (say, a nurse specialist) is welcome, as long as she really knows the language and is prepared to explore new paths.

As Dr Rosy Daniel said at a seminar on Integrated Cancer Care hosted by HRH the Prince of Wales at Highgrove House on 19 March 1999, the patient is the one who integrates the various aspects of the route. The patient, not the healthcare provider, has to make the journey. Everybody will tread a slightly different path. For one, music therapy will have healing properties; for the next, yoga, for the next, massage, or Chinese herbs. Some will explore many therapies, some only one. The choice is individual. So healthcare providers need to make sure that what is on offer is clearly signposted, and then leave the patient to devise his own programme and to integrate its different parts. The doctor does not need to understand or even approve of all that the patient does: but should not block the way, by dismissive remarks or refusal to refer. At the same time, doctors should try to be knowledgeable about what is on offer, and particularly to make friendly contact with local cancer support groups and complementary therapists (Calman and Hine 1995).

The cancer journey is an adventure. It is possible, even desirable for some, to join the guided tour. But for those who wish to find their own path, explore the mountains, shoot the rapids, doctors have a vital role in helping to make the process easier. Some might even wish to explore these paths themselves. At least they start off with the advantage that they know the country and the language.

When doctors get cancer

When doctors develop the disease they will feel and behave in exactly the same way as their patients: they will want to try anything and everything to improve their prognosis. It is even possible that, knowing more about the track record of orthodox treatments, they will be even less inclined than lay people to put their entire trust in them. In a recent Observer Review was a report by Jerome Burne of a doctor who explored alternatives (Burne 1999):

> One morning last month, Dr William Fair downed the Chinese herbal remedy he believes has helped keep his cancer at bay for 18 months, and went to give a lecture to his colleagues on the value of meditation, prayer and vitamins in fighting cancer. What makes this remarkable is that Fair is a leading cancer surgeon at one of America's most hi-tech specialist cancer hospitals, Memorial Sloan-Kettering in New York, where the merest mention of herbs or meditation is heresy.

In my case I was extremely lucky that my general practitioner supported me in my visit to the Bristol Cancer Help Centre. He took the trouble to learn about what I was trying to do for myself, and encouraged me all along the way. I began to feel better, and ready to start work again as a freelance publisher's editor. In fact I felt so well that I took on too much work and became stressed, and on the verge of falling back into depression. I consulted my doctor. 'Are you doing your relaxation and meditation?' he asked. I had to admit that it had slipped a bit. 'Well, there's no point in going to Bristol and not following the programme,' he said. He prescribed a week off work, an outing to Portsmouth to see the Tall Ships re-enactment of the First Fleet sailing to Australia (an event connected with my brother's involvement with sail training, which I had thought I was too busy to fit in), and rededication to the way of life I had learned at Bristol.

The fact that my GP was supportive meant that I could then embark on my journey knowing that if I needed to discuss anything to do with complementary therapy I could go back to him without fear of being ridiculed or dismissed, whatever the views of my consultants. By the time he retired a few years later I was strong enough to stand on my own feet (though his successor was also supportive). Unfortunately this is not always the case in primary care, and newly diagnosed cancer patients are often very vulnerable and lack the energy and persistence to pursue even slightly unorthodox ways of helping themselves.

As the years progressed I became stronger both mentally and physically, and contributed in various ways to the self-help network, enrolling as a volunteer visitor for Breast Cancer Care, becoming the Secretary of my local cancer support group, and serving on the Council of CancerLink. I had just started my translation of *Psychologie et cancer* (Guex 1989) and embarked on a postgraduate counselling diploma (having relinquished my previous work as an editor) when a bombshell hit the world of complementary medicine: the interim report in the *Lancet* of the study of women with breast cancer attending the Bristol Centre (Bagenal *et al.* 1990), in which I had been involved as a patient. The story has been told elsewhere (Goodare 1996): suffice it to say here that it set back the cause of integrated medicine a good few years. In spite of my greatly increased workload I had no choice, it seemed, but to become involved in the patients' struggle to set the record straight. However, once again in a strange way we were able to use the lessons we had learned at Bristol to tackle this new threat.

Fighting to save the Bristol Cancer Help Centre

The Bristol Centre had taught us that every crisis brings its opportunity: that the crisis of cancer could lead to renewal, to changing things in our lives that were unsatisfactory, to find ways of living more creatively. The crisis of the *Lancet* report forced some of us to question the medical and research establishment in a way never before done by research 'subjects'. This led to new opportunities. The small support group formed among the women in the study to challenge its results found mutual strength to do things never before dreamt of. We wrote our own letter to the *Lancet*, held a press conference, sent a formal complaint to the Charity Commission about the way in which the two cancer charities who had sponsored the study had publicized it without ensuring that it was soundly based, and made a television film for Channel 4. Finally we put together our own stories in the book *Fighting Spirit* (Goodare 1996).

When the Charity Commission upheld our complaint in January 1994 we wrote again to the *Lancet*, who did not publish our letter, and also to the *British Medical Journal*, who did (Goodare 1994). In fact the editor actually asked me to expand the letter. He later invited me to join with him in writing an editorial on the patients' rights in research (Goodare and Smith 1995). The wheel had come full circle, and the poacher had turned gamekeeper.

Relapse and renewal

All this work took its toll, and by September 1995 I was feeling exhausted, and ready for a refresher at the Bristol Cancer Help Centre. I booked for a conference there in October on

'The Question of Hope', and also for a two-day seminar for counsellors and psychotherapists led by Lawrence LeShan. Shortly before I was due to leave I went for one of my regular check-ups with my oncologist. She found a lump in my left breast and ordered a mammogram. The radiologist was not satisfied with the first film and asked me to attend for a repeat session. This could not be fitted in before my visit to Bristol, so I made a booking for after my return.

At Bristol I was greatly inspired by the conference, especially by the contribution of Candace Pert, who talked about her research on the interaction of mind and body at the cellular level. Here was a scientific explanation of those things that some of us as cancer patients knew well from our own experience, but which had been so often dismissed by doctors as not scientifically proven and therefore non-existent. We 'knew' that our emotional histories had contributed to our illness: here was scientific evidence that this might in fact have been the case. Moreover, if emotional factors had played a part in our disease we could actually use our minds to help heal our bodies, as LeShan and others had shown. In 1997 Pert published *Molecules of Emotion*, an account of her research for the general reader (Pert 1997, 1999).

This conference was followed by LeShan's seminar, which was largely focused on the emotional self-care of the therapist rather than the presentation of case studies, and was exactly what I needed. I stayed with an old friend, one of the healers working at the Cancer Help Centre, and I mentioned to her my new lump. Confidently and calmly she gave me healing. While I was staying with her came another wonderful event: my husband telephoned to update me with the home news and correspondence, which included an invitation from the editor of the *British Medical Journal* to join his new editorial board as the only 'patient representative'. That Sunday I dropped in to a Clifton church for morning service and joined in the singing of 'Amazing Grace' with tears in my eyes. By the time I went on to Harrogate, where I had been invited to give a talk to the National Association of Theatre Nurses on 'A holistic approach to breast cancer', I was walking on air.

When I went back home and attended the hospital for my repeat mammogram, the radiologist showed me the first film, and there, obvious in the middle of the picture behind the nipple, was a walnut-sized white mass. That, she said, was the thing she wanted to have another look at. She persuaded me that she needed two more pictures — and then yet another. But the lesion had disappeared. And when I felt my breast, indeed it had gone.

I shall never know for sure whether or not that mass was cancerous, since no needle biopsy had been performed. But whatever it was, my visit to Bristol, the healing, the conference, the seminar, the inspiration of meeting old friends, and the buzz from the *BMJ* invitation, had somehow wrought a change in my body. The problem had been resolved. From that day I decided that I would discharge myself from further visits to the oncologist. I now have an annual mammogram, which has so far been clear.

So what have been the essential elements in my cancer journey? To what extent have complementary therapies helped?

The contribution of complementary medicine

At the time of diagnosis my prognosis, though not dire, was not particularly good. I did not know this at the time (nobody told me and I didn't think to ask). I did however see the form filled in by my oncologist before I went to the Bristol Cancer Help Centre stating that I was

'Stage II'. The histology report was not included, and it was only much later, when I asked for an oestrogen-receptor (ER) test to be done on the stored tissue did I discover that it was ER-poor, and that the tumour had been 'poorly differentiated'. All I knew was that I had had a big lump the size of a Victoria plum and that I'd better make sure I did everything possible to help myself.

Yes, I had a fistful of risk factors for breast cancer that I could now do nothing about: a family history (both grandmothers and an aunt); early menarche, late menopause, late childbearing, two years on hormone replacement therapy, and long-term use of hair dye. But those things I could modify, I did: diet, exercise, a graceful acceptance of grey hair, a more creative way of dealing with stress, and now that both my own and my husband's family were more or less grown up, in LeShan's admirable phrase, I could 'sing my own song' (LeShan 1989). What did I really want to do with the rest of my life? When I was myself diagnosed there was no psychological support available for cancer patients through the NHS in my local area. The self-help movement and the Bristol Centre filled the gap for me, and I soon realized that if I was going to be any use at supporting others, which I now wanted to do, I needed training.

It is important to stress that people with cancer rarely need psychiatric help: they are going through a life crisis and they need crisis counselling, though sometimes, as Dafter puts it so elegantly (Dafter 1996), this gives them the opportunity to deal with long-buried issues.

> 'Because serious illness often activates unfinished life issues, the 'toxic' emotions that naturally arise during these unsolicited life reviews can actually provide energy and motivation for important inner and outer changes.'

By the time I had completed two years of counselling skills training and a further two years of a postgraduate diploma in counselling, I felt ready to work with cancer patients in the knowledge that my own health would not be adversely affected. There was a further element, touched on by LeShan. Though the self-abnegation characteristic of the 'cancer-prone personality' was not helpful, and the phrase of Christ's second commandment so often forgotten by Christians was its second part, 'Love your neighbour *as yourself*, a certain healthy altruism was actually life-enhancing. This seems to have been a good recipe for survival so far. I am convinced that had I not visited the Bristol Centre I would have been at serious risk of slipping back into depression, and possibly suicide. So I have good reason for thinking that the Bristol Centre saved my life.

Towards integration

Finally, some thoughts on how clinicians can help patients to integrate for themselves what is on offer.

1. Listen to the patient, and work in partnership with him or her. Whatever their theories about what caused their cancer (British Nuclear Fuels, the mother-in-law, or the contraceptive pill), please listen, and don't dismiss these ideas as unscientific. The patient may be right, and in any case these ideas are part of the patient's search for meaning, which in itself may be therapeutic.

2. If at all possible, provide complementary therapies — reflexology, aromatherapy, acupuncture, counselling, even healing — as part of your primary care package. When

patients are undergoing aggressive cancer treatments (particularly chemotherapy) they may well sink into depression: at this point they may simply need loving support rather than referral to a psychiatrist and yet more drugs. 'Palliative care' should start from the time of diagnosis, not be reserved for the last few days.

3. Any psychological support should be offered routinely, without any suggestion of stigma, in the same way as bereavement counselling.

4. The informal carer and other family members also need support.

5. Make sure that any complementary therapists employed by you or referred to by you are professionally qualified.

6. If the patient asks for assistance with some complementary treatment — for instance, Iscador injections — do your best to help if you can: above all, don't undermine patients' efforts to help themselves by dismissive remarks. The placebo effect is very powerful. So is the 'nocebo' effect.

7. The person with cancer is the one to make the choice as to which therapies, if any, are appropriate for him or her.

8. Make use of your local cancer support group. Many such groups have their own network of complementary therapists, and some offer free treatment. These groups are a valuable resource that you cannot afford to ignore. If you wish to check their credentials, ask if they follow CancerLink's 'Declaration of Good Practice'. These groups spring up to fill gaps in statutory services, so it might be helpful to find out from them what they perceive the local gaps to be.

9. Don't be afraid to touch, with the greatest tact, discretion, and respect.

10. When death approaches, don't regard it as a defeat. Sometimes great work is done in the last weeks and days, and the doctor who can accompany the patient and not push for useless and unpleasant treatments will be honoured and respected by the whole family. Don't just do something—BE there.

References

Bagenal, F. S., Easton, D. F., Harris, E., *et al.* (1990). Survival of patients with breast cancer attending Bristol Cancer Help Centre. *Lancet*, **336**, 606–10.

British Medical Association (1986). *Alternative therapy*. BMA, London.

British Medical Association (ed. F. Fisher) (1993). *Complementary medicine: new approaches to good practice*. Oxford University Press, Oxford.

Burne, J. (1999). He thought he knew all there was to know about cancer . . . *The Observer Review*, 21 March, 3.

Calman, K. and Hine, D. (1995) *A policy framework for commissioning cancer services*: a report by the Expert Advisory Group on Cancer to the Chief Medical Officers of England and Wales. Department of Health, London.

Dafter, R. E. (1996). Why 'negative' emotions can sometimes be positive. *Advances*, **12**, 6–19.

Dennison, A. (1990). What do I want from my cancer doctor? In *Cancer and the mind* (ed. M. Slevin and R. Short), pp. 53–6, British Journal of Hospital Medicine, London.

Goodare, H. (1994). Wrong results should be withdrawn. *British Medical Journal* **308**, 593.

Goodare, H. and Smith, R. (1995). The rights of patients in research. *British Medical Journal* **310**, 1277–8.

Goodare, H. (ed.) (1996). *Fighting spirit: the stories of women in the Bristol breast cancer survey.* Scarlet Press, London.

Guex, P. (1989). *Psychologie et cancer, manuel de psycho-oncologie.* Payot, Lausanne.

Guex, P., trans. H. Goodare (1994). *An introduction to psycho-oncology.* Routledge, London.

Hennezel, M. de, trans. C. Janeway (1997). *Intimate death.* Warner Books, London.

LeShan, L. (1989). *Cancer as a turning point.* Gateway Books, Bath.

Main, J. (OSB) (1985). *The present Christ: further steps in meditation.* Darton, Longman and Todd, London.

Pert, C. B. (1997). *Molecules of emotion: why you feel the way you feel.* Scribner, New York. British paperback edition (1999). Simon & Schuster, London.

Walshe, W.H. (1846). *The nature and treatment of cancer.* Taylor & Walton, London.

Chapter 17

Complementary care in oncology: a patient-led revolution?

Hilary Thomas

Hilary Thomas is Professor of Oncology at the University of Surrey and the Royal Surrey County Hospital. Her main clinical interest is in gynaecological cancers. Her main research interest is biological therapy for cancer, in particular cytokine therapy and monoclonal antibodies. She is also involved in work relating to the relevance of cytokines in ovarian cancer and strategies for overcoming resistance to cancer therapy.

Complementary medicine is just that — an attempt to complement and not thwart conventional care. Complementary medicine considers the whole person and not simply the disease and is based on the belief that your attitude and state of mind have a great influence on your physical health. If you are happy, relaxed and optimistic your physical health is likely to be better than if you are miserable and depressed. With cancer, emphasis is placed on the use of complementary medicine for self-healing and the wide range of therapies available means that most patients can find an acceptable option which at worst will cause no harm and at best may prove beneficial.

There can be few experiences more devastating than a diagnosis of cancer. No matter how the patient receives that news — as a thunderbolt from the blue or as a gradual process of realization — there are often weeks of uncertainty and it is likely to be a defining moment in their lives.

Yet as doctors we are trained to comprehend, interpret, and integrate facts and then deliver information. We are not well educated in supporting the whole patient or even seeing their point of view.

As the taboo associated with a diagnosis of cancer has gradually dissolved, patient expectation has increased. Patients want and expect more information as well as being involved in their management to a greater extent. This does not simply relate to decisions about their treatment but also in being able to take control of their lives. They want to help themselves and sometimes this need overrides the often patronizing and condescending way in which their treatment is co-ordinated.

An individual diagnosed with cancer may well be setting off on an evidence-based journey along a heavily protocolized route for the treatment of — say — lymph node positive breast cancer. The pre-menopausal woman with the diagnosis may have a whole series of choices ahead of her in terms of the nature of her treatment, her own attitude to risk, whether she wants every possible treatment available or whether she wants to be able to pick and choose. Her 'choices' about conventional treatment may be quite limited when faced with the statistics about the benefits of adding together three treatments where one was previously considered sufficient. For example — the use of chemical castration with antioestrogen therapy (e.g. Tamoxifen) and adjuvant chemotherapy. Similarly the choice about alopecia during chemotherapy may be a stark one given the evidence about the benefit of those agents which cause alopecia.

Availability of complementary care in the conventional oncology setting

There can be no doubt that there has been a patient-initiated growth in the availability of complementary medicine within the conventional setting of cancer therapy (Ernst and Cassileth 1998). The first complementary care centre in the UK for patients with cancer was the well-known Bristol Cancer Help Centre. Initially this concentrated largely on diet to the point that the Bristol Diet in itself became well known (see below).

More recently a number of complementary cancer care centres have been established and it is now frequently the case that therapies such as aromatherapy, massage, visualization, T'ai Chi and other techniques are available at the same time as conventional radiotherapy or chemotherapy. Along with this there has undoubtedly been an increased uptake and perhaps an increased demand. There is wider use of homoeopathic medicine and herbal medicine, and indeed some herbal remedies are actively encouraged by professional staff involved in the treatment of cancer patients. One example is the greater use of aloe vera tablets and gel for patients who might have a radiation reaction.

A close relative, when faced with inflammatory breast carcinoma, received chemotherapy and radiotherapy. She had widespread disease which progressed relentlessly with relatively short periods of remission; as a result she spent long periods as an in-patient. Yet through all of this she never gave up her hope and the most obvious manifestation of this was her correspondence with a faith healer. At the time I had not yet started on my own career path in oncology but I have not changed my underlying view — that the patients should be allowed access to whatever they require to make their journey more tolerable and, hopefully, more successful. I would not necessarily measure success in terms of outcome such as survival, but more in terms of the patient and family's ability to come to terms with the diagnosis of cancer and resolve conflicts and difficulties along the way.

It would be inappropriate to list individually all of those disciplines which fall within complementary care and which may be advantageous to the cancer patient. I have focused on a few notable areas, but clearly you may find treatments referred to elsewhere which are beneficial and have a role either treating the symptoms or the psychological effects of the diagnosis of cancer.

Herbal treatments

Plant materials have been used to treat cancer for many centuries. Indeed a relatively high proportion of chemotherapy agents are derived from plants even today. Many are synthetic derivatives from a compound which was originally derived from plant material. A well-known drug named taxol (paclitaxel) is derived from the Pacific yew tree and felling these trees has now had an impact on the environment and survival of the screech owl. The Madagascan periwinkle has been used to make the drugs vinblastine and vincristine, which have been in use for three or four decades.

Aromatherapy

Often the role of plants in complementary care is within aromatherapy oils used for massage. Although there has been some suggestion that massage could actually spread cancer there is little evidence to support this contention except perhaps in a limited group of patients where the massage is clearly taking place in an area of disease. Aromatherapy massage is not deep massage and is usually superficial, often being applied to the limbs and the back. This is not advocated over the tumour site. Aromatherapy can be useful in the treatment of nausea, constipation, depression, lymphoedema, radiation reaction, and even insomnia. All of these may be side-effects of conventional treatment for cancer or may be experiences during the terminal phase of illness (Wilkinson 1995).

Often complementary treatments have spin-offs which are unexpected. One good example of this is the patient who does not respond to conventional antiemetics. In one case, severe nausea during radiotherapy to the abdomen did not respond to the 5-HT3 antagonists, but responded very well to once weekly aromatherapy (although the radiotherapy was given on a daily basis). Consequently if aromatherapy is effective it is a very useful alternative and one which should be encouraged.

It is said that one third of patients with cancer experience nausea and vomiting. This is now less of a problem with the advent of antiemetic drugs such as the 5HT3 receptor antagonists, but nevertheless these are accompanied by constipation and hence many patients may find aromatherapy more acceptable for mild nausea. Oils which can help to reduce nausea include peppermint (*Mentha piperita*), ginger (*Zingiber officinale*), and cardamom (*Elettoria cardamomum*). When applying essential oils they should always be contained within a carrier oil. Oils should not be applied during radiation to the area being treated but can be used subsequently for dryness. Those oils which are good for skin conditions include lavender (*Lavandula angustifolia*), German chamomile (*Matricaria recutitia*), and Roman chamomile (*Chamaemelum nobile*). It is probably wise to avoid essential oils with oestrogen-like properties, particularly for those tumours which may be hormone sensitive. This would rule out fennel, aniseed, clary sage, and geranium (Buckle 1997). There is no scientific data to support this view but it seems wise in the absence of data either way.

Studies have been undertaken, such as one at the Marie Curie Centre in Liverpool, where patients received massage with and without Roman chamomile. The group receiving the aromatherapy were found to have statistically significant improvement of quality of life and reduced anxiety compared with the group receiving massage alone (Wilkinson 1995).

Aromatherapy is a means of enhancing quality of life and improving the situation overall for the cancer patient. It should always be considered, particularly where conventional therapy gives rise to problems (McNamara 1994).

One subtype of herbalism is the flower remedies of Dr Edward Bach. He worked in the early part of the twentieth century preparing 38 remedies from wild flowers. He was a pathologist and bacteriologist who had switched to homoeopathy at the turn of the century. He believed the negative emotions in cancer patients needed to be treated and by holding his hand over a plant he was able to experience the properties of that plant and use it to treat the individuals' emotions appropriately. This treatment is without side effects.

Limitations of massage

Massage will not cure cancer, indeed it is unlikely that it will change the outcome of the disease itself in any way. Many people find massage difficult for cultural or religious reasons; they may be inhibited by exposing their bodies to another person or about being touched. It should be undertaken in an airy, warm, private space without interruptions and many people find dim light beneficial. Massage sessions usually take around an hour and it can be difficult to find such time within the busy schedule of a hospital setting. The cost of the sessions and the oil may be prohibitive for some people but there are an increasing number of centres which offer a subsidized service within the National Health Service.

Visualization

Biofeedback is a technique which draws on the mind. Many believe that it utilizes the hidden power of the mind to heal. Visualization, through imagination, is part of this strategy. The patient is encouraged to view the growth as evil and the cancer cells as disorganized and open to attack. At the same time they can visualize the immune system, for example as a knight in shining armour who enables them to demolish the 'big C'. Patients are encouraged to repeat this process daily or even twice daily at the same time as they undertake breathing exercises and relaxation.

I will never forget the patient under my care with a relapsed ovarian cancer who was being treated in an experimental trial of a monoclonal antibody radiolabelled with a radioactive isotope. This patient found great strength in visualization, a technique which she had learnt from reading. When thinking about the monoclonal antibody therapy she visualized goldfish dressed up in bib and tucker circulating around her abdomen and hoovering up all the cancer cells. She called her cancer Fred and would refer to how well she was feeling as to whether Fred was doing well or not. Such a technique is now more widely taught and more likely to be widely adopted.

Stress and cancer

The association between stress and cancer is contentious (McGee 1999). There is some evidence that 'fighting spirit' predicts a better outcome than 'giving in' to the diagnosis. However this may not be stress related, indeed people who are used to stress may be more likely to respond positively when faced with a diagnosis of cancer and be able to cope with the treatment and the implications of the diagnosis (Protheroe *et al.* 1999).

The first summary of the psychological characteristics of patients with breast or uterine cancer were presented by Snow (1893). 250 of these women were described as having 'general liability to the buffets of ill fortune'. The association of stress and cancer remains a preoccupation and a study has recently been published which has been questioned because of recall bias (i.e. the women with cancer knew their diagnosis by the time they were interviewed). This is clearly a very difficult area for research as the hypothesis being tested, that stress causes cancer, is rather vague. Literature reviews have concluded that there is no good evidence for any relation between stressful life events and breast cancer (Petticrew *et al.* 1999).

Nutrition

The environment of a hospital is often high-tech and impersonal, and for many people it increases their anxiety. They may consequently find it difficult to communicate, and bottle up their emotions until they are back at home in a familiar and comfortable atmosphere. The Cancer Help Centre at Bristol pioneered a well-organized approach which many patients have found helpful and supportive. This was one of the first such centres in the world and offers day or week-long residential courses for patients and their carers. In early years the Bristol Diet was highly restricted and often interfered with patients' quality of life because of the need to adhere to a very limited number of foods, and in particular the lack of red meat and alcohol, both of which might prove to be a comfort for some patients newly diagnosed with cancer. It may be a part of their everyday lives, the absence of which will be noticed. Nowadays a broader range of options is available. Counselling takes place with doctors and nurses to identify a treatment programme suitable for the particular individual. A range of complementary therapies is available and special diets are now optional rather than obligatory as when the centre was first established. Another similar centre is the Gerson Centre in Mexico which also has an international reputation and clientele.

Increasingly, patients are attempting to help themselves by purchasing nutritional supplements. This is in many cases to decrease their risk of cancer, but sometimes to enhance their chance of responding to treatment or improve their long-term outcome after the diagnosis of cancer has already been made. Dietary measures such as decreasing consumption of calories, fat, alcohol, and smoked or pickled foods may reduce the incidence of specific adult cancers. Increased dietary fibre does appear to have a protective role although this is not clear-cut. A large percentage of adult and child cancer patients take unproven therapies during their illness and alternative nutritional therapies are the commonest of these, reflecting an increasing public interest and awareness of 'natural remedies' (Weitzman 1998).

Tumours in children have not been shown to be influenced by diet and the evidence about the role of diet in the development of cancer is often epidemiological and sometimes conflicting. Although breast cancer is a disease of the Western world, attempts in case control studies and other smaller studies to show that fat intake correlates with the development of breast cancer have been unsuccessful, and it is not clear whether this is an effect of total calorie intake or specifically related to lipids. Veganism and macrobiotic diets are highly restricted and can lead to complications such as reduced bone mass or anaemia, particularly in children. Children, pregnant and lactating women, and those with chronic illness should undertake major dietary changes only with professional supervision. The social disruption which such restrictive diets can bring about may make it difficult for a patient to share meals with friends and family, which would have further impact on the quality of life. The macrobiotic diet philosophy, the Gerson diet among others, as well as the use of high dose vitamin C and mineral therapy to combat cancer or reduce the risk of developing it are among a range of strategies. Although they may differ in the details, many involve fresh whole foods with a strong emphasis on a low-fat vegetarian diet. However there is no clear scientific evidence that dietary manipulation is a successful therapy for established cancer.

Complementary medicine — what is available?

Counselling
Acupuncture
Aromatherapy
Homoeopathy
Herbalism
Meditation
Visualisation
Healing
Relaxation
Massage
Osteopathy
Reflexology
Hypnosis
Dietary treatments

The extremists

Doctors in the National Health Service may be cynical and negative about the use of complementary medicine, but by the same token complementary practitioners may pour scorn on conventional treatment. Both extremes are equally unhelpful for patient and doctor. They may undermine the patient's confidence in their conventional treatment, or compromise their relationship with their doctor by offering unproven therapy which has not been shown to alter the outcome of a cancer as opposed to proven therapy which has been subject to greater scientific scrutiny. One example of a poor combination of complementary medicine and conventional treatment is the use of radiotherapy to the abdomen in a patient who is religiously adhering to a strict vegan diet which contains no meat, eggs, milk, or cheese. The intake of largely raw food and high roughage may stimulate the bowel and make the side-effects of the conventional treatment much worse. A middle road must be adopted, and the best way for most patients is probably to be completely open to their conventional and complementary specialists about the approach which they are adopting.

Counselling

Counselling may be helpful not only to discuss the situation which has arisen and its implications, but also to take a view on life which is more objective, to assess your reaction to the situation and the contribution which this reaction itself makes. It is not uncommon for families experiencing the intense emotions brought about by a diagnosis of cancer to vent them by expressing anger or resentment towards another individual. A professional counsellor has had formal training and will have experience of cancer sufferers and their families. A GP or partner in the same doctor's surgery may have experience and training in counselling and psychotherapy and may be able to provide a preferable alternative for many people as an approach to them may be more discreet. Half the battle is accepting that there is a problem and seeking help. Once you can face the problem directly you are in a position to overcome it.

The organization CancerBACUP was established by a doctor who herself had ovarian cancer. It was not until she was diagnosed that she realized that there was a dearth of support for patients and a lack of information. CancerBACUP provides free telephone advice to cancer patients and their families (tel 0808 8000 1234). It is staffed by specially trained nurses who can give specific information about different cancer types. Perhaps even more importantly it has a wealth of literature which has been well reviewed by both patients and professionals and which can often provide information which your doctor may not have time to provide or the infrastructure in your hospital may not offer. Information itself is often an important form of complementary therapy for cancer patients who find themselves in a whirl after their recent diagnosis.

Conclusion

If becoming completely absorbed by complementary therapy makes you feel that life is worth living then why not? The important message from me as an oncologist is not to choose complementary medicine as an alternative to conventional medicine but as an added benefit. Anybody advocating that conventional medicine is discontinued, without the blessing of your oncologist and team, should be avoided. All of us should have open minds to the possibility that all of these therapies, both conventional and complementary, have a role in the treatment of the cancer patient. Anybody with a mind which is closed to that possibility could not be of benefit to the cancer patient.

References

Buckle, J. (1997). *Clinical aromatherapy in nursing*. Arnold Publishers, London.

Ernst, E. and Cassileth, B. R. (1998). The prevalence of complementary/alternative medicine in cancer: a systematic review. *Cancer*, **83**, 777–82.

McGee, R. (1999). Does stress cause cancer? Editorial *British Medical Journal*, **319**, 1015–6,

McNamara, A. P. (1994). *Massage for people with cancer*. Wandsworth Cancer Support Centre, London.

Petticrew, M., Fraser, J. M., and Regan, M. F. (1999). Adverse life events and risk of breast cancer: a meta-analysis. *British Journal of Health Psychology*. **4**, 1–17.

Protheroe. D., Turvey, K., Horgan, K., Benson, E., Bowers, D., and House, A. (1999). Stressful life events and onset of breast cancer. Case control study. *British Medical Journal*, **319**,1027–30.

Snow, H. L. (1893). *Cancer and the cancer process*. Churchill, London.

Weitzman, S. (1998). Alternative nutritional cancer therapies. *International Journal of Cancer Supplement*. **11**, 69–72.

Wilkinson, S. (1995). Aromatherapy and massage in palliative care. *International Journal of Palliative Nursing*, **1**, 21–30.

Chapter 18

A new chance in life

Sally and Edward Baldwin

Sally Baldwin, after being diagnosed with breast cancer, combined orthodox and complementary treatments and went to the Gerson Clinic in Mexico. She is involved in setting up The Speedwell Trust, an integrated health advisory service in Oxford, to offer hope and help to the seriously ill. Sally's husband, Edward, is principal spokesman for complementary medicine in the House of Lords, and has served on the Research Council for Complementary Medicine and as Chair of the British Acupuncture Accreditation Board.

It was a sweltering day on 22 July 1993 when I was diagnosed with breast cancer — a 5 cm tumour which had spread to the lymph nodes under my right arm. Yet I was shivering as Edward and I returned to break the news to our three sons, then aged 19, 17, and 13. A later biopsy showed it was a Grade II, Stage 3 infiltrating ductal carcinoma (there are three grades and four stages).

Tears and eerie silences followed. Friends held my hand and cried, while I tried to assure them I was not about to die. I was bombarded with confusing advice and my emotions fluctuated wildly. I was fifty-one, far too young to die. I had a young family and a busy, interesting life. Surely not me, cancer was something that happened to other people.

I became a cancer victim, no longer a woman — no more innocent flirtation and charming compliments. A dear family friend sent a book written for his octogenarian friends, as he considered me an honorary octogenarian. I felt very vulnerable, especially when an elderly clergyman said I must realize I was very threatening. Many people over about sixty considered cancer taboo. Mostly, however, we basked in warmth and kindness.

My initial reaction was surprisingly one of relief as I had had a number of previous biopsies and I knew all was not well. I had had a lifetime of illness — low fevers, allergies, and ten miscarriages. I had been on lithium for four years for manic depression (though since doing the Gerson therapy I am now mercifully free from depression).

The malignant area was so large — a hard, hot, uncomfortable mass and not a lump — that I never suspected cancer. But there was a history of cancer in the family and my mother had died of it not long before.

I had been a manuscript expert at Sotheby's and had then been involved with the arts, especially a club for children. I had also become involved with complementary therapies, had an International Therapy Examination Council qualification in massage and was practising in Oxford. I was interested in iridology, counselling, nutrition, and natural healthcare and was well aware of how to look after myself. However, I did far too much, was permanently exhausted and survived on willpower. People turned to me and I spent most of my time trying to help them, often neglecting my family and my own needs.

So I was glad to be at home with the family. At last I could do what I wanted for a change. I needed only to see my favourite people and it was all right to rest and do nothing without feeling guilty. I had faith that all would be well.

Edward, who was Joint Chairman of the Parliamentary Group for Alternative and Complementary Medicine, had read much of the latest research and was well informed. He saw the situation as a challenge and I feel I owe my life to his constant support and encouragement. Immediately we decided on a treatment devised by the German doctor Max Gerson, who had worked with the renowned thoracic surgeon Dr Sauerbruch in Munich.

Gerson found a successful diet for his own migraines and discovered it cured his patients of a wide variety of diseases. Albert Schweitzer, whose wife was cured by him of TB, described him as 'one of the most eminent geniuses in medical history'. He had remarkable successes with so-called incurable cancers which he described in his *A Cancer Therapy — Results of Fifty Cases* (Gerson 1990) which has now become the handbook for those on the therapy. He later moved to the USA, but his unconventional methods fell foul of the authorities, and after his death his dynamic daughter Charlotte set up a clinic in Mexico, just over the border in Tijuana. Although we knew about the clinic, we felt we could carry out the programme successfully at home.

Gerson saw cancer as an accumulated disease of the whole organism, so that concentrating on the removal or destruction of the tumour, which he saw as only the symptom of an underlying condition, was insufficient. The body must be detoxified and the immune system built up.

The aim of his programme is to restore the metabolism. The treatment is demanding, expensive, and time-consuming but I was impressed by the radiant *joie de vivre* of the people I knew who had recovered on it, even from stage 3 melanoma. It takes a good two years — preferably with rest, support, a peaceful, unpolluted environment and no direct sunshine in the heat of the day — to restore the liver and get the body working normally again, but it can be done. Surgery to remove the toxic load is sometimes recommended.

The idea of the regime caused consternation because of its *outré* nature. Somebody asked whether I would do it 'right to the bitter end?' I was tempted to reply 'No, I'm saving two chocolate bars for the last day'.

My consultant wanted to start on orthodox treatment but agreed to complementary medicine in addition. However, Edward and I chose not to accept orthodox treatment at this point, particularly the aggressive chemotherapy on offer. It does not combine well with the natural approach of the Gerson regime which has no side-effects and which we thought offered my best chance of survival.

I had just started the therapy when I went in for the biopsy/lumpectomy and to have two lymph nodes removed from my axilla. The nurses were fascinated with what I was doing, which was new to them, and were very co-operative.

The programme consists of fresh organic carrot/apple and green vegetable juices to build up the immune system and three square meals; plus coffee enemas which stimulate bile, detoxify the liver, and act as painkillers and antidepressants.

My day used to begin at 6.30 a.m. and end at 10.30 p.m. or later, though I snatched as much rest as possible during the day. It started with fruit, and a coffee enema — not nearly as unpleasant as one would imagine — which provided a chance to read. There were five enemas a day. Apparently the caffeine reaches the liver via the portal system and increases the flow of bile, which allows toxins to be evacuated.

Initially the diet is vegan, consisting solely of organic vegetables and fruit, and no fat, oil, salt, refined sugar, caffeine, alcohol, soy products, sprouted, pickled or smoked foods. A pure unrefined form of flaxseed oil called Omegaflo is allowed, which provides polyunsaturates and linoleic acid. To restore the sodium–potassium balance, which is severely disturbed in cases of cancer, salt is totally excluded and large amounts of potassium administered, to release sodium from the cells and prevent oedema.

Breakfast consists of a fresh orange juice, porridge, stewed dried and/or fresh fruit and peppermint tea. For lunch and supper there is a potassium broth called *Hippocrates Soup* (*), baked potatoes, interesting salads, gently cooked vegetables and plenty of fruit. Protein (white fish and pulses) and very low fat organic yoghurt are only introduced when the body is sufficiently detoxified after several weeks, as protein is thought to encourage tumour growth. I noticed no ill effects of the vegan regime.

Starting at 9 a.m., a freshly made juice is drunk every hour on the hour — thirteen daily, including the earlier orange. Four are green — made from an equal quantity of mostly green vegetables, lettuces (not iceberg which has little chlorophyll), watercress, green pepper, Swiss chard, red cabbage, and apples. The remaining nine are made from carrots and apples. The combination makes the fresh enzymes even more effective. It would be impossible to eat that many carrots in a day.

Juicing takes a considerable time. Our juicer, a powerful Norwalk, was lent by the Debra Stappard Trust. We bought a large water distiller and put a filter in our bathroom as most tap water is far from pure.

Medication includes self-administered liver and B12 injections, iodine which is applied as thyroid tablets in organic composition and as lugol drops in inorganic compound, which are added to the juices. Niacin, acidoll, and pancreatin are added too, mainly with meals.

Most of the day is taken up with the regime as juices, soup and meals have to be made regularly and the coffee concentrate boiled up for the enemas. Help is necessary, especially as one is likely to feel very tired and to suffer from 'flare-ups' which are rather like a short bout of 'flu and are in fact a sign that the therapy is working. They can be unpleasant and alarming and sometimes people give up at this stage because they think it is not working, but after this 'healing crisis' the cancer or other illness will often have receded quite remarkably.

....

(*) 1 1/Ĭ2 lb (675g) or more tomatoes, 1 1b (450g) potatoes, 2 small leeks, 2 medium onions, 3–4 stalks of celery or a knob of celeriac, plenty of garlic and fresh herbs, especially parsley. The unpeeled vegetables are chopped up and put in a large saucepan, covered with water, simmered gently for about 1 1/2 hours and liquidized on a low setting. Serve with lemon juice, freshly pressed raw garlic and garnish with more herbs.

Uncomplainingly our boys learned how to make the juices and cook for themselves, and we had outside help. However, after two months the tumour had increased to 10 cm and eventually I agreed sadly to have a mastectomy. Even so, the cancer continued to spread as plaque and nodes on the chest wall and in the axilla and it was then we were told the outlook was 'gloomy'. At the worst I might only have three months.

When this time had elapsed I had taken to my bed. I felt I was dying and people had lowered their voices to an ominous whisper.

We decided to set off for Mexico, into the unknown, with less than two days' warning, having hastily packed a minimal amount for two weeks. Our departure was cheered by my 82-year-old father, sporting a barrister's wig and a false nose with battery-operated eyebrows.

There, after a harrowing journey, I discovered I had been making serious mistakes in the regime, especially by not drinking the juices fresh enough and so missing most of the vitamins and enzymes. Putting the necessary potassium in the juices meant that they had gone off more quickly — and we had not been putting the right green vegetables into the juices, which is very important. I had also forgotten to take some medications.

Six months had been lost and I had to start the two years all over again. I was among the 15% of patients most difficult to treat and even the Gerson Clinic could not promise to help me at this stage. How I wished I had gone out at once.

I was determined to live and from then onwards I have visualized myself fully well, especially first thing every morning. I began to recover, thanks to daily visits from my wise, experienced doctor who was a qualified surgeon and familiar with orthodox medicine as well. I had innumerable treatments, such as hyperthermia — carefully regulated baths reaching up to 110F which produced fevers of up to 103F (cancer cells do not like heat), insulin injections, laetrile, ozone therapy, clay packs on the chest wall and castor oil poultices.

Active exercise was discouraged if one was very ill — the body needed rest in order to deal with detoxifying, but I enjoyed mini-trampolining on the terrace to stimulate the lymph system. Mostly we relied on herbal teas when needed — peppermint to combat nausea, chamomile to soothe and help with sleep, valerian for depression, and pau d'arco for candida, viruses etc. And very effective they were.

We decided I should stay longer but Edward had to return to the family and parting was painful. I had virtually nothing with me, the minimum of clothes, and a few tapes and books but I was never bored. I loved the ever changing view of the Pacific, and the Mexican life and music in the street below.

I spent hours either sleeping or reading in bed with claypacks on my chest. I painted, and had superb concerts in my room listening to music in the dark looking out over the twinkling lights along the bay. Gradually I came to feel intense joy, alone in my whitewashed room with a view of mountains and sunsets over the Pacific, grateful to be given the chance to start my life again.

It was immensely inspiring, more like a holiday than being in hospital, and Charlotte Gerson, still handsome and vibrant in her seventies, gave us uplifting talks quoting innumerable success stories with the regime. I made friends with some interesting people from all over the world. Many were far from wealthy; for example a talented English conductor was being paid for by donations from his devoted orchestra.

Many patients seemed to be making astounding recoveries. One arrived in a wheelchair and after three weeks was able to walk — no, dance out to her car. Visibly my area of plaque became smaller and less 'angry' and the cancer regressed. I stayed for eight weeks and then Edward returned to collect me.

Unfortunately, the day before we were due to come home I discovered I had a nasty bladder infection. In order to prevent the cancer spreading it was necessary to have antibiotics. The journey — thirty-one hours without sleep — was too much for me and I came home worn out, with a pulse which reached 120. I have rarely felt so ill. I started to turn yellow as I was so liverish and I could not eat or sleep properly. I was no longer in my safe cocoon and to make things worse I felt spiritually bereft. All this confirmed the doubters' worst fears. However, my consultant noticed a change for the better and was impressed.

I was almost housebound for two years, living quietly from day to day. I found the routine reassuring. Except for some angry outbursts, I was profoundly happy being at home with the family and appreciating the smallest things — walking to the river in the early morning, listening to the radio, mostly music, and reading. Art books and painting were particularly uplifting and prayer and meditation were a great comfort, especially in the early hours. (Friends would keep me in mind every evening at 10.00 p.m. and the effect seemed tangible and heartening.)

At first it was hard to ask for help, but though a few close friends vanished, most people were wonderful, especially the family and our dedicated living-in helper, Hugh — who was with us for a year — the ever-reliable organic farm-shop and a rota of faithful juice-making friends, all of whom stood by me however scary things became.

Life during those two years was like a game of snakes and ladders. I fell downstairs onto my coccyx and an MRI scan showed I had fractured my sacrum. However, my coffee enemas plus arnica and the Bach flower rescue remedy prevented me needing painkillers and later the doctors were surprised that the pain had only lasted one week instead of an expected six.

The shock brought on new nodes daily. The outlook began to look dismal again and my doctors said they thought they could do nothing for me. I lost the will to live and wrote farewell letters, which was devastating for the family who had been so brave and cheerful.

A healing service at a cathedral nearby was a crucial turning point. The Provost, a remarkable, inspiring man, felt that I had just lost my sense of direction. He gave me the Myers-Briggs personality test to help me find out my strengths and I realized I needed to be much more creative. He gave me a sense of purpose, raised my spirits once more, and we went regularly to his simple healing services.

Despite this the malignant area progressed slowly — but the surgeon noticed a change. The area was no longer so diffuse and he now felt he could operate. (Later on he told me that something that he could not put his finger on had happened and it was at this time that he began to think that perhaps I could recover after all.)

He decided on a complex *latissimus dorsi* operation, which involved replacing $15 \times 9 \times 3$ cm of cancerous plaque from my chest with a large flap of skin from my back. He did a skilful job and it 'took'. Friends brought juices and food to the hospital and I even gave myself five enemas a day. This time I was in a larger NHS hospital with poor morale. The nurses refused to help me with the unpleasant job of clearing up the enemas, which I had to give myself in bed starting on the day after my major operation when I still had my long drainage tubes in. I even had to find and change my own bedding.

Although I had been warned I could be in excruciating pain, once more I relied on the enemas and had almost none. My consultant was impressed with the enemas as painkillers — as he was that the histology showed that the cancer was now only Grade I instead of the Grade III he had feared. My GP said that my rapid healing was 'the best example of complementary medicine he had seen'.

However, there was a small node which the surgeon was not able to remove as it was separate from the main area of plaque. Before the operation this had begun to ulcerate, which was worrying. The operation cut off the blood supply, and it improved but still remained. Soon a second small lump appeared and it was obvious the cancer was not yet contained. I had another operation to remove some lymph nodes from under my arm, as it had not been possible to do this during the recent operation.

About this time I started taking the promising natural remedy CoEnzymeQ10, encouraged by favourable trials with breast cancer in Denmark, and the drug tamoxifen. This had become appropriate because my oestrogen receptors had now become positive, which had also pleased the consultant.

In January 1995, a fortnight later, the two remaining lumps disappeared suddenly. Blood tests confirmed that everything was within the normal range. At first we hardly dared to believe the good news and to be on the safe side I had radiotherapy. For a while unpleasant side-effects were exhaustion, burning, and depression. We waited anxiously for results of a mammogram and X-rays in September 1995, but they were still clear, my consultant gave me ten out of ten, and we were all overjoyed.

Although sceptical, the excellent medical team here did all they could to enable me to do the therapy along with their orthodox treatment of surgery, radiotherapy, and tamoxifen. I visited my GP for regular examinations and extensive blood tests — for liver function and blood chemistry, plus thyroid and urine tests. I faxed the results to my doctor in Mexico and she decided how I should proceed with reducing the programme during our periodic telephone consultations. It was consoling to be able to talk with her whenever the outlook was bleak.

For twenty-two months I kept up the full regime of thirteen juices and five enemas — far longer than usual because of my earlier mistakes and the fact that I had seemed to be getting worse. (Some people manage to return to work, with help, while still on the therapy.) Gradually the regime was reduced and I returned to a normal life. After three years I noted that I had clocked up over 10 000 juices and 4000 enemas and now, nearly seven years since the diagnosis, it must be thousands more.

Coming back to the world was exhilarating but daunting (I felt like Rip Van Winkle) and I was frustrated by my fluctuating energy levels. I could not keep up with my friends and what seemed to me their hectic pace and had to live within my limits. I felt indecisive, unconfident, and frumpy, with nothing whatsoever to contribute. It was as though I was lacking my outer skin.

What I had not expected was what my doctor called the Lazarus Effect. Once, I was excited to be going to the opera, but four friends walked past and when I spoke they rushed away, clearly wondering if they had seen a ghost. Over and over it happened. I longed to be included in whatever was going on but I kept being left out because, as people later explained, they did not want to put me in the awkward position of refusing. They did not mean to be unkind, but could not see me as well. (It would have been so boosting to be invited.)

I told a medical friend about this and later met him on a coach. He said he had mentioned the Lazarus Effect at a conference for nurses and we laughed about how anyone could behave like that. I said I had been clear for several years and so was taken aback when he shouted out as I was getting off the coach 'Good to see you looking so well. Have you got any secondaries yet?' Since then I have been wary of the expression 'in remission'. It implies that it is only a matter of time, however well one is doing.

I had homoeopathy, in particular the mistletoe remedy Iscador and a remedy to counteract radiation. I tried a number of other treatments including applied kinesiology, vega-testing, osteopathy and cranial osteopathy, reflexology, acupuncture, electrocrystal therapy, radionics, dowsing, hydrogen peroxide, ascorbic acid (vitamin C), essiac, royal jelly, and herbs (Western and Chinese), in particular for parasites — also an ozone generator, plus a RadiTech bar and crystals for geopathic stress. We decided to explore every approach, however bizarre, and met a number of healers who seemed caring and sincere. One was convinced that a crusader was speaking through him and his voice would become a reedy falsetto as he administered the healing. Another 'materialized' sweet-smelling oil from his hands onto my forehead. Yet another was a psychic surgeon who performed an 'operation' on me.

I visited a Jungian psychotherapist and explained that as I might have only three months I did not want to explore what could have happened in the woodshed, but wanted to make the best possible use of the remaining time. He asked me how I got on with my father and when I explained that he had been a great support he said that showed deep denial and that there were years of work to be done. When I said I found spiritual things a great solace he told me to 'come down off the ceiling' — and charged me £300 in advance. I decided to write to him saying that I did not wish to be treated like this and would like my money back — an empowering experience.

Then I went to a delightful person who had worked with the dying for twenty years. She seemed ideal until she said she had grave doubts about the Gerson therapy as she felt it made people die sooner. I said when I got better I would … but before I could finish my sentence she replied, 'but you may *not* get better.' I realized she was planning to give me a beautiful death. It was doubly difficult having to deal with other people's hang-ups when I longed for help and was getting weaker all the time.

One person who was helpful was a friend who had been active in the Bristol Cancer Centre. She was always positive and encouraging and made a visualizing tape for me to make the radiotherapy less daunting. Another friend in Jersey, who treated me with her own remarkable flower remedies, always said that she felt I could recover. I hung onto this encouragement, when most people held out little hope.

I had problems with acceptance. Should I accept the situation or not? I was saddened to hear someone say that her sister, who had had six children, had been diagnosed with a tumour the size of a pea. She had accepted this (as a death sentence) from the beginning and had eventually died, without a single complaint. Did she really have to die, or was she conditioned to think that there was no alternative? I believe that many people die unnecessarily through lack of encouragement and support.

Another thing which saddens me is when people embark on the gruelling Gerson regime but decide, for example, that they do not fancy the enemas. The programme is so carefully worked out that if one alters it one may not succeed. I have often seen this happen. Or people tell me they would only take such drastic action if the situation became serious, by which time it is too late to start, especially after extensive chemotherapy and radiotherapy. It is possible to succeed on the therapy after these but there is so much more toxicity to deal with. People often say they wish they had had all the options explained instead of being told they should start chemotherapy, or else.…

I was fortunate to have such a supportive husband and we became close as a family. It must be daunting enough to be diagnosed with cancer without finding one's family in a panic, adamant that one must follow orthodox treatment, so that if one wants to try other things one is even up against those nearest and dearest. I often think of the many women whose husbands leave them if they get breast cancer, with children to bring up and very little money.

I found creative things inspiring and music was especially healing — violin lessons (very good physiotherapy) gave me something to work for and to look forward to. Whenever I was *in extremis* I found painting lifted my spirits. In the beginning I used to draw symbols for the cancer and the healthy cells overcoming it each day, and I would date them. They were a revealing way to tell which was winning, and I would alter the symbols accordingly to strengthen the opposition. I kept a taped daily diary which now provides an interesting record. I also experimented with delicious, colourful vegetable and fruit dishes and I started compiling a healthy cookery book. A good haircut helped, and occasional visits to the opera or theatre were a great treat.

Forgiveness was very important, especially towards myself, and avoiding feeling guilty at the slightest opportunity. Making time to do something I really wanted each day, living in the present and setting short and long-term goals were helpful. Keeping things simple was vital.

Friends came up with imaginative ideas to help — making donations towards our expenses in Mexico, coming regularly to make juices, bringing cups to drink them from, and paints, brushes, art books, flowers that could later go in the garden, frivolous, funny things, a pile of CDs, meals for the family, good books, books on cassette, poetry, cards and letters.

I had some poignant letters. People told me about their lives in a way they never had before, because they felt I would understand. One friend kept a holiday diary in Provence with photographs, so that he could be my 'eyes and ears'. Best of all these letters kept me in touch with normality and what was going on in the world outside. I was greatly supported by friends in the same situation (though it was tragic to see so many of them die). I yearned to talk about facing death but found most people unwilling. They were clearly afraid. At last I found a clergyman who used to come and discuss the deepest things, and laugh a great deal too. I was very grateful.

What were not helpful were anger and frustration. I hated to see the house and garden becoming run down. Some people were surprisingly insensitive in their use of language and I found myself feeling absurdly hurt, and bewildered. Often people stayed too long, especially in hospital after operations. I avoided negative people and surrounded myself where possible with cheerful optimists.

Many people succeed on the Gerson without going to Mexico. There is a trained Gerson doctor in London, and a lively support group which can offer advice on Disability Allowances etc. For me it has become a way of life and I try to keep it up even though it still takes up to 1 1/2 hours a day. I aim to start the day with a brisk walk and an enema and to make four fresh juices. 80% of the time I live mostly on organic vegetables and fruit but 20% of the time I eat more freely, still avoiding meat. When out I try to buy fresh carrot juices and mix them with apple juice. Plenty of sleep makes all the difference.

My kind of cancer can be aggressive and I want to do everything I can to prevent recurrence. I believe the therapy has kept me healthy, optimistic, and free from distant metastases. I feel better than ever and my doctor says I look ten years younger. I take responsibility for my own life and listen to my 'inner voice'. I speak out, laugh, and enjoy things much more.

It has been sobering, but enriching. Whenever I feel stressed and anxious, I try to recapture the joy I felt in that minimalist whitewashed room in Mexico, and everything falls into perspective. As a friend with cancer said 'Now you can begin living'.

Postscript

Since Sally wrote this, the cancer has returned, causing fluid in the pleura (lining of the lung) affecting her breathing. She is now trying the new Plaskett regime, similar to the Gerson with juices and enemas, but utilising current research allowing the therapy to be more focused. It is less arduous, as some juices are replaced by nutritional supplements, in her case specifically targeting hormone-related cancers. She is also pleased to have discovered the Buteyko breathing method. Her outlook is still very positive.

Edward Baldwin

Why the Gerson regime? I am sure there are people who believe we opted for this for purist natural medicine reasons. This is not, however, the way the mind works when confronted by possible imminent death. After nearly 30 years of the 'war on cancer' orthodox treatment has made remarkably few inroads into the mortality figures, whatever the fund-raising charities may like to claim. It was a matter of comparing the strongly based research evidence for the tried and tested, but largely failed, methods of mainstream medicine with the far more slender but in our view promising evidence from Gerson, which is probably the best known of the dietary alternatives. Unlike chemotherapy it aims to rebuild a healthy body rather than just attack the tumour, and thus has valuable spin-offs in general health. Early trials have not dented the optimism generated by over 60 years of case histories of recovered patients.

My role in Sally's battle against her illness — and few patients know what a battle it is until they have cut loose from the medical system in a life-threatening situation and fought their own way through the jungle — was firstly as research adviser. Her chances under orthodox treatment were bad, whereas under Gerson they appeared more than reasonable. When her surgeon, in advocating radiotherapy, cited a particular study, it was I who would get hold of it, read it up, and come back with any questions. In one instance we were astonished when we found that with her cancer type, mortality went up after radiotherapy. A year later a subsequent meta-analysis corrected this downwards, and we were able to change our minds and agree with Sally's surgeon that radiotherapy could be valuable.

I also helped to investigate a whole range of other complementary therapies, many of which we were already familiar with in outline, as a strategy to support mind, body, and spirit. Because there is no clear map of the territory this is not always easy. Also, because of medical and family pressures when the going gets tough, it is important that patients take on only what feels comfortable for them. Sally in fact pursued a number of avenues while doing the Gerson, and it is a powerful argument for the path on which she decided that we never ran out of options, however unlikely some of them may have seemed. This was a strong factor in maintaining hope, and this itself was therapeutic. The medical notion of 'false hope' can be deeply harmful to patients.

As well as being Sally's research and information officer, I was her buffer against the world. Nowhere was this more important than in her meetings with her surgeon, caring though he clearly was. Friends of ours who have gone to appointments without a husband or friend by their side have suffered considerably from the poor interpersonal skills of the modern specialist, and a cancer patient cannot afford this extra stress. I also tried to protect Sally against casual callers at a time when I felt she needed rest, and in this I was not always popular. A wife who thrives on talk and human contact can easily feel that her lifeline to the world is being cut off.

A key domestic role was that of overseer of all things administrative. A regime like the Gerson takes a lot of running — that will remain one of its drawbacks until it is harnessed within a mainstream healthcare setting — and there were medications and equipment to order, therapists to keep in touch with, household tasks to see to, and above all juicing and cooking to be organized on a relentlessly constant basis.

As Sally emerged from her cancer I spent more time, as Chair of the Parliamentary Group for Alternative and Complementary Medicine, in publicizing the Gerson and other regimes. My attempts to interest leading oncologists in this approach have been a 'qualified failure' (see papers by Bailar and Smith 1986 and Bailar and Gornik 1997 dealing with the 'war against cancer'). There is a belief system in mainstream medicine in this country that nutrition as a potentially curative modality is only one step above astrology. I say this advisedly, because most of the arguments I have met with rest in the final analysis on the belief that it would be absurd to do serious research in this area. There is already enough evidence for some of these approaches to warrant proper pilot studies, and in fact a prospecive study of a similar nutritional regime has recently received official funding in the United States.

It has been, as they say, a learning experience. Helpers of cancer patients, as well as the patients themselves, tend to appear as heroes. It is not (always) so, as John Diamond points out in his book (Diamond 1998). We go on, mostly, because we must go on. There were times of terror, and times of despair. It is not true, as some people claim, that it is worse for the helper than the patient. But comfortable it is certainly not, and the important thing (at which I was not always successful) is to be there at all times. When you have to research and take the treatment decisions yourselves, often in opposition to medical advice, this is doubly crucial.

Note:

There are about 200 patients in the UK doing the Gerson therapy for cancer, ME, arthritis, and other degenerative diseases. The Debra Stappard Cancer Trust lends out juicing machines and other equipment. The Gerson Support Group (PO Box 74, Leatherhead, Surrey KT22 7YD, tel. 01372–817652) supplies information and literature. The Gerson Institute has been offering intensive short training courses in California for doctors and nurses to make the protocol more widely available; it can also be approached by patients at Box 430, Bonita, CA 91908, USA, tel. 00 1 619 585 7600 (www.gerson.org). Charlotte Gerson has recently amalgamated her clinic with another well-established clinic in Tijuana, Mexico and she is training another team of young doctors there. Some of the methods have changed since our visit in 1994. An excellent first-hand account of the therapy can be found in the book *A Time To Heal* by Beata Bishop.

Details of the Plaskett regime can be obtained from the Nutritional Cancer Therapy Trust, tel 01483-202264. www.webangels.co.uk/cancertherapy/

References and further reading

Bailar, J. C. and Smith, E. M. (1986). Progress against cancer? *New England Journal of Medicine*, 314, 1226–32.

Bailar, J. C. and Gornik, H. L. (1997). Cancer undefeated. *New England Journal of Medicine*, 336, 1569–74.

Bishop, B. (1996). *A time to heal.* Penguin Arkana, London.

Diamond, J. (1998). *Because cowards get cancer too.* Vermilion, London.

Gerson, M. (1990, 5th edition). *A cancer therapy: Results of 50 cases.* Gerson Institute, PULSE, PO Box 430, Bonita, California 91908.

Hale, T. (1999). *Breathing free.* Hodder and Stoughton, London.

Hildenbrand, G., *et al.* (1995). Five-year survival rates of melanoma patients treated by diet therapy after the manner of Gerson: a retrospective review. *Alternative Therapies in Health and Medicine*, 1, 29–37.

Chapter 19

Complementary care and the sceptical surgeon

Michael Baum

Michael Baum is a Professor of Surgery at the Royal Free and University College Medical Schools, and Consultant Surgeon to the University College London Hospitals Trust. Prior to this he served as Professor of Surgery at King's College, London and the Royal Marsden Hospital, London. His research interests include clinical trials in the development of treatment for early breast cancer. He chairs the largest collaborative group for clinical trials in this country. He was recently appointed chairman of a national steering committee to introduce arts and humanities into the undergraduate curriculum, and has written extensively on the social anthropology of alternative medicine and the philosophy and ethics of clinical research.

Unlike science which is concerned with the general, the repeatable elements in nature; medicine, albeit using science is concerned with the uniqueness of the individual patients. In its concern for the particular and the unique, medicine resembles the arts (Calman and Downie 1996).

Introduction

The art and science of the practice of surgery in patients with cancer have the twin objectives of improving length of life and quality of life. All other outcome measures must be considered surrogates and discounted from this discussion. The objective of this chapter is to illustrate how the surgeon himself can be a holistic practitioner contributing much to the quality of life, even amongst those patients who are predetermined to die of the disease, but also to recognize the limits of his skills, at which point the role of complementary therapist has to be defined. At the outset, for the sake of clarity of thought, I believe it is essential that we can reach some agreement about the very meaning of the words; art, science, complementary, and holistic. Having attempted to define these often ephemeral or slippery words,

I will then describe in some detail the practice of a surgical oncologist, as a clinical scientist and a humanist who should recognize the limitation of his skills and the point at which complementary care should be integrated.

What is art? What is science?

In John Keats' famous letter to Benjamin Bailey dated 22nd November 1817, he writes 'I am certain of nothing but of the holiness of the heart's affections and the truth of imagination — what the imagination sees as beauty must be truth … the imagination may be compared to Adam's dream — he awoke and found it truth'. This is often misquoted as the statement 'beauty is truth, truth is beauty'. In a way this could be one definition of the meaning of art in its broadest sense — the pursuit of truth about the human condition through the acts of imagination via poetry, literature, music, or the visual arts. Science, the second pillar, upon which Western civilizations stand, has been described by Allen Cotrell, FRS, as the disciplined search for truth (Cotrell 1997), in other words a search for objective realities based on sound philosophical principles which is complementary to the pursuit of 'artistic truth'. It would certainly be out of place in this chapter to digress at length about the philosophy of science, but in its simplest terms the principles of modern science concern the elaboration of an hypothesis to explain observed facts, and then the testing of that hypothesis by experimentation in an attempt to falsify the hypothesis (Popper 1992) The hypothesis is allowed to stand as a conditional 'truth' for as long as it can withstand robust attempts at falsification. Central to the practice of science is measurement and if the only outcomes of importance in the practice of oncology are length of life and quality of life, then it is essential that these can be measured. The date of a patient's death is seldom a controversial issue, but the measurement of quality of life is based on an instrumentation which is relatively new (Fallowfield 1990). It is my intention to demonstrate how the practice of clinical science in the hands of a surgical oncologist can improve both length and quality of life.

What is complementary care?

There are a wide range of disciplines already described in this book which are intended to complement the skills of the clinician in the totality of the care of a patient with cancer. Some are bizarre, some have little if any scientific credibility, whilst many have an important role in making the patients feel better in the corporeal domain, or live better in the spiritual domain at the time the clinician is attempting to cure or palliate the disease. I have no problem whatsoever with these concepts but some practitioners of complementary medicine are intellectually dishonest and claim that they can 'heal' the patients without providing the objective evidence required by a scientist. If challenged they will often claim to be healing the spirit, at which point the arguments get metaphysical and spiral like smoke from an extinguished cigarette!

Holism as a word and a concept

The English language has a rich and beautiful vocabulary. My *Oxford English Dictionary* weighs several kilograms and occupies a whole shelf on my bookcase. All these wonderful words have precise meanings. It saddens me to witness how English words are being debased by a pop-culture that encourages transient values and transient meanings to our vocabulary.

Two small examples which I find intensely irritating are the modern usage of the words 'clinical' and 'organic'. Clinical is now used to imply a dispassionate and heartless approach to a subject where the opposite is true in that a good clinician in medical tradition is taken to mean the wise and compassionate elder. Organic, a word with precise meaning in chemistry describing substances whose building blocks are hydrocarbons, is now a slippery word conveying a vague notion of that which is ecologically sound. The same worry concerns the use of the word 'holistic' when applied to the practice of medicine. The word 'holism' was coined in 1926 by Jan Smuts who used it to describe the tendency in nature to produce wholes from the ordered grouping of units. The philosopher and author Arthur Koestler developed the idea more fully in his seminal book '*Janus: A Summing-Up*' (Koestler 1978) in which he talks about self-regulating open hierarchic order (SOHO). 'Biological holones are self-regulating open systems which display both the autonomous properties of wholes and the dependent properties of parts. This dichotomy is present on every level of every type of hierarchical organization and is referred to as the Janus phenomenon' (Janus is the Roman God that looked in both directions at the same time). *Chamber's 20th Century Dictionary* describes holism in a precise and economical way as follows: 'Complete and self-contained systems from the atom and the cell by evolution to the most complex forms of life and mind'.

Thus the concept of holism is complex and exquisite, and as an open system lends itself to study and experimentation. In my opinion, the hijacking of the word 'holistic' by proponents of alternative medicine is another example of debasing the currency of our language in order to prop up primitive and closed belief systems. The holism described by alternative medicine is a purely metaphysical construct where the mind, body, and spirit are bound together by vital forces or energy fields. The self is perceived as the platform on the three-legged stool of the mind, body, and spirit and if the glue that sticks one of the three legs to the platform softens, then the structure collapses. This glue, this vital force, these paranormal energy fields, are not open to the experimental method of study and, therefore, have to be considered a surrogate for faith whose popularity increases in our society.

Holism in the organization of organic systems

To do justice to General Jan Smuts' definition of the word holism, we have to start with a reductionist approach to the molecular level, and then from these basic building blocks attempt to reconstruct the complex organism which is the human subject living in harmony within the complex structure of a modern democratic nation state. Since Watson and Crick described the structure and function of DNA in 1953, the development of biological holism has grown way beyond anything Jan Smuts might have envisaged. The basic building block of life has to be a sequence of DNA, that codes for a specific protein. These DNA sequences or genes are organized within chromosomes forming the human genome. The chromosomes are packed within the nucleus with an awe-inspiring degree of miniaturization. The nucleus is a holon looking inwards at the genome and outwards at the cytoplasm of the cell. The cell is a holon that looks inwards at the proteins which guarantee its structure and function contained within its plasma membrane, and at the energy transduction pathways contained within the mitochondria which produce the fuel for life. As a holon, the cell looks outwards at neighbouring cells of a self-similar type which may group together as glandular elements, but the cellular holon also enjoys cross-talk with cells of a different developmental origin communicating by touch through tight junctions, or by the exchange of chemical messages via short-lived paracrine polypeptides. These glandular elements and stromal elements group together as a functioning organ which is holistic in looking inwards at the exquisite functional integrity of itself, and outwards to act in concert with the other organs of the body. This concert is orchestrated at the next level in the holistic hierarchy through the neuroendocrine/immunological control mediated via the hypothalamic pituitary axis, the thyroid gland, the adrenal gland, the endocrine glands of sexual identity, and the lympho-reticular system that can distinguish self from non-self. Even this notion of selfness is primitive compared with the next level up the hierarchy where the person exists in a conscious state somewhere within the cerebral cortex, with the mind, the great unexplored frontier, which will be the scientific challenge of doctors in the new millennium.

The role of the surgeon in the palliation of cancer

With those semantic and philosophical discussions behind me I would like to elaborate on the pragmatism of the surgeon literally at the cutting edge of the team responsible for improving the length and quality of life of patients with cancer.

In spite of an enormous financial commitment into the research and treatment of cancer there is little evidence that the mortality from the common cancers in the developed world is decreasing. Admittedly this might be a paradox resulting from an ageing population, which in itself will increase the incidence of the disease, together with refinement in diagnosis which may artificially enhance the prevalence of the disease. Furthermore, more accurate classification of causes of death within our Cancer Registry might artificially inflate mortality from cancer, but whichever way you look at it, it is very difficult to determine that modern cancer treatment is contributing to a major *reduction* in mortality for cancer. Does this mean therefore that the activity of surgeons, radiotherapists, and other oncologists over the last century has been in vain? Nothing could be further from the truth because crude cancer statistics as generated by the National Cancer Registries take no account of the way cancer therapy improves the quality of life and the dignity of dying.

Nowhere is this seen more clearly than in the role of surgery for the palliation of cancer. The surgical oncologist must always play a leading role in the multidisciplinary approach to the management of the disease. Surgeons more than anyone have a clear idea of the natural history of cancer as they are most often involved in the initial evaluation of patients with the commonest malignancies. 30% of the work of any general surgeon involves cancer.

The surgeon has five essential roles in the palliation of cancer; local control of the disease, the control of discharge or haemorrhage, the control of pain, reconstruction, and rehabilitation. Even if not curative, surgery is essential to gain control of the local disease or for the relief of obstruction to hollow viscera such as the gut, the biliary tract, and the genito-urinary system. In addition, even in the presence of distant metastases, removing a primary tumour may control discharge, fistula, and haemorrhage. Once a primary tumour has already infiltrated nerve roots it is extremely difficult for surgery in itself to relieve pain but this complication of advanced cancer should always be anticipated and attempts to control the cancer before it infiltrates nerve roots, especially around the brachial and sacral plexus, may prevent the development of intractable pain in the future.

Just because the patient is facing a limited expectation of life, does not mean that he or she should carry the added burden of physical or functional morbidity. Reconstructive surgery, involving the head and neck region and the breast, may be of vital importance in allowing a patient to face an uncertain future with equanimity. Furthermore, preserving an intact gastrointestinal and urogenital tract may spare the dying patient the additional burden of a colostomy, ileostomy, or urostomy bag. The essential role of the surgeon in the palliation of cancer will be illustrated using the specific examples of the breast, as this is my particular speciality.

The quality of life of patients with breast cancer

Breast cancer is the commonest female malignancy in the Western world and the commonest cause of death in the age group 35–55. In the United Kingdom alone there are 25 000 cases registered annually, resulting in over 15 000 deaths from the disease each year. Approximately 5% of all cases that present are in the advanced stages, where cure is an unrealistic expectation and of those cases presenting at an early stage (potentially curable) about a half will relapse with metastatic disease over a 20 year period of follow-up (Baum and Schipper 1998). Breast cancer is almost unique in its potential for very late relapse, for which prolonged vigilance is necessary.

It is fashionable these days to dismiss the achievements of William S. Halsted at the turn of the century, losing sight of the fact that he introduced the radical mastectomy predominantly to achieve local control of locally advanced disease (Halsted 1898). It also has to be remembered that there is one thing worse than a radical mastectomy and that is an ulcerated, fungating, and malodorous tumour on the chest wall. The radical mastectomy in the days before the availability of radiotherapy or chemotherapy achieved this objective in approximately 70% of cases. These days, locally advanced breast cancer is conventionally managed by chemotherapy, endocrine therapy, or radiotherapy. However, radical surgery still has a role. There are occasional rare patients where local control of the disease has not been possible with combinations of systemic therapy and radiotherapy yet the patient is not obviously dying of distant metastases. Under these circumstances a radical operation, removing the breast, the affected surrounding skin, and the underlying muscles, together with clearance of involved axillary lymph nodes, may in itself be palliative. Reconstruction of the defect is possible using myocutaneous flaps.

Patients with 'early stage' disease, even though they might ultimately relapse with systemic metastases may avoid the disgusting and painful results of uncontrolled local disease, by either a modified radical mastectomy or a quadrantectomy, axillary node dissection, and radiotherapy to the breast. The decision over which approach is to be preferred is determined by the size and position of the original primary, in relation to the size of the breast and to some extent the preference of the individual patient. An initial failure to control the disease in the axillary nodes can result in the very worst complications of breast cancer, where the uncontrolled disease grows to obstruct the lymphatics, the axillary vein, and the brachial plexus. This can lead to a painful, useless, and swollen arm. Any woman who has been submitted to a mastectomy, however poor her long-term prognosis, should be offered reconstruction as part of her psychological rehabilitation. At the same there are no good empirical data to support the common-sense notion that breast conservation in itself necessarily improves psychological morbidity of the treatment of the disease (Fallowfield *et al.* 1986). These outcomes are more significantly influenced by the skills of the surgeon and the support of the complementary therapist (Fallowfield *et al.* 1987).

Techniques for reconstruction have improved enormously over recent years and this has largely depended upon the availability of implantable prostheses. For relatively small-busted women, having had a simple or modified radical mastectomy in the past, a sub-pectoral tissue expander can produce pleasing results that will satisfy most patients. However, women who have been submitted to radical mastectomy or mastectomy plus radiotherapy in the past usually fare better with a myocutaneous flap to produce sufficient volume to match up with the contralateral breast. Occasionally a reduction mammoplasty of the contralateral breast is necessary to achieve a perfect outcome.

Finally, we treat the patient as an individual with her own symptomatic problems and be flexible with regard to the primary therapy and thus treat the patient first and the cancer second.

Team work and the cancer surgeon

A modern surgical oncologist is one member of a team. Any self-respecting team these days includes a clinical oncologist and a medical oncologist, diagnostic radiologist, histopathologist, and clinical nurse specialist. It is my particular prejudice that the clinical nurse specialist (nurse counsellor) bridges the gap between the clinical scientist and those other disciplines that offer complementary care. My own team has immediate access to a clinical psychologist, as well as counsellors and I have made brave attempts in the past to evaluate this service according to scientific principles, with the development and use of psychometric tools (Fallowfield *et al.* 1987). When I was Professor at the Royal Marsden my patients had direct access to art therapy (*vide infra*), therapeutic massage, and relaxation classes within the adjacent institute for complementary care. However, I have never recognized a role for homoeopathy, special diets, or any other new age 'hocus pocus' which have become more and more popular in the age of postmodern relativism. I do have a soft spot, or call it a personal prejudice, in favour of art therapy, and was instrumental in developing this service at the Royal Marsden Hospital. Camilla Connell, the art therapist at this institution published a beautiful book on the subject '*Something understood — art therapy and cancer care*' (Connell 1998). I would like to freely quote from the preface that I was invited to write for the book, because I think it truly illustrates a recognition of the limitations of my surgical science and the importance of the integration of complementary care. 'My interest and enthusiasm (for art therapy) can be described at two levels, first there is an uncanny thematic similarity running through the works of many of these patients who face serious disease. It is as if the experience of cancer stimulates some deeply hidden communal memory to evoke the symbolism of life and death, fear and hope. The tree, for example, is a recurring theme in these works of art, one that can be traced back through many cultures to its origin, Etz Chaim (tree of life) of the Old Testament. At the individual patient level what I found so moving is the obvious cathartic value of using art to express hidden fears, the progression of the imagery from fear to hope as a sign of recovery, and sadly in the reverse direction as a sign of deterioration. There is no doubt that art is a powerful medium for self-expression for frightened patients who do not have the words or will to express themselves verbally. Good medicine is not only the practice of the science of the subject but also the practice of the humanities of the subject; central to the humanitarian practice of medicine is the development of good communication skills. Central to the development of good communication skills is the development of empathy. Strictly speaking, empathy means trying to get inside the patient's head to feel his or her fears and pain, a task that even the most empathetic of doctors can find extremely difficult. As far as I am concerned, art therapy is the most direct line to the patient's experience of illness.'

Conclusion

Complementary medicine is practised at the highest level in the hierarchy that governs the human organism. Providing the complementary specialist concentrates on making the patient feel better and spiritually at ease, then its position is secure into the new millennium. I would also urge proponents of complementary medicine to appreciate that the holistic system is an open system which lends itself to the experimental method. There is much research that is urgently required to investigate the psychosomatic aspects of disease and the spiritual dimension to care. Complementary therapists, therefore, should resist complacency and join forces with clinical scientists to explore the domain between the mind and the neuroendocrine levels of the human organism. Who knows? I might one day be convinced that a mind at peace with its body might enhance the powers of self-healing, as a biological adjunct to the skills of a surgeon. This is a subject worthy of research, but at this point an unsubstantiated but plausible hypothesis.

References

Baum, M. and Schipper, H (1998). *Fast facts: breast cancer*. Health Press, Oxford.

Calman, K. and Downie, R. (1996). Why arts courses for medical curricula? *Lancet*, **347**, 1499–500.

Connell, C. (1998). *Something understood. Art therapy in cancer care*. Wrexham Publications, London.

Cotrell, A. (1997). Letter to *The Times*.

Fallowfield, L. (1990). *The quality of life. The missing measurement in healthcare*. Condor Book Souvenier Press (E & A) Ltd. London.

Fallowfield, L. J., Baum, M., and Maguire, G. P (1987). Addressing the psychological needs of the conservatively treated breast cancer patient. *Journal of the Royal Society of Medicine*, **80**, 646–700.

Fallowfield, L. J., Baum, M., and Maguire, G.P. (1986). Effects of breast conservation on psychological morbidity associated with the diagnosis and treatment of early breast cancer. *British Medical Journal*, **293**, 1331–4.

Halsted, W. S. (1898). The radical operation for the care of carcinoma of the breast. *Johns Hopkins Hospital Reports*, **28**, 557.

Koestler, A. (1978). *Janus: A summing up*. Picador, London.

Popper, K. (1992). *The logic of scientific discovery*. Routedge, London.

Chapter 20

Complementary therapies in palliative care

Mandy Barnett

This chapter will consider the place of complementary therapies in palliative care, focusing on the use of particular therapies, the evidence base for their use in the palliative care setting, and the problems encountered in evaluating their benefit.

Parallels and paradoxes

The field of palliative care has developed rapidly in the UK over the last 30 years or so [1], in recognition of the need for a more holistic approach to patients who are facing death. The aim within palliative care is to offer optimum care for a patient's physical condition, and in addition to address psychological, social, and spiritual issues, in order both to maximize the quality of life remaining and to achieve a dignified and peaceful death. This is summarized by the definition from the European Association of Palliative Care: the active total care of a person whose disease is no longer amenable to curative therapy. Initially much of the development of palliative care took place in the voluntary sector, but there has been a steady increase in NHS involvement and funding. Alongside these developments has come the recognition of palliative medicine as a medical subspecialty[2], with the subsequent creation of standards of practice and training programmes to improve the provision of specialist care across all regions.

Within palliative care, the emphasis on enhancing quality of life and helping the patient to achieve the goals that are important to them clearly requires the recognition of patient autonomy as a central concept. This is not always comfortable for healthcare professionals, particularly when patients' wishes appear to dictate a course of action (or inaction) which

---

[1] Starting from the establishment of St Christopher's Hospice in South London in 1967, there are now upwards of 230 in-patient units distributed throughout the country, plus a further 120 services, comprising either freestanding day units, or homecare or hospital support teams.

[2] In 1987, as a subspecialty within medicine and thereby regulated by the Royal College of Physicians.

does not seem to be in their best interests. This can be further complicated by the multi-disciplinary make-up of palliative care teams, which leads to a variety of professional perspectives, requiring a high degree of interdisciplinary collaboration and trust if the best outcomes are to be achieved (Speck 1998).

Reflecting back to Chapter 1, there are interesting parallels in the development of both complementary therapies and palliative care within mainstream healthcare, which are reflected in the degree to which they are also integrated.

Current practice experience

Anecdotally, there is widespread acceptance and use of complementary therapies in palliative care settings in the UK. However, reported work is extremely sparse, and largely unpublished.

Wilkes (1992) reported on a questionnaire survey carried out by Trent Palliative Care Centre in collaboration with Help the Hospices. This produced a response from 108 units: 37 larger in-patient units (>12 beds); 17 medium units (8–12 beds), and 54 smaller units, including those comprising nurse-led day-care facilities or home or hospital support teams only.

Of the responders, 75 offered at least some form of arts, crafts, or diversional therapies, with 33 providing extremely active programmes. Only 7 provided no activities, of which 5 were hospital-based support teams. Attitudes among the staff were generally positive, although doctors were more sceptical than other professionals (however, this did not impinge on the availability of therapies).

Considering specific therapies offered, by far the most common were combinations of massage (76), aromatherapy (73), and relaxation (71). Acupuncture and reflexology were equally prevalent but provided less often overall (28). Hypnotherapy and healing involving laying on of hands also had a place (14). A few units (6 or less) reported on a wide range of other therapies or techniques: meditation (6); Bach flower remedies (5); visualization, Yoga, healing crystals, Alexander technique, energy balancing, and acupressure (1–3).

Historically, many hospice and palliative care units in the UK have accessed practitioners locally according to availability, often on a voluntary basis, or have relied on skills developed independently by in-house staff, particularly nurses but occasionally doctors. Salaried complementary practitioner posts or sessions are less common, as they fight for priority alongside other developments.

This was demonstrated by a more recent survey of 190 hospices providing in-patient services (all those listed in the Hospice Directory at the time of the survey) (Lee and Whitehead 1998). They obtained a high response rate of 88%, although not all questionnaires were adequately completed. They found that 91% of respondents provided some form of complementary therapy, and those who didn't were considering it for future development. Among their respondents, the most common therapies reported were aromatherapy, reflexology, massage, and relaxation, but a wide variety were employed in smaller numbers, including acupuncture, reiki, dream therapy, and homoeopathy. The high percentage offered may reflect some confusion over terminology, as some units also included music and art therapy and counselling in their responses. In the latter case, while 22% cited counselling, it is likely that others offered it but did not consider it a complementary therapy.

The question regarding who provided the therapy revealed a diversity of arrangements: 26% only used paid therapists, while 34% only used volunteers and 40% used a combination of both. However, interpretation of these responses was complicated by the factor that many of the therapists were nurses already employed by the hospice, rather than salaried as therapists. It was also not clear whether volunteers were professional therapists offering one or two free sessions on altruistic grounds, or semi-trained practitioners. Given the lack of regulation and standardization of training in many therapies any combination is possible.

Evaluation of complementary therapies

Although complementary therapies are generally viewed as beneficial to patients in the palliative care setting in psychosocial terms, there has been little formal evaluation of their effects. One problem is in defining the aims of complementary therapies in palliative care — are they being offered simply as some form of diversional therapy or with specific aims — are these aims clearly set down, and is any mechanism in place to evaluate the effectiveness of the service? If the latter, is this in the context of general patient satisfaction, or using specific measures such as pain relief, reduction of anxiety, etc. Given the historical position of voluntary service provision, cost effectiveness has not been an issue and has therefore provided little stimulus for assessment. This has a number of potential disadvantages:

1. Therapies are likely to be accessed by patients who already know or use them, rather than across the board — this tends to be the younger, female, higher socio-economic group patient, rather than the symptomatic frail elderly who make up the majority of palliative care referrals.

2. Possible treatment benefits specific to individual therapies are not being clearly defined — for example differences between relaxation and visualization techniques in anxiety reduction.

3. Symptom control issues that may be helped by specific therapies are not being targeted at client groups — for example massage and acupuncture are both relatively widely available, thus it would be useful to consider the specific role of each approach in different pain scenarios.

4. Evaluation by anecdotal reports of enhanced patient satisfaction alone can prove a weak bargaining point when there are competing financial priorities.

In other words, the very acceptability of complementary therapies within the palliative care setting may prove to be a disservice both to patients and practitioners if it prevents efforts at targeting interventions to particular client groups rather than relying simply on patient demand. In addition, as many of the voluntary sector hospices come under increasing pressure to justify their expenditure when contracting their services to multiple primary care groups, the employment of complementary therapists may be seen as a luxury when they could be demonstrated to be cost-effective if properly evaluated.

For example, a problem of clinical accountability was reported recently in an oncology department (personal communication) where an aromatherapist was employed to offer sessions to patients attending the department, who could either self-refer or be referred by professionals involved in the patients' treatment, but only for undefined psychosocial benefit. The problem arose when a well-intentioned and possibly well-informed health professional referred a patient for a specific treatment (reduction of lymphoedema); the therapist felt professionally vulnerable because this was outside her remit in the context of her work in the department and the clinicians in the department had too little knowledge of the possible therapeutic applications of aromatherapy to determine if this was a valid treatment outcome, although such evidence does exist (Kirshbaum 1996). The patient was treated in the end with reference to non-specific psychological benefits, but this misses both the point and a valuable opportunity.

Palliative care outcomes — problems with definition and measurement

Within the palliative care setting, difficulties have been encountered in all areas of formalized research, extending well beyond the evaluation of complementary therapies. Palliative care outcomes, be they issues of quality of care or cost-effectiveness, are notoriously difficult to define and measure (Rinck *et al.* 1997; Bruera and Suarez-Almazor 1998).

In the global context, quality of life has proved elusive to define (van Knippenberg and de Haes 1988). First, quality of life can refer to certain aspects of life or life as a whole, and secondly the difference between measurements made 'subjectively' and 'objectively'.

Both of these issues have particular resonance in the palliative care context: how to judge what makes for a 'good' quality of life for any one individual, particularly in the face of advanced and progressing disease states (Fowlie and Berkeley 1987; Donnelly and Walsh 1996). Calman (1984) made one of the best early attempts at definition with this group in mind, when he proposed that quality of life was represented by the differences between reality and expectations for any one individual, depending on present lifestyle, past experiences, hope for the future, dreams, and ambitions. Thus the larger the gap between the reality and the expectations, the poorer the quality of life. Conversely, where an individual can find a sense of meaning even in the face of physical limitation and deterioration, quality of life may still be positively perceived (Cohen and Mount 1992).

This leads into the second measurement issue of 'objective' versus 'subjective' evaluation. Early instruments were observer-rated, simple assessments of performance status (Karnofsky 1949), the modern consensus is that the best and most consistent judge of both physical and psychological dimensions is the patient (Slevin *et al.* 1988), and this has been the focus of more recent work (Bullinger 1992).

However, this ideal may not always be achievable, particularly in the last few days of life when patients are too unwell to complete even brief instruments (Morris *et al.* 1986). This makes instrument design and application difficult, although some aimed at process of care have demonstrated consistent correlations between self-ratings and observer-ratings (Higginson and McCarthy 1993). The problem is knowing what to measure.

Physical symptoms and functional ability scores have proved most accessible and thereby form the basis of much reported work. For example, the EORTC Quality of Life Study Group developed a modular approach to measuring both physical symptomatology and global aspects of quality of life among cancer patients (Aaronson *et al.* 1988). Even here patients' deteriorating condition can lead to poor accrual, high attrition rates, and problems with establishing reliability of measures, which makes the measurement of effectiveness of therapeutic strategies difficult. Nevertheless, work continues on developing and improving appropriate instruments, and including more existential elements (Cohen *et al.* 1997).

In the psychosocial context, outcomes and methods of measurement have proved equally difficult to adapt to the palliative care population. The gold standard applied to definitions of psychiatric disorder is the DSM criteria (American Psychiatric Association 1994), which groups 'affective disorders' into several separate domains: major depression, anxiety, and adjustment disorders. However, this assessment may not easily be extrapolated to physically ill patients, and dying patients in particular, for two reasons:

1. The fundamental issue of distinguishing between 'appropriate distress' and 'affective disorder' — at what point does sadness at approaching the end of life become pathological (Mayou and Hawton 1986)?

2. The confounding effects of physical illness and concurrent treatment on somatic symptoms which normally form an integral part of the psychiatric diagnostic pattern.

Looked at from the opposite point of view, physical symptoms can themselves exacerbate psychological distress, particularly if the person's condition is deteriorating (Barnett 1995). This is not a linear relationship: Fowlie *et al.* (1989) found that physical symptoms were less important in determining overall quality of life than the extent to which the individual had come to terms with his condition and reached peace with himself.

A number of standardized psychological questionnaires have been developed specifically to use with physically ill patients, and have been validated among patients with cancer in various settings. In the UK, the Rotterdam Symptom Checklist (de Haes *et al.* 1990) and Hospital Anxiety Depression scale (Zigmond and Snaith 1983) have been especially popular, and have been validated among advanced cancer populations (Hopwood *et al.* 1991). However, these still may not be sufficiently sensitive or specific for patients with deteriorating symptoms (Ibbotson *et al.* 1994), and studies using them among palliative care populations have raised concerns about interpretation of results based on such questionnaires (Faull *et al.* 1994; Barnett 1995).

Research questions and outcomes in complementary therapies

Paradoxically, the problems experienced in palliative care research could prove advantageous to researchers working at the complementary therapy/palliative care interface: health professionals in the palliative care setting have embraced complementary therapies more wholeheartedly than many others. They are used to dealing with nebulous outcome concepts in their own field and are struggling to find ways of proving their effectiveness in the modern world of clinical governance and evidence-based medicine which may be brought to bear both on individual practice and purchasing decisions.

This brings us back to the question of how complementary therapies may be most valuable and best used in the palliative care setting. From the patient's viewpoint, a survey of preferences among cancer patients carried out from the Royal London Homoeopathic Hospital indicated that the primary outcome sought was psychological benefit (Stevensen 1995). However, a number of other benefits may be obtainable in terms of global quality of life or more specific physical symptom control, and trials are beginning to be conducted in this patient group to assess the effects of specific complementary therapies.

One problem has been attracting resources and suitably trained personnel to carry out research (RCCM Tenth Anniversary Report 1992; Zollman and Vickers 1999), given that much of the financial backing within orthodox medical research originates from the pharmaceutical industry or large cancer charities.

Despite this, there have been a number of positive developments: several institutions and charities have appointed staff with a specific remit for developing and evaluating complementary therapies with reference to cancer care and palliative care.[3] Alongside this, a number of studies have set out to evaluate particular therapies from a quality of life viewpoint using defined scales and outcomes, although these have been limited in the palliative care setting to those few therapies which are widely offered. This will be discussed briefly in the following section.

Studies of complementary therapies relevant to palliative care

Aromatherapy and massage

Given the popularity of aromatherapy and massage in the palliative care setting and the fact that many of the therapists involved are also nurses, it is not surprising that this is one of the most investigated areas to date, although studies have been hampered by small subject numbers. Wilkinson (1995) reviewed the relevant literature on aromatherapy and massage used in a variety of settings, and went on to describe one of the first randomized trials among palliative care patients, comparing aromatherapy massage with massage alone. The trial was carefully designed to control for confounding variables, and used standardized questionnaires to measure psychological, physical, and global quality of life dimensions; in addition a semi-structured self-report questionnaire was designed to assess patients' views on the experience of massage and aromatherapy itself. Results from the first 51 patients entered in the study demonstrated significant benefits on all dimensions for the aromatherapy group, whereas in the massage group scores on each dimension showed positive changes but did not reach significance, suggesting that while massage alone was helpful, the use of essential oils in the aromatherapy group conferred additional benefit. Patient responses on the semi-structured questionnaires similarly indicated a variety of perceived benefits, particularly reduced tension and pain relief.

Kite *et al.* (1998) report an ongoing assessment of the aromatherapy service provided at the Cancer Support and Information Centre at Mount Vernon Hospital. The practitioner developed a specific quality of life evaluation tool (similar in item content to the EORTC QLQ-30 (Aaronson *et al.* 1988)) and also used the Hospital Anxiety Depression (HAD) Scale, which was completed by patients before and after their course of six sessions. The patient group was largely women with breast cancer undergoing primary treatment with radiotherapy, referred because of symptoms of anxiety and depression. Out of 89 initial referrals, 58 completed all six sessions, and among this group HAD scores were significantly lowered (indicating improved mood).

A combination of subjective and objective benefits were obtained in a study of aromatherapy used in a general hospital among elderly patients (Cannard 1996). Here the use of aromatherapy massage led to improved sleep patterns and a concomitant reduction in night sedation requirements.

----

[3] Hammersmith Hospitals NHS Trust has run an integrated complementary therapy service since the late 1980s and appointed a Team Leader in 1996 with a lecturing focus.

Cancer Relief Macmillan Fund appointed a research fellow in complementary therapies in 1999.

Sara Lee Trust is a charity set up to provide and evaluate complementary therapies, affiliated to St Michael's Hospice in East Sussex.

These examples are illustrative, not an exhaustive picture.

Reflexology

A small but potentially significant study was reported at conference level of a randomized trial of reflexology versus placebo reflexology. Although patient numbers were small ($n = 12$), reported differences using a quality of life visual analogue scale reached significance (Hodgson, conference abstract, Royal College of Nursing Conference on *Complementary Therapy and Pain Control*, May, 1999). Clearly further evaluation is both possible and warranted.

Acupuncture

Despite increasing literature on acupuncture, developments in palliative care have not been widely evaluated. One recent study reported on the use of auricular stud acupuncture to treat a variety of types of pain among 28 patients attending a hospice either as in-patients or out-patients. Significant reduction in pain scores was achieved despite the small number of subjects, and the authors recommend further investigation (Dillon and Lucas 1999).

Relaxation

There are few reports of the use of relaxation techniques alone, but one impressive randomized trial included relaxation techniques among a variety of non-pharmacological approaches aimed at managing breathlessness among lung cancer patients (Bredin *et al.* 1998). Results demonstrated significant reduction in physical and emotional distress combined with improved coping strategies, despite deteriorating performance status.

Hypnotherapy

Clearly this is not a treatment modality amenable to controlled trial methods, but a retrospective survey of patients receiving hypnotherapy in a palliative care setting did suggest improved coping as a positive outcome (Finlay and Jones 1996).

Herbalism

Studies specific to the palliative care setting are lacking, but in some instances results from other populations may be useful to palliative care patients. For example, the reported benefits of St John's Wort (Linde *et al.* 1996) as a treatment for mild depression could provide a useful alternative to antidepressants, whose side-effects combined with a delayed onset of action often poses a dilemma for doctors offering treatment to patients who are already consuming a cocktail of drugs and whose prognosis is likely to be short.

Multicentre trials and patient involvement in trial design

As complementary practitioners increasingly recognize the need to regulate their own professions, more structured evaluation becomes both necessary and more possible. In the palliative care setting, multicentre trials have begun to be developed in a variety of therapeutic areas, as few units are large enough to carry out such work alone, and this can be applied to complementary therapies equally as to other symptom control measures. The validity of such an approach was highlighted in a recent report of a study attempting to evaluate the effect of aromatherapy on mood among a hospice day centre population, using a rigorous randomized controlled design (Mew *et al.* 1999a, 1999b). The authors report that all patients wished to continue with treatment after the study concluded, although measured mood improvements did not reach significance — however patient accrual was slow and attrition high. The authors concluded that a multicentre approach would help to overcome these methodological issues.

This is indeed the approach of Wilkinson, who has followed on from her initial work to set up a multicentre randomized trial comparing aromatherapy massage with relaxation therapy on quality of life. This study aims to evaluate over 500 advanced cancer patients attending palliative care and clinical oncology departments over a two year period (S. Wilkinson, personal communication).

Although the randomized controlled trial may be viewed as the gold standard, other robust methodologies exist which may be adapted more easily to complementary therapies (Levin *et al.* 1997; Vickers 1996).

Conclusion

Both complementary therapies and palliative care can be considered to have come of age at the beginning of the new Millennium. The move towards evidence-based practice should be viewed not as a threat but as a creative challenge to researchers and therapists, which will lead to both increased and improved use of therapies for palliative care patients.

References

Aaronson, N. K., Bullinger, M., and Ahmedzai, S. (1988). A modular approach to quality-of-life assessment in cancer clinical trials. *Recent Results in Cancer Research*, 111, 231–49.

American Psychiatric Association (1994). *Diagnostic and statistical manual of mental disorders* (4th edn) (DSM IV). American Psychiatric Association, Washington DC.

Barnett, M. (1995). *The doctor–patient relationship in advanced cancer*. MD Thesis, University of Bristol.

Bredin, M., Krishnasamy, M., Corner, J., *et al.* (1998) Multicentre randomized controlled trial of a nursing intervention for breathlessness in patients with lung cancer. *Palliative Medicine*, 12, 470.

Bruera, E. and Suarez-Almazor, M. (1998). Cost effectiveness in palliative care. Editorial. *Palliative Medicine*, 12, 315–16.

Bullinger, M. (1992). Quality of life assessment in palliative care. *Journal of Palliative Care*, 8, 34–9.

Calman, K. C. (1984). Quality of life in cancer patients — an hypothesis. *Journal of Medical Ethics*, 10, 124–7.

Cannard, G. (1996). The effect of aromatherapy in promoting relaxation and stress reduction in a general hospital. *Complementary Therapies in Nursing and Midwifery*, 2, 38–40.

Cohen, R. S. and Mount, B. (1992). Quality of life in terminal illness: defining and measuring subjective well-being in the dying. *Journal of Palliative Care*, 8, 40–5.

Cohen, S. R., Mount, B. M., Bruera, E., *et al.* (1997). Validity of the McGill Quality of Life Questionnaire in the palliative care setting: a multi-centre Canadian study demonstrating the importance of the existential domain. *Palliative Medicine*, 11, 3–20.

De Haes, J. C. J. M., Knippenberg, F. C. E., and Neijt, J. P. (1990). Measuring psychological and physical distress in cancer patients: structure and application of the Rotterdam Symptom Checklist. *British Journal of Cancer*, 62, 1034–8.

Dillon, M. and Lucas, C. (1999). Auricular stud acupuncture in palliative care patients. *Palliative Medicine*, 13, 253–4.

Donnelly, S. and Walsh, D. (1996). Quality of life assessment in advanced cancer. *Palliative Medicine*, 10, 275–83.

Faull, C. M., Johnson, I. S., Butler, T. J. (1994). The hospital anxiety and depression (HAD) scale: its validity in patients with terminal malignant disease. Abstract published in *Palliative Medicine*, 8, 69.

Finlay, I. G.and Jones, O. L. (1996). Hypnotherapy in palliative care. *Journal of the Royal Society of Medicine*, 89, 493–6.

Fowlie, M. and Berkeley, J. (1987).Quality of life — a review of the literature. *Family Practice*, 4, 226–34.

Fowlie, M., Berkeley, J., Dingwall-Fordyce, J. (1989). Quality of life in advanced cancer: the benefits of asking the patient. *Palliative Medicine*, 3, 55–9.

Higginson, I. J. and McCarthy, M. (1993). Validity of the support team assessment schedule: do staff ratings reflect those made by patients or their families? *Palliative Medicine*, 7, 219–28.

Hopwood, P., Howell, A., and Maguire, P. (1991). Screening for psychiatric morbidity in patients with advanced breast cancer: validation of two self-report questionnaires. *British Journal of Cancer*, 64, 353–6.

Ibbotson, T., Maguire, P., Selby, P., Priestman, T., and Wallace, L. (1994). Screening for anxiety and depression in cancer patients: the effects of disease and treatment. *European Journal of Cancer*, 30A, 37–40.

Karnofsky, D. A. and Burchenal, J. H. (1949). The clinical evaluation of chemotherapeutic agents in cancer. In *Evaluation of chemotherapeutic agents* (ed. C. M. McCleod), pp.191–205. Columbia University Press, New York.

Kirshbaum, M. (1996). Using massage in the relief of lymphoedema: *Prof Nurse*, 11, 230–2.

Kite, S. M., Maher, E. J., Anderson, K., *et al.* (1998). Development of an aromatherapy service at a Cancer Centre. *Palliative Medicine* 12, 171–80.

Lee, S. and Whitehead, D. (1998). *Survey on complementary therapies.* The Sara Lee Trust. St Michael's Hospice, St Leonard's on Sea, East Sussex, UK. Unpublished.

Levin, J. S., Glass, T. A., Kushi, L. H., *et al.* (1997). Quantitative methods in research on complementary and alternative medicine. A methodological manifesto. NIH Office of Alternative Medicine. *Medical Care*, 35, 1079–94.

Linde, K., Ramirez, G., Mulrow, C. D., *et al.* (1996). St John's wort for depression — an overview and meta-analysis of randomised clinical trials. *British Medical Journal*, 313, 253–8.

Mayou, R. and Hawton, K. (1986). Psychiatric disorder in the general hospital. *British Journal of Psychiatry*, 149, 172–90.

Mew, J., Clarke, D., Wilcock, A., *et al.* (1999a). Use of the Profile of Mood State (POMS) to assess the effect of aromatherapy on mood in patients with cancer. *Psycho-Oncology*, 8, 1–13.

Mew, J., Clarke, D., Wilcock, A., *et al.* (1999b). Practicality of carrying out a controlled trial of aromatherapy in patients with cancer attending for hospice day care. *Psycho-Oncology*, 8, 1–13.

Morris, J. N., Suissa, S., Sherwood, S., *et al.* (1986). Last days: a study of the quality of life of terminally ill cancer patients. *Journal of Chronic Disease*, 39, 47–62.

Research Council for Complementary Medicine, Tenth Anniversary Report (RCCM, London 1992)

Rinck, G. C., van den Bos, G. A., Kleijnen, J., *et al.* (1997). Methodologic issues in effectiveness research on palliative cancer care: a systematic review. *Journal Clinical Oncology*, 15, 1697–707.

Slevin, M. L., Plant, H., Lynch, D., *et al.* (1988). Who should measure quality of life, the doctor or the patient? *British Journal of Cancer*, 57, 109–12.

Speck, P. (1998). Power and autonomy in palliative care: a matter of balance (Editorial). *Palliative Medicine*, 12, 145–6.

Stevensen, C. (1995). Surveys in complementary therapies: assessing the needs of people with cancer. *Complementary Therapies in Nursing and Midwifery*, 1, 110–2.

van Knippenberg, F. C. E. and de Haes, J. C. J. M. (1988). Measuring quality of life of cancer patients: psychometric properties of instruments. *Journal of Clinical Epidemiology*, 41, 1043–53.

Vickers, A. (1996). Methodological issues in complementary and alternative medicine research: a personal reflection on 10 years of debate in the United Kingdom. *Journal of Alternative and Complementary Medicine*, 2, 515–24.

Wilkes, E. (1992). *Complementary therapy in hospice and palliative care*. Unpublished study available from Trent Palliative Care Centre, Sheffield, UK.

Wilkinson, S. (1995). Aromatherapy and massage in palliative care. *International Journal of Palliative Nursing*, 1, 21–30.

Zigmond, A. S. and Snaith, R. P. (1983). The hospital anxiety and depression scale. *Acta Psychiatrica Scandinavica*, 67, 361–70.

Zollman, C. and Vickers, A. (1999). ABC of complementary medicine — What is complementary medicine? *British Medical Journal*, 319, 693–6.

Acknowledgements

I would like to thank Catherine Zollman, Director Medical Education Services, Research Council for Complementary Medicine; Michelle Kohn, Complementary Therapies Medical Advisor, Macmillan Cancer Relief; Deborah Whitehead, Coordinator, Sara Lee Trust; Susie Wilkinson, Head of Caring Services Research, Marie Curie Cancer Care.

Chapter 21

Nursing perspectives

Caroline Stevensen

Caroline Stevensen is a private Holistic Healthcare Consultant and
Practitioner, Senior Lecturer in Clinical Aromatherapy at Oxford Brookes
University, and Director of Services for the Haven Trust. Her background
includes a degree in social work and she is a registered nurse. She
specializes in body therapies and is qualified in acupuncture, shiatsu,
aromatherapy, massage, reflex zone therapy, and iridology. She has
published research on the effects of aromatherapy massage on post
cardiac surgery patients. She is deputy editor of *Complementary Therapies
in Nursing and Midwifery: An International Journal.*

Cancer nursing care has benefited from the expertise of specialist nurses world-wide.
Generally, specialist cancer nurses assist patients receiving surgery, chemotherapy, radiotherapy, needing pain relief, suffering from lymphoedema, those requiring psychological
support, and they support patients who are dying and their carers. These roles are vital for
patients to receive optimum care with conventional treatments. In recent years there has
been a new breed of nurse specialist emerging in the field of cancer care. These nurses are
specializing in the use of complementary therapies or are incorporating the use of complementary therapies into their existing practice with patients (Stevensen 1996; Corner *et al.*
1995). This chapter will explore issues surrounding the inclusion of complementary therapies into cancer nursing practice.

The development of complementary therapies in nursing practice

Interest in complementary therapies within nursing has grown at a rapid rate, particularly
during the past ten years. This has happened mostly in the western world with the development of professional interest groups and journals in the subject. As examples of these, the
United Kingdom's Royal College of Nursing has a Complementary Therapies in Nursing
forum which in 1999, its ninth year, had 10 000 members (Royal College of Nursing 1999)

and the journal *Complementary Therapies in Nursing and Midwifery* reached its sixth year of publication in 2000. The UK has taken a lead in the comprehensive professional developments in complementary therapies practice within nursing and other countries such as Australia and New Zealand have followed closely behind. The area of holistic nursing which embraces the idea of treating the patient in body, mind, and spirit has been a growing movement in the USA for many years and the *American Holistic Nursing Journal* has been published for over ten years.

Interest in these nursing practices may be in response to the fact that medicine is seen to have become so technologically orientated, increasingly isolating the patient (Stevensen 1994*a*, Sayre-Adams and Wright 1995). Nursing is often described as the art and science of caring, but as the following quote (Lanara 1984) reflects, it does not always manage to live up to this image in all its aspects:

> Nursing today is at a critical and one might say, tragic crossroads. The nurse is better educated, more knowledgeable and science-orientated. Yet the patient, for all the superb physical and technical improvements in his environment, feels lonely and even abandoned, because nobody cares for him as a person.

The need to redress this balance and rediscover the heart of nursing through caring and touch has led much of the professional interest in complementary therapies. There is also a need to harness the therapeutic potential of nursing and a desire by nurses to 'humanize' healthcare (Wright 1995). Nurses, through their large numbers and unique position at the bedside, are able to lead other healthcare professions in the incorporation of complementary therapies into practice, for example using complementary ways to manage pain and microbial infections when methods from orthodox medicine have failed. Acupuncture is now commonly used in pain clinics and essential oils, such as tea tree and lemon with their chemical constituents, are increasingly incorporated in the management of wounds and infections.

Personal support and psychological care are aspects where nurses are assisted by using complementary therapies in clinical practice. The saying that 'actions speak louder than words' may have some truth in that many nurses are attracted to practise complementary therapies that employ a therapeutic as compared to a technologically orientated form of touch as a means of offering appropriate care. In cancer care, for example, a distressed patient may be offered a form of touch therapy to relieve the stress and pain and to regain a centred and calm state.

It is difficult to describe the boundaries of complementary therapies within nursing as many different therapies have been used by nurses throughout the world. These include acupuncture, Alexander technique, aromatherapy, autogenic training, breathing techniques, biodynamic massage, Chi Kung, counselling, guided imagery, hands on healing, healing touch, herbal medicine, homoeopathy, humour and laughter therapy, hypnotherapy, massage, reflexology, reiki, relaxation techniques, shiatsu, healing with sound and music, Tai Chi, therapeutic touch, visualization techniques, yoga. An informal survey of members of the Complementary Therapies in Nursing forum concluded that those nurses used massage, aromatherapy, and reflexology as the main complementary therapies in their nursing practice (Rankin-Box 1997). It also showed that more nurses practised these therapies in the private than the public sector, possibly reflecting the relative amount of nursing resources in both areas. In the public healthcare sector, nurses often had to practice these therapies in their own time, in addition to an already full day of nursing care.

In many settings it is still considered a luxury rather than a necessity for nurses to practise complementary therapies as an integral part of their care. It is believed that this attitude will remain until the benefits of these therapies are better understood by nurses generally.

In the USA, nurses have been practising different forms of hands-on therapies: therapeutic touch, introduced by Krieger (1975), and healing touch are two of the most common. Due to the legislation in the USA, there are problems with the open practice of complementary therapies for nurses in certain states. Australian nurses are adopting a variety of techniques including forms of hands-on treatments that originated with their Asian neighbours including Chinese massage (Tuina) and Thai massage as well as aromatherapy.

The current use of complementary therapies

Cancer nurses have embraced the use of complementary therapies in response to the needs of patients. To the knowledge of the author, there is no large or recent analysis of cancer nurses in terms of therapies practised. As cancer is one of the most prevalent diseases amongst the population of the world today, it seems fair to presume that many of the therapies mentioned previously in this paper are also practised by nurses in cancer care. All the above mentioned therapies have been practised in the UK with cancer patients.

As each year passes there is a trend for an ever-widening band of complementary therapies to be employed. This is not to say that patients necessarily have choice. Service development may be *ad hoc* and a complementary therapy service in most cancer units will only be offered by one or two nurses or therapists, each of whom are trained in a single therapy. Larger and more specialized complementary therapy units are able to offer a wider range of therapies such as massage, aromatherapy, reflexology, counselling, shiatsu, relaxation, and art therapy. In the cancer nurses' role, the complementary therapies may offer holistic care, symptomatic relief, self-help, and hope. Nurses practising complementary therapies are trying to offer a more complete form of caring for the patient rather than replacing other methods of conventional cancer care.

Symptomatic relief

Symptoms which may be helped with complementary therapies include physical and emotional pains, side-effects from radiotherapy and chemotherapy, fatigue, stress, low mood, anxiety, insomnia, nausea, constipation, oedema, wounds, hot flushes, and infections to name a few. Some examples are listed here. The homoeopathic medicine called Radium bromide (Rad. brom) can offer relief from the fatigue that accompanies radiotherapy and another called Cantharis can be helpful to treat any heating or burning of the skin. Women with hot flushes as a side-effect of Tamoxifen may find that a combination of homoeopathy and acupuncture or shiatsu is helpful in reducing their number and intensity. In these cases, homoeopathy is prescribed according to the individual constitution and symptoms of the patient. Appropriate gentle yoga exercises may be helpful in the management of lymphoedema wherever its location in the body as each yoga posture is designed to open and relax the body in a different way. Shiatsu, a form of Japanese massage performed with pressure on the acupuncture points and their pathways can be very beneficial in relieving stress and pain, revitalizing the general level of energy. It is calm and relaxing in its effects, more deeply than other forms of bodywork.

Reflexology is another energizing treatment that patients find useful in the relief of symptoms. One 32-year-old woman who had four recurrences of Hodgkin's lymphoma found reflexology to be the best method of revitalizing her energy whilst on chemotherapy. Another women who had suffered from shoulder pain for two years following a mastectomy was amazed to find that she was pain free when shiatsu pressure was placed on SI 11, an acupuncture point on the shoulder blade. She was puzzled why this point was not known to physiotherapists and other therapists when she had received such an instantaneous effect. Another woman with a very late stage of breast cancer and severe arm pain and emotional pain found a combination of relaxation, supported exercises, and gentle manual lymphatic drainage massage the only relief for severe emotional and physical pain which stayed with her until death.

Self-help

Self-help is one of the most valuable gifts that can be offered to a person living with cancer. It empowers the patient and carer alike. In terms of complementary therapies, a nurse may offer a patient a massage and then be able to teach their carer a simplified form of massage to continue the treatment at home. This is not only beneficial to the patient, but allows the carer to develop an active role in the care of their loved one.

For patients and carers, breathing, relaxation, visualization, and guided imagery techniques may be taught by the nurse, then may be continued at home with the help of an audio or video tape. Patients should be offered enough freedom in these techniques and be allowed to choose the images, colours and scenarios that help them individually. One woman with breast cancer chose a knight on a white charger to gallop through her body mopping up any errant cancer cells in its path whilst another chose a more gentle image of dolphins swimming through her system quietly and lovingly rebalancing her physical and chemical energies. The use of sound has appealed to patients and the ability to hum, sing or chant a single or variety of notes to help rebalance and revitalize the body's system has appealed to different patients. At a simpler level, nurses can allow patients to explore the realm of music and sound by having a variety of soothing and uplifting music available for patients to listen to either during other therapeutic treatments or on their own. Personal stereos have gone a long way to making this possible in a busy ward environment.

Cancer nurses have a unique role to support patients and their carers in a wide variety of environments as in- and out-patients, in clinics, hospices, and in their own homes. Time is a rare commodity for nurses. The pressure of spending sufficient time with patients to perform complementary therapies is believed to be one of the main reasons that more cancer nurses have not adopted these therapies into practice. However, the skilled use of complementary therapies in cancer nursing practice may actually save time and enhance the quality of nursing care. Working with groups of patients doing relaxation, breathing, and visualization may enable individuals to perform this task for themselves, for example with the help of a tape in their own time and environment. The use of relaxation and relaxation with guided imagery can relieve stress and anxiety (Bridge *et al.* 1988) as well as nausea, vomiting, and anxiety in patients receiving chemotherapy (Lyles *et al.* 1982). Nurses can also offer skilled help and advice in group work and group therapy which offers the therapeutic advantage of sharing and not feeling so isolated.

Offering hope

What could be a more valuable part of the nurse's role than to be at the bedside 24 hours a day, offering hope, comfort, and support to patients? Still too often there are people with late stage cancers who live in fear of pain and death. These patients may have been told that nothing more can be done to help them from conventional medicine.

The more fortunate of these patients may find themselves in a position where there are forms of support, possibly including complementary treatments. Dr Anne Clover, medical consultant in homoeopathic medicine in the UK sometimes says to patients, 'We don't know exactly what starts or stops the cancer process ... there are many unknown factors ... so let's go on in hopes' (personal communication). At this level, complementary medicine can offer hope to patients for a better quality of life and symptomatic relief when conventional medicine has no more to offer. With the increasing availability of complementary therapies provided by nurses in clinical areas, it is hoped that doctors may never have to say to patients that there is nothing more that can be done. Nurses need to take their share of responsibility in informing patients about potential complementary therapies that may be both appropriate and beneficial, so in turn offering hope as well. The ability to show patients that they are worthy of care and comfort is an important aspect of offering complementary therapies in the later stages of cancer care. To assist patients to a peaceful, comfortable, and cared-for death is one area where nurses using complementary therapies can make a big difference. It is also a way that communication between patient and carer, who may otherwise feel helpless with their loved one who is dying, may be nurtured. The use of simple comforting massage, including soothing and holding techniques, beautiful music, and aromas may be ways to make these difficult times more uplifting and tolerable for all concerned.

Holism in complementary cancer nursing

In recent years nursing has embraced the idea of holism. Within this approach, nurses care for the patient as a whole — body, mind, and spirit. There has been much discussion around the idea of holism and complementary therapies. Is the practice of complementary therapies necessarily holistic or are they just another task? (Bay 1995). For example, using P6 acupuncture for the relief of nausea or offering aromatherapy essential oil based mouthwash for the relief of mouth ulcers following chemotherapy, are these offering holistic care or are they merely techniques? In these contexts, most people would argue the latter. In general, it is in the approach to the patient where holism is important, that all their needs are considered. In this sense, offering holistic care should be part of every nursing role. The nurse may need to make appropriate referral to other healthcare professionals, complementary therapists, or carers as appropriate. Holism may best be described as meeting the most appropriate needs of the patient, whatever they may be. In itself, the issue of holism does not need to be a professional problem for the cancer nurse, more one of recognition and definition.

The management of change

Change is a constant and inevitable aspect of life. In order for nurses to introduce complementary therapies into cancer nursing practice, they need the skills to practise the therapy and to understand the management of change. Knowledge of the process of change enables nurses to be more in control (Rankin-Box 1995). This allows a smooth process with the knowledge, co-operation, and collaboration of the multiprofessional team and the management. The need of healthcare organizations to cut costs in the public sector seems to be a global experience, certainly true in the UK, USA, and Australia in the late 1990s. Financial restraints may also hamper the ability of nurses to introduce complementary therapies within their practice. Additionally, the smaller the organization and the fewer the nurses, the more difficult it may be for nurses to affect this change due to the pressures of their other responsibilities. The management of change and the introduction of complementary therapies into cancer nursing practice are inextricably linked. The acceptance of the chosen complementary therapy into mainstream cancer care will govern the ease with which this process may occur. Other issues that affect this process are research, safety and efficacy, policy development, and standard setting.

The lack of research evidence in the field of complementary therapies within cancer nursing is another reason often given by management and sceptics for not introducing complementary therapies into practice. Without new innovations however, nursing care generally would not progress.

Research basis for complementary therapies

Evidence-based practice in healthcare has become a catch phrase as the new millennium begins. In spite of the problems with quality of information and research methodology, cancer nurses practising complementary therapies are just as much affected by this issue as the rest of the healthcare community. For new innovations such as complementary therapies within nursing care, the lack of research evidence may be used as a reason by managers and other professionals to prohibit their use in clinical practice. There is also the question of the ability to transfer research findings. How much of the research evidence from health settings outside the cancer field can be applied directly to the work with patients with cancer? The answer to this is far from clear. Let us examine a sample of the research that has been performed by nurses directly with people with cancer.

Acupuncture and related treatments such as acupressure and transcutaneous electrical nerve stimulation (TENS) are well known as a treatment in pain clinics. From a small pilot study performed by Gadsby *et al.* (1997), initial results suggest that acupuncture-like transcutaneous electrical nerve stimulation offers beneficial effects in quality of life and fatigue symptoms, warranting further investigation.

In the USA, research has been performed looking at the effectiveness of therapeutic touch in a variety of settings since the initial work of Krieger (1975). So far there have been no specific studies focusing on people with cancer, although it is known that there are patients with cancer who are experiencing this therapy (Sayre-Adams and Wright 1995 p13). However, there are reports of nurses using therapeutic touch (TT). As part of its method, TT enables patients to mobilize their own inner resources so that self-healing can take place. It is at this point that deep relaxation can occur and anxiety, physical, and emotional pain can be relieved (Krieger 1979). This observation seems to be the key to the effect of many hands-on complementary therapies compared to methods of conventional pain relief.

Sims (1986) performed a small-scale study with positive but statistically non-significant results measuring the effects of massage on the well-being of six patients receiving radiotherapy for breast cancer. Patients reported less symptom distress, higher degrees of tranquillity and vitality and less tension and tiredness compared to the control group. However, as with so many of the massage studies, this one was hampered by poor methodology that limits the ability to generalize these results. Wilkinson (1995) in a hospice setting gave cancer patients body massage with and without the essential oil of camomile at 1% dilution. Camomile is known for its calming properties. The results showed that the addition of the essential oil to the base oil of sweet almond not only improved anxiety, but brought about moderate and persistent improvements in anxiety, physical symptoms, and quality of life. Corner *et al.* (1995) randomized 24 cancer patients to massage or aromatherapy massage with 18 patients acting as controls. Blended essential oils at 2% of lavender, rosewood, lemon, rose, and valerian were used. Both forms of massage led to a moderate improvement in anxiety scores over the course of treatment. Reductions in depression scores were small and not significant.

As an example of cancer nursing research into other complementary therapies, a Canadian nurse (Perry 1996) examined the influence of nurse gender on dialogue in silence, mutual touch, and sharing the lighter side of life with patients with cancer. One of her findings was that a light-hearted attitude was common amongst the exceptionally competent nurses, both male and female. Despite some tragic circumstances in their work lives, these nurses deliberately chose, most of the time, to see the positive and humorous side of situations for the benefit of both their patients and themselves. She concludes that silence and touch both expose a basic honesty. This opening up of the spirit of nurse and patient allows care to be given and received, no matter what the sex of the nurse. Fritz (1988) found that laughter was rated as the most effective way of relieving pain compared to other self-initiated non-invasive techniques with 53 oncology outpatients. Laughter is often described as internal jogging in the sense that the release of endorphins in the brain may be similar in its effects of real jogging or running.

In Europe, particularly Germany and Switzerland, some nurses practise anthrosopophy, defined by its founder Dr Rudolph Steiner (1861–1925) as a path of knowledge that aspires to guide the spiritual within the human being to the spiritual in the universe. Steiner describes humans in terms of the four-fold man: physical body, etheric body, astral body, and ego. In this model Steiner described illness as malfunction of four bodies of man and aimed to reintegrate the rhythms of the four bodies. Much of the work done with people with cancer with anthrosopophy is around boosting the patient's immune system with substances such as iscador, from the mistletoe plant, as well as balancing the four bodies with rhythmic movements, called Eurythmy and artistic therapies to balance body and mind (Trevelyan 1997). Patients at the Royal London Homoeopathic Hospital have been treated with iscador for many years. In a pilot study, Clover *et al.* (1995) found that there was a potential for patients to be helped in terms of quality of life using a variety of therapies including homoeopathy, iscador therapy, massage, and relaxation techniques provided by the multiprofessional team.

Stevensen (1994*b*) performed a survey examining the complementary therapy needs of 120 patients with cancer attending the Royal London Homoeopathic Hospital. She found that most patients wanted complementary therapies to help with stress and anxiety, much more than pain, fatigue, nausea, and other symptoms that may be expected by this group of patients.

Cancer nurses, like other health professionals, draw on the research performed on complementary therapies outside cancer care and evaluate their potential benefits to patients with cancer. The few examples mentioned above illustrate the degree of diversity of complementary therapies practised by cancer nurses and acknowledge that, as with every other field of healthcare, there is a need for more quality research.

Standards of training and practice

For nurses to practise any complementary therapy they must be adequately qualified. A full professional training in the complementary therapy is preferable, but a shorter course may be enough to be competent to practise in a limited way. For example a one-day course to learn hand and foot massage alone is sufficient to practise those skills, but not to practise a full body massage. Limits of training and competence must be understood and respected for the safety of the patient. Bay (1995) asks 'How can nurses be truly accountable if they learn only the basics of reflexology, aromatherapy, and massage?' Nurses in the UK are bound by the regulations of the United Kingdom Central Council Code of Professional Practice (UKCC 1992) which states that nurses must be competent in every aspect of the nursing care that they perform. This applies to complementary therapies as well. Several UK universities and colleges are now offering courses in complementary therapies for nurses and other health professionals. The extent of these has grown so much that there are now too many courses available to mention here. These specialist courses are appropriate for nurses as they can take prior knowledge and learning into account and are able to have academic discussions about the integration of these therapies into the clinical environment.

It is recommended that nurses using a complementary therapy in their cancer care practice are registered with, and members of, the professional body governing the therapy being practised. In this way, the best interests of the patient are safeguarded. In the event of litigation regarding the practice of complementary therapies within nursing, the expert witnesses would be called from both nursing and the complementary therapy in question. Cancer nurses offering complementary therapies need to be aware of this, especially as the patients that they are working with are often receiving strong drug therapies and radiotherapy. The interactions of the particular complementary therapies with orthodox treatments need to be understood as far as research and common practices will allow. For example, the use of certain essential oils may be inappropriate with some chemotherapy or radiotherapy treatments. Patients need careful assessment due to the associations of smell and nausea, and the way that certain chemicals within the citrus essential oils are light sensitive.

Ongoing clinical supervision and professional updating are crucial for nurses practising complementary therapies. People with sufficient experience to perform these supervisory roles may be scarce at present, this will be resolved over time as more experience is gained. The onus for professional updating in complementary therapies is on the individual as with other areas of nursing. Being a member of a professional body for complementary therapies can be useful for this purpose.

Obstacles to the inclusion of complementary therapies

Time, money, belief systems, and a poor evidence base are factors that may all limit the way in which complementary therapies may be included in cancer care. Some health authorities have banned the use of therapies such as aromatherapy due to fears about these potent and highly volatile substances. No therapy or medicine is without its potential risks, but in skilled hands it is there to help and heal. More than once over a 20 year career in complementary medicine, the author has had letters concerned about her spiritual welfare as some believe that complementary medicine is somehow dangerous to the spirit. Let us remember that it is in the Bible that Jesus had herbs brought to him at his birth by the three wise men, his feet anointed or massaged with oil, and he performed healing to the sick. The real fears expressed by staff and patients about complementary therapies may come from a lack of knowledge. Fortunately these are slowly disappearing as therapies become more widely practised. It is almost impossible to pick up a popular magazine or a professional journal, cancer related or otherwise that does not have some reference at some point to one of the therapies that we now refer to as complementary or alternative.

The future

The rate and growth of complementary therapies in nursing generally is not just a fad, it is here to stay. As cancer nurses look for complementary and alternative methods of help and healing patients, the complementary cancer nursing of today will become the integrated cancer nursing of tomorrow. It will soon be the norm for complementary therapy programmes to be found in every cancer nursing environment. As much of the development of these therapies in cancer care has been in response to patient demand, so the rate of growth in this area will continue to be far ahead of the ability of research to evaluate its effectiveness.

As world-wide research progresses and nurses reclaim their caring and healing roles, patients will probably be offered an ever widening selection of therapies to alleviate symptoms and offer comfort, hope, and self-healing. With the innovations of these therapies by cancer nurses and other professionals and in collaboration with ongoing holistic and pharmaceutical research, it may be from the so-called complementary methods offered today that components may be found to arrest the cancer process itself in the future.

References

Bay, F. (1995). Complementary therapies — just another task? *Complementary Therapies in Nursing and Midwifery*. 1, 34–6.

Bridge, L. R., Benson, P, Pietroni P. C., and Priest, R. G. (1988). Relaxation and imagery in the treatment of breast cancer. *British Medical Journal*, 297, 1169–72.

Clover A., Last, P., and Fisher, P. (1995). Complementary cancer therapy: a pilot study of patients, therapies and quality of life. *Complementary Therapies in Medicine*. 3, 129–33.

Corner, J., Cawley, N., and Hildebrand S. (1995). An evaluation of the use of massage and essential oils on the wellbeing of cancer patients. *International Journal of Palliative Nursing*, 1, 67–73.

Fritz, D. J. (1988). Non-invasive pain control methods used by cancer outpatients. *Oncology Nurses Forum* (supplement). p. 108.

Gadsby, J. G., Franks, A., Jarvis, P., and Dewhurst, F. (1997). Acupuncture-like transcutaneous nerve stimulation within palliative care: a pilot study. *Complementary Therapies in Medicine*, 5, 13–18.

Krieger, D. (1975). Therapeutic touch: The imprimatur of nursing. *American Journal of Nursing*, 5, 784–7.

Krieger, D. (1979). *The therapeutic touch: how to use your hands to help or heal.* Prentice-Hall, Englewood, Cliffs, New Jersey

Lanara, V. (1984). *Heroism as a nursing value.* Sisterhood Evnikin, Athens.

Lyles, J., Burish, T., Krozeley, M., and Oldham, R. (1982). Efficacy of relaxation training and guided imagery in reducing the aversiveness of cancer chemotherapy. *The Journal of Consulting and Clinical Psychology.* 50, 509–24.

Perry, B. (1996). Influence of gender on the use of silence, touch and humour. *International Journal of Palliative Nursing*, 2, 7–14.

Rankin-Box D. (1995) Managing change in the workplace. In *The nurses handbook of complementary therapies.* (ed. D. Rankin-Box), p. 13. Churchill Livingstone, Edinburgh.

Rankin-Box D. (1997). Therapies in practice: a survey of nurses' use of complementary therapies. *Complementary Therapies in Nursing and Midwifery*, **3**, 92–9.

Royal College of Nursing (1999). *In Touch*, newsletter of the Complementary Therapies in Nursing Forum.

Sayre-Adams, J. and Wright, S. G. (1995). *The theory and practice of therapeutic touch*. p. vii. Churchill Livingstone, Edinburgh.

Sims, S. (1986). Slow stroke back massage for cancer patients. *Nursing Times*, **82**, 47–50.

Stevensen, C. J. (1994*a*). The psychophysiological effects of aromatherapy following cardiac surgery. *Complementary Therapies in Medicine*, **2**, 27–35.

Stevensen, C. J. (1994*b*). All things considered: a survey of the needs the complementary therapy needs of patients with cancer. *Nursing Times*, **91**, 44–45.

Stevensen, C. J. (1996). Complementary therapies in cancer care: An NHS approach. *International Journal of Palliative Nursing* , **2**, 15–18.

Trevelyan, J. (1997). Anthroposophical medicine: a nursing perspective. *Complementary Therapies in Nursing and Midwifery*, **3**, 152–5.

UKCC (**United Kingdom Central Council**) (1992) *Code of professional conduct*. UKCC, London.

Wilkinson, S. (1995). Aromatherapy and massage in palliative care. *International Journal of Palliative Nursing*,**1**, 21–30.

Wright S. G. (1995). Bringing the heart back into nursing. *Complementary Therapies in Nursing and Midwifery*, **1**, 15–20.

Chapter 22

Complementary therapy and paediatric cancer

Sheila Weitzman

Sheila Weitzman is Senior Staff Oncologist and Associate Director of Clinical Affairs, Division of Haematology/Oncology, Hospital for Sick Children, Toronto and Associate Professor, Department of Paediatrics, University of Toronto. She has a long-standing interest in alternative/complementary therapy for paediatric malignancy.

Cancer remains the second commonest cause of death in childhood and the commonest cause of death from disease, none the less approximately 75% of children with cancer are being cured with traditional therapy (Fig. 22.1; Robison 1997). For some cancers such as Hodgkin's disease, non-Hodgkin's lymphoma, germ cell tumour, retinoblastoma, hepatoblastoma, and Wilm's tumour, the cure rates now approach 90% or better. For the most part, the common tumours of childhood are significantly more sensitive to chemotherapy

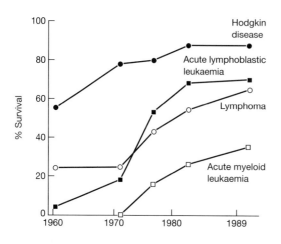

Fig. 22.1 Cancer specific trends in 5-year survival for children younger than 15 years of age, determined in the Surveillance Epidemiology, and End Results program. (Adapted from *Cancer statistics review 1973–88*, ed. L. A. Ries, B. F. Hankey, B. A. Miller, *et al.* (1991). NIH publication no 91-2789. National Cancer Institute, Bethesda.)

than are the adult epithelial malignancies (carcinomas), and children have the added advantage of being able to tolerate chemotherapy better. With a few exceptions, mostly metastatic cancers, every child with cancer has at least a chance for cure with conventional therapy and clearly, whatever else we do, *nothing should be done or given to a child with cancer that will interfere with the traditional therapy*.

The worst thing a parent or practitioner can do is to refuse or delay conventional therapy. This does not mean however, that parents and patients should have no choices in their treatment.

Complementary therapies have not been shown to improve the survival rates of children with cancer, but childhood cancer patients and their parents can work within the framework of traditional therapy to improve the quality of survival. The concept of the 'Wellness Community' (Benjamin 1995), that cancer patients who participate in their fight for recovery improve the quality of their lives, and may possibly enhance their chance of recovery, is an important one for children as well as adults. Although it is difficult to prove, it appears to make intuitive sense that one's emotional and mental state is important in recovery from a physical disease. Unquestionably those children with a healthy and positive attitude appear to tolerate not only chemotherapy better, but also other aspects of their treatment such as recovery from limb salvage surgery.

Complementary medicine

Many terms have been used to describe complementary medicine including alternative, unorthodox, unconventional, holistic, homoeopathic, Eastern medicine, and natural medicine. In a recent survey of paediatric cancer patients the term alternative therapy was used for those remedies that lack scientific testing and lack recognition of effectiveness by conventional medicine (Fernandez *et al.* 1998). Examples included naturopathy, homoeopathy, and herbal and Chinese remedies. Complementary therapies were defined as those used in addition to conventional therapy, to improve the well-being of the child and to relieve symptoms, and included the psychological and behavioural approaches. Both terms are frowned on by some non-traditional therapists however, and in much of the literature they are used interchangeably to describe any therapy that has not undergone rigorous scientific testing.

The use of complementary therapies has greatly increased in recent years, and the number of visits to alternative practitioners now exceeds those of visits to physicians (Sawyer *et al.* 1994). In the study by Fernandez, 25% of parents who gave complementary therapies to their children spent between $1000–10 000 and 5% spent more than $10 000 (Fernandez *et al.* 1998).

Why parents choose complementary therapies

Two studies, from Canada (Fernandez *et al.* 1998) and Australia (Sawyer *et al.* 1994), found that 42–46% of all paediatric cancer patients receive alternative or complementary therapies at some point in their disease, and many studies have shown that the same is true of adult patients (Lerner and Kennedy 1992; Cassileth *et al.* 1984).

There appear to be many reasons for this phenomenon. Public distrust of government and 'profit-driven' pharmaceutical companies has led to the belief that a conspiracy exists to suppress a cancer cure. This is added to by the limited success, and toxicity, of traditional

Table 22.1 Reasons indicated by parents for the use of alternative and complementary therapies in paediatric oncology patients (*n*=156)

To do everything possible for their child	82%
To 'boost' the immune system	77%
To cure the cancer	40%
To give 'softer' treatment	38%
To slow the progression of the cancer	35%
To use a more holistic approach	33%
To use psychologic forces	30%

Adapted with permission. Fernandez *et al.* (1998)[3]

therapy, as well as the belief that alternative therapies are 'natural' and therefore better. There is also a belief that bad diet causes cancer and therefore dietary manipulation must be able to cure it.

The reasons some parents chose complementary therapies for their children are shown in Table 22.1 (Fernandez *et al.* 1998), with the commonest being that they wanted to do everything possible for their child, a reason with which it is difficult to argue. Pendergrass in addition, found that complementary therapy was used to alleviate symptoms such as pain and nausea, because of religious beliefs or because the parents were advised to do so (Pendergrass and Davis 1991). As would be expected, more children with advanced disease, and those at high risk of death, were found to receive complementary therapy.

As soon as the diagnosis is confirmed, parents are inundated with material on complementary therapies by concerned friends and relatives, by complementary therapists, through newspapers, books, pamphlets and increasingly today through the internet. It is extremely difficult for parents to judge the merits of the claims made.

Helping parents make informed decisions

In general, the concepts on which traditional methods are based such as 'evidence-based care', and 'statistical significance being essential to demonstrate efficacy', are not nearly as convincing to the lay-person, particularly one whose child is facing death, as anecdotes of apparently successful therapy.

Cancer patients, and the parents of children with cancer, believe that they should take an active role in their healthcare and that they should have the freedom to choose their therapy. For this freedom of choice to be meaningful, however, it is vital that the relative merits of the choices with which they are faced are clearly understood. Parents therefore need to be taught to assess critically the available evidence.

During a recent conference, a parent of a child with a brain tumour asked why an anecdote about the successful use of a complementary therapy in a child of similar age, with the same tumour in the same position as his own child's tumour, should not be more meaningful to him than the results of a trial of traditional therapy.

The answer is simple; taking an anecdote as evidence, does not take into account positive and negative reporting biases whereby successes are usually reported but failures are not. Without knowing the number of children treated on a specific therapy, it is impossible to judge the efficacy of the therapy. A report of one good success does not mean that the drug did not fail in the remainder of the patients to whom it was given. Two other examples illustrate other important problems with anecdotes.

A patient at HSC was diagnosed with Hodgkin's disease, treated with conventional methods and did well. A year later, the patient was seen by a different physician for node enlargement and was diagnosed with a relapse. The primary physician, returning from leave, felt that a viral infection was a more likely cause, and asked for a biopsy. The parents refused as the patient's nodes had shrunk. They attributed the shrinkage to 2 weeks of herbal therapy.

Before judging the outcome of an intervention, it is important to be sure that the patient actually had the disease for which he was treated.

An adult patient received radiation therapy to the floor of the mouth for a carcinoma. He then went to Mexico for alternative therapy and for the rest of his life publicized the alternative therapy as curing his cancer. Radiation therapy to that particular cancer in that position is, however, curative in 90% of cases.

It is important that no other therapy, that may have affected the outcome, was given prior to or concomitantly with the therapy being evaluated. To judge the value of an anecdotal therapy, parents should attempt to answer the questions outlined in Table 22.2. If they cannot, the testimonial is valueless.

Understanding placebo effects

Any intervention given to a randomly selected group of individuals who are assured that it will 'work', may result in improvement in up to 50% of cases (Rosenfeld 1996a). Placebos do not shrink tumours or cure cancer, but they may affect subjective symptoms such as pain, fatigue, nausea, hunger, anxiety, and depression. The more empathetic and trusted the prac-

Table 22.2 Questions for a parent to ask about any therapy being considered

How many children have been treated with the therapy?
How many were successful and how many failed?
How many had the same disease as your child?
Was the disease proven by biopsy (X-ray is not enough) within a reasonable time period of the therapy?
Did the child have any other treatment before or during the therapy ?
How was the response demonstrated?
If it was demonstrated radiologically was it the same method, at the exact same location as the pre therapy scan?
What was the toxicity of the therapy, both immediate and long-term?

titioner prescribing the placebo, the better it works. When judging testimonials/anecdotes, the placebo effect needs to be remembered.

In general one would hope for more than a placebo effect when treating a patient, but the usefulness of such an effect in reducing symptoms is both underestimated and underutilized.

Avoiding the unscrupulous practitioner

A recent publication on alternative medicine defined a 'quack' as someone who, for personal or financial gain, regardless of qualifications, sells, prescribes, or performs treatments that he or she knows to be ineffective, dangerous, or both (Rosenfeld 1996b). Unfortunately a medical degree is no guarantee of good faith, as all too many licensed physicians are only too ready to 'rip off' patients to make money. Reasons for parents to be suspicious include the following:

- practitioner who claims the existence of a conspiracy to withhold cures. One out of 3 oncologists and their immediate families will develop cancer. They would scarcely be part of a conspiracy to hide a cure. In fact any oncologist would give up a great deal to be the first person to discover the 'cancer cure';
- demands for payment up-front;
- selling a product that promises to cure a wide variety of ailments — cancer, arthritis, skin diseases, dropsy, AIDS, gastric complaints all with the same easy remedy;
- instant fix;
- testimonials and 'case histories' to bolster claims but no studies;
- the therapist recommends stopping conventional therapy, or refers to it as 'slash, poison, and burn';
- the therapist has excuses for a tumour that is getting worse, such as, 'it appears to be bigger but it has changed in size so treatment is working', 'the tumour is growing out of the leg so that's good', 'the leukaemic blast count has risen but so have the lymphocytes (immune cells) so the vaccine is working'.

These therapists, however empathetic they may seem, should be avoided.

Current complementary cancer therapies

It is not possible to discuss all the contemporary complementary practices in any single text. The commonest types of complementary therapies used in children appear to have changed since Pendergrass' earlier study in which faith healers, megavitamins, metabolic therapies, immune therapies, and mind control of cancer were most frequent (Pendergrass and Davis 1981). Dietary therapies in this early study were reported to be used rarely, but the results of a more recent survey suggests an increased frequency (Fernandez *et al.* 1998). The types of complementary therapies used tend to reflect the current social and cultural interests, and to mimic what is popular in the conventional therapy of a particular era. In the Fernandez series shown in Table 22.3, 60.8% of children were given herbal teas, while the second commonest therapy was given to stimulate the immune system. Most parents used a combination of pharmacologic therapy and mind-body interventions, of which the commonest was relaxation/imagery techniques (Fernandez *et al.* 1998).

Table 22.3 Alternative and complementary therapies used by paediatric oncology patients

Therapy	no	%	95%CI (%)
Alternative therapies (n=130)			
Herbal teas	79	60.8	52–69
Plant extracts	73	56.2	48–65
Therapeutic vitamins	71	54.6	46–63
Diet	64	49.2	41–58
Essiac tea	60	46.2	38–55
Shark cartilage	25	19.2	12–26
Homoeopathy	23	17.7	11–24
Lactobacillus	20	15.4	9–22
Chinese medication	20	15.4	9–22
Ozone therapy	7	5–40	2–9
Complementary therapies (n=97)			
Relaxation/imagery	73	75.2	67–84
Massage	64	66.0	57–75
Therapeutic touch	41	42.2	32–52
Chiropractic	19	19.6	11–28
Hypnosis	3	3.1	0–6

Adapted with permission. Fernandez et al. (1998)[3]

Herbal therapies

The finding that herbal teas were the commonest alternative therapy used in paediatric cancer patient, reflects the prevailing view that these preparations are 'natural' and therefore harmless. This perception is false. Many commonly prescribed pharmaceuticals are extracts from different species of plants including several anticancer drugs such as vincristine (periwinkle plant) and paclitaxel (western yew). The problem is to know which herbs are useful, which are toxic, and in particular, when treating a paediatric cancer, to know which may interfere with and reduce the effects of the traditional therapy. In North America, the production remains unregulated, the potency of preparations may vary even within brands, there may be ingredients other than those listed, and additional chemicals may have been added. Some have been deliberately fortified with steroids, non-steroidal anti-inflammatories and even tranquillizers. One of the foremost advocates of the use of herbal medicine has been quoted as calling the North American market 'a minefield of hyperbole and hoax' (Rosenfeld 1996b).

This problem is confounded when a child is taking a mixture of herbs such as is found in herbal teas. Fortunately European countries have established better standards with respect to purity and potency, none the less patients, parents, and caregivers need to consider the active ingredients in herbal preparations to be drugs and to demand that they be regulated as such. The ease with which Noni juice remains obtainable, despite reports of potential lethal toxicity (Lewis 1998), clearly illustrates the problem. Regulation is unlikely to occur however, because of the conception that traditional practitioners are deliberately trying to hide useful therapies, as well as the conception that people have the right to choose their therapy even if it has been proven to be useless.

Parents should be aware of the problems and should limit the use in their children to herbs that have some basis in science, and which have been found to be non-toxic. All medication given to a child with cancer, traditional and non-traditional, should be subjected to the same scrutiny (see Table 22.2), before the drug is used. Unfortunately the few clinical trials that have been done, for example with Essiac (Jacobs 1997) have failed to show an effect on survival. The high incidence of use of herbal therapies in children with cancer however, means that herbal preparations must become the focus of more trials. Herbal therapy may well have a role in supportive care of childhood cancer patients, but efficacy, lack of toxicity and lack of interference with traditional therapy must be clearly shown.

Immune therapies

Several complementary drugs are used in an attempt to stimulate the immune system to fight cancer cells. Two examples are echinacea and mistletoe extracts. Both are said to stimulate the immune system through several mechanisms. Mistletoe, for example has been shown to stimulate T-cell migration, increase spleen cell responses to phytohaemagglutinin and concavalin A (Kuttan and Kuttan 1992) and to stimulate natural killer cell cytotoxicity (Schink 1997), amongst other activities. Trials in cancer patients have shown mixed results with some trials demonstrating a prolongation of survival (Moss *et al.* 1996), while others have shown no responses (Friess *et al.* 1996; Gabius *et al.* 1994).

Clinical trials, particularly in paediatric patients, should be done to establish the true usefulness of this drug in childhood cancer patients. As there is no information on the interaction with conventional therapy and at least one recent alternative text lists it as very toxic and a herb to be avoided (Pressman 1999), mistletoe cannot be recommended until proper trials are done.

Several children seen recently at HSC have been on echinacea at the time of diagnosis. Although it certainly failed to prevent the onset of cancer in these young patients, little can be said about it outside of a trial. Even theoretically however, although there is some evidence of its effectiveness in patients with influenza and coryza, the use of a drug that stimulates the immune system on a chronic basis in a normal child can only be deplored.

Similarly although a recent study at HSC showed that it is probably safe taken in pregnancy as far as fetal malformations are concerned (Koren, personal communication), the use of any drug that is not essential during pregnancy cannot be supported. It points, once again, to the fact that these substances are not thought of as drugs, a mind-set that needs to change.

Mind-body interventions

Faith healing

In its traditional form, faith healing involved the use of prayers and incantations associated with laying on of hands to get rid of the evil spirit which occupied the body and caused the disease, a combination of healing through divine intervention and exorcism (Achterberg *et al.* 1994). Today it is equally commonly used to mean spiritual healing through prayer, without the other interventions. In the series by Pendergrass and Davis (1991) it is quoted as the most commonly used complementary practice in paediatric cancer but the authors feel that most parents included simple prayer in this category. The only real disadvantage of this and other mind-body interventions is that patients are taught that they can control their disease and they therefore feel responsible if it does not work.

Support groups and psychotherapy

The oft quoted study by Spiegel et al. (1989) showing that women with breast cancer who took part in support groups lived on average 18 months longer than a control group who did not, has lent credence to the belief that treatment of emotional and mental health can affect physiological function and is an important part of cancer therapy. Psychotherapy has been shown to be important in alleviating symptoms such as expectant vomiting and pain. It also has the advantage of being cost-effective and non-invasive. These methods should be considered to be part of the overall therapy of patients who are old enough to participate.

Biofeedback

Biofeedback is a treatment method that uses monitoring instruments such as electrodes attached to various parts of the body to feed back to patients information about their body of which they are normally unaware. With the help of mental exercises and through trial and error, the patient learns to control certain bodily functions such as heart rate, blood pressure, mood, and so on. The greatest use is in relaxation and reduction of stress (Pressman 1999).

Meditation

Meditation is defined as a self directed method of relaxing the body and calming the mind. Today it is a well-accepted technique for reduction of stress and has been shown to allay anxiety and reduce the severity of chronic pain. Adverse effects have been reported in a small number of patients including feelings of disorientation and negativity, and even induction of schizophrenic episodes.

Music therapy

Music therapy is an important part of complementary therapy in childhood cancer because of its universal applicability even to infants and very young children. A large body of research has documented its usefulness in reducing fear and anxiety, and inducing relaxation, in ill and hospitalized children. It has also been useful in reducing stress associated with painful procedures in selected patients (Achterberg et al. 1994).

Art therapy

Art therapy is also particularly useful in young children, enabling them to express fears and concerns that they cannot express by other means. In addition it can often be used by trained practitioners to assess how children are coping with the illness and its therapy. Art therapists are trained in diagnosis and in helping patients with specific problems, including in the area of childhood bereavement (Zambelli et al. 1989).

Many other mind-body therapies including hypnosis, aromatherapy, and guided imagery are available and all have their proponents. As far as paediatric cancer is concerned, 50% of paediatric malignancies occur in children less than 5 years of age in whom the majority of these therapies have limited or no benefit.

There is absolutely no evidence that any of these therapies, including faith healing and psychotherapy, cure paediatric cancer. Their usefulness lies in their ability to improve the quality of life of children who are old enough to understand and to participate, and to help them cope with the rigors of curative conventional therapy.

Nutritional therapy for cancer

During the past two decades there has been considerable scientific study of the relationship between nutrition, calorie and fat consumption, and the development of cancer. Sufficient evidence has been found that alteration in diet can reduce the risk of certain adult cancers that the National Institute of Health in the United States has now published suggested dietary guidelines (Weinhouse *et al.* 1991). These recommendations are not meant to be applied indiscriminately to children where excessively restricted diets may impair normal growth and development. The recommendations are also not intended to suggest that dietary manipulation can cure established cancer (Ca 1993). However during the past decades there has been a resurgence of nutritional therapies involving diet, herbal, and vitamin supplements. Amongst the commonest are the macrobiotic diet, the Gerson diet, the Livingston diet, and vitamin and mineral supplementation.

The macrobiotic diet

This was modified and popularized in the USA by Michio Kushi and it is now the most commonly used unconventional nutritional approach to cancer (Dwyer 1990). Apart from the diet it offers also a 'spiritual philosophy'. The diet, which is primarily vegetarian, high complex carbohydrate, and low-fat, is based mainly on cereal grains, vegetables, seaweeds, and beans. Nutritionists feel that the diet does not conform to any accepted theory of nutritional support and is not helpful in maintaining nutritional status amongst cancer patients since the diet is high in bulk, low in several essential nutrients such as vitamins D, B12, iron and calcium, and relatively low in calories.

The Gerson diet

The patient eats mainly a raw vegetarian diet and drinks freshly prepared vegetable and fruit juices every hour, takes four types of enemas, including coffee enemas for 'detoxification' of the body and as originally prescribed, consumes 2–3 glasses of fresh calf's liver serum, now replaced by carrot juice. Other elements include salt restriction and potassium supplementation, extreme fat restriction, temporary protein restriction, iodine and thyroid administration, and vitamin C (Lerner 1994*a*).

Livingston therapy

The program of the Livingston-Wheeler Clinic includes a primarily vegetarian wholefood diet. The therapy also includes fresh whole-blood transfusions preferably from a family member, gamma-globulin, splenic extract, and a variety of vaccines including an autologous vaccine prepared from the patient's own blood, BCG, and other non-specific vaccines. Antibiotics are also given and supplemental megadose vitamins including A, C, E, B6, and B12. Purging with enemas including coffee, frequent hot tubs with vinegar in water, and a program to acidify the blood are also included (Lerner 1994*b*). In a prospective study, Cassileth and colleagues (1991) randomized patients with metastatic cancer to standard therapy with or without Livingston therapy, and found that there was no difference in survival between the 2 groups, and unexpectedly also no improvement in the quality of life of patients receiving the diet.

There is no evidence that nutritional therapies produce dramatic survival benefits. They may however, as shown by a British review of the Gerson diet, improve the quality of survival by improving mood and confidence. The nature of the Gerson and other dietary therapies 'requires an active contribution by the patient and family to his/her state of health and meets a need not satisfied by conventional therapy' (Reed *et al.* 1990). This involvement of the patient and family may be the most important part of any of the dietary therapies described.

Careful assessment of the popular diets shows that these so-called successful diets vary from each other in a number of significant ways. However, they all have a central theme which is a low fat, high fibre diet, high in fruits and vegetables, the same diet which is recommended to decrease the incidence of several adult carcinomas.

Lerner summarizes the scientific evidence, case reports, and clinical assessments by physicians by stating that these dietary programs are clearly not definitive cures for any cancer, but that survival may be enhanced by *any* healthy vegetarian diet as well as the will to live and a healthy attitude towards life (Dwyer 1990).

There is no evidence that these diets have any role in the therapy of paediatric tumours. Strict application of these diets may indeed be nutritionally harmful in young patients (Dwyer 1992). There is also no evidence for the role of 'detoxification' and apart from other side-effects such as death from electrolyte imbalance, bowel necrosis and perforation, toxic colitis, and hypochloraemia (Pendergrass and Davis 1981), coffee or other enemas are strongly contraindicated in a population that is frequently neutropenic.

From a dietary point of view, the most important role a parent can play is to maintain good nutrition of the child, however possible. The addition of fruits and vegetables is desirable if it can be acheived while maintaining a balanced intake, without giving a diet too high in bulk. Involvement of parents and patients in this area has the added advantage of satisfying their need for active involvement and for some degree of control.

Vitamin therapy

Vitamin C

This functions as a chemical reducing agent and antioxidant, and many studies have suggested that it reduces the incidence of gastric cancer, bladder cancer, and possibly other epithelial cancers such as lung and breast cancer (Howe 1990). A study by Sinks and Wilkins in children with brain tumours found that a statistically significant threefold risk of delivering a child who later developed a brain tumour was associated with low maternal intake of vitamin C during pregnancy, an effect that remained after adjustment for other factors (Block 1991). High-dose vitamin C was touted by Cameron and Pauling (1978) as a means of prolonging life in cancer patients, but controlled studies have found no difference in outcome among patients taking Vitamin C or placebo either in heavily pretreated patients or in patients who received no previous therapy (Creagan *et al.* 1979; Moertel *et al.* 1985). The potential adverse effects include the possibility that in *pharmacologic* amounts vitamin C is both pro-oxidant and cancer-promoting, by releasing cancer promoting, highly oxidant catalytic iron from ferritin (Herbert and Kasdan 1993). High dose vitamin C has no role in the therapy of paediatric cancer patients.

Vitamin A and carotenoids

A large body of evidence suggests that foods high in vitamin A and carotenoids are protective against the development of a variety of epithelial cancers (Mettlin 1984; Mettlin *et al.* 1979). No association has been published in paediatric cancer. Trans-retinoic acid has been effective in the treatment of acute promyelocytic leukaemia in children and adults, and cis-retinoic acid is being tried as a differentiating agent in advanced stage neuroblastoma.

The use of high-dose Vitamin A as a nutritional therapy in advanced malignant disease has been disappointing. In addition, large amounts of retinoids in the blood or tissues can be toxic to skin, liver, and brain and may cause birth defects (Olson 1983), although it appears that beta-carotene can be given safely.

Vitamin E

Biochemical studies suggest that vitamin E functions as a lipid soluble antioxidant and free radical scavenger and may be important in reducing the incidence of epithelial cancers. The only toxicity reported is due to interference with platelet aggregation and bleeding in patients on anticoagulants (Hildenbrand *et al.* 1992).

Selenium

Evidence suggests that there is a strong inverse correlation between selenium intake and selenium levels in the blood and cancer risk in adults (Bertram *et al.* 1987), although no studies exist in paediatric malignancy. Selenium is among the most toxic essential elements and the narrow range of safe levels of intake of this nutrient suggest that the use of selenium as a food supplement cannot be recommended. American Cancer Society guidelines suggest that a varied diet should ensure adequate selenium intake, with selenium being mainly found in seafood, meat, and cereals.

A recent review found that although observational studies indicate that diet high in antioxidants may prevent certain adult cancers, results from prospective studies of antioxidant supplementation have failed to demonstrate efficacy in preventing cancer for any of the antioxidants tried, with the exception of a trial in the Chinese population who had significant nutritional deficiencies (Mayne 1997).

It appears that supplementation should be limited at present to people with low levels of antioxidants. There is little disagreement, on the other hand, about the importance of a high intake of antioxidants in the form of fresh fruits and vegetables.

Refusal of conventional therapy

By far the most significant problem related to complementary therapy is parental refusal of potentially curative traditional therapy. In the Fernandez (1998) study, only 2% of the parents who responded refused conventional therapy. However, this problem is being seen with increasing frequency in paediatric cancer centres. This year alone there have been 6 cases seen at 3 children's hospitals in Canada. Potential cure rates ranged from 60–90%. Four of these children subsequently died, while the other two accepted therapy only after disease progression to a stage requiring considerably more therapy.

Parental right to choose their child's therapy is an extremely controversial topic, but fortunately the law is clear on the issue. Parents can make that decision for themselves but not for their underage children. Paediatric oncologists should make every effort to persuade parents of the value of therapy including using the 'survivors' who have been through therapy for the same tumour. They are often the most vocal and certainly the most persuasive proponents of the traditional therapy. In the end, oncologists are required by law to assume that the interests of the child supersede those of the parents.

Conclusion

An appraisal of the literature makes it obvious that there remains a clear gap between the conventional cancer therapist with his/her belief in evidence-based medicine and the purveyors of alternative therapies. What is equally obvious is that the parents of paediatric cancer patients have demonstrated a clear need for therapies other than the conventional, which will allow them some degree of control over their children's treatment, particularly when conventional therapy fails. Possibly the most important way to fulfil this need is a caring attitude on the part of the oncology team which includes dealing with not only the medical concerns but all aspects of the patient's life. If cancer patients do not receive this type of treatment and support from their oncologist, they will seek it elsewhere and often pay large sums of money to do so.

On present evidence, alternative therapies do not offer hope of cure of an established paediatric malignancy, but judicious attention to diet and to the general well-being of the patient, as against the purely medical concerns, can lead to improved quality of life.

When one considers the wide variety of complementary therapies available, all of which have their avid and vocal proponents, it is evident that money and time needs to be spent on testing the most promising of the complementary therapies. We need to be able to offer parents some guidance in their quest to do the best they can for their child. Because it is patently impossible to test all available therapies, parents too need to learn to judge the value of a therapy and to look past unsubstantiated testimonials in order to make the best choices. By so doing, the extreme portions of alternative programs such as unnecessary blood transfusion therapy, unproven immune manipulations, extreme food restrictions (to name a few) can be avoided. For the patient or parent to be allowed to feel that they are seen as individuals with individual needs and that they play an active and important role in the care, may be the most important lesson that traditional therapists can learn.

The dying patient, or their parents, will always seek a miracle and complementary therapies will always abound. The demand of medical practitioners for evidence of efficacy will, and should, always exist, but the realization that efficacy does not only refer to prolongation of survival, but also to quality of life, should allow for integration of the best of the conventional with those areas of the unconventional that seem safe, reasonable, and desirable.

References

Achterberg, J., Dossey, L., Gordon, J. S., *et al.* (1994). Mind-body interventions. In *Alternative medicine. Expanding medical horizons* (ed. B. M. Berman and D. B. Larson), pp. 3–43. A report to the NIH on alternative Medical systems and Practices in the United States.

Benjamin, H. H. (1995). *The wellness community guide to fighting for recovery from cancer.* GP Putnam's sons, New York

Bertram, J. S., Kolonel, I. N., and Meyskens, F. L. (1987). Rationale and strategies for chemoprevention of cancer in humans. *Cancer Research,* **47,** 3012–31.

Block, G. (1991). Vitamin C and cancer prevention: the epidemiologic evidence. *American Journal of Clinical Nutrition,* **53,** 270S–82S.

Ca (1993). *CA—A Cancer Journal for Clinicians,* **43,** 309–19.

Cameron, E. and Pauling, L. (1978). Supplemental ascorbate in the supportive treatment of cancer: Prolongation of survival times in terminal human cancer. *Proceedings of National Academy of Science,* **75,** 4538–42.

Cassileth, B. R., Lusk, E. J., Strause, T. D., and Bodenheimer, B. J. (1984). Contemporary unorthodox treatments in cancer medicine. A study of patients, treatments and practitioners. *Ann Intern Med,* **101,** 105–12.

Cassileth, B. R., Lusk, E. J., Guerry, D., *et al.* (1991). Survival and quality of life among patients receiving unproven as compared with conventional cancer therapy. *New England Journal of Medicine,* **325,** 1180–5.

Creagan, E. T., Moertel, C. G., O'Fallon, J. R., *et al.* (1979). Failure of high-dose vitamin C (ascorbic acid) therapy to benefit patients with advanced cancer. *New England Journal of Medicine,* **301,** 687–90.

Dwyer, J. (1990). The macrobiotic diet: no cancer cure. *Nutrition Forum,* **7,** 9–11.

Dwyer, J. (1992). Unproven nutritional remedies and cancer. *Nutrition Reviews,* **50,** 106–9.

Fernandez, C. V., Stutzer, C. A., MacWilliam, L., and Fryer, C. (1998). Alternative and complementary therapy use in paediatric oncology patients in British Columbia: Prevalence and reasons for use and nonuse. *Clinical Oncology,* **16,** 1279–86.

Friess, H., Beger, H. G., Kunz, J., *et al.* (1996). Treatment of advanced pancreatic cancer with mistletoe: results of a pilot trial. *Anticancer Res,* **16,** 915–20.

Gabius, H. J., Gabius, S., Joshi, S. S., *et al.* (1994). From ill-defined extracts to the immunomodulatory lectin: will there be a reason for oncological application of mistletoe. *Planta Med,* **60,** 2–7.

Herbert, V. and Kasdan, T. S. (1993). Ferritin iron and vitamin C as cancer promoters (meeting abstract). *Molecular biology of hematopoeisis,* 8th symposium, Basel, Switzerland, pp. 118, July.

Hildenbrand, G., Collin, J., Gaby, A., *et al.* (1992). Diet and nutrition in the prevention and treatment of chronic disease. In *Alternative medicine. Expanding medical horizons* (ed. B. M. Berman and D. B. Larson), pp. 207–70.

Howe, G. (1990). Dietary factors and risk of breast cancer: Combined analysis of 12 case–controlled studies. *JAMA* **82,** 561–9.

Jacobs, J. J. (1997). Unproven alternative methods of cancer treatment. In *Cancer: principles and practice of oncology.* 5th edn, (ed. V. T. Devita, S. Hellman, S. A. Rosenberg), pp. 2993–3001. Lippincott–Raven, Philadelphia.

Kuttan, G. and Kuttan, R. (1992). Immunological mechanisms of action of the tumour reducing peptide from Mistletoes. *Cancer Lett,* **66,** 123–30.

Lerner, I. J. and Kennedy, B. J. (1992). The prevalence of questionable methods of cancer treatment in the United States. CA, **42,** 181–91.

Lerner, M. (1994*a*). *Choices in healing.* pp. 261–283, MIT Press, Cambridge, Mass.

Lerner, M. (1994*b*). *Choices in healing.* pp. 319–333. MIT Press, Cambridge, Mass

Lewis, R. (1998). Walk safely in four directions, *Canadian Journal of Herbalish*, **19**, 12–13.

Mayne, S. T. (1997). Antioxidant nutrients and cancer incidence and mortality: an epidemiologic perspective. *Adv Pharmacol.*, **38**, 657–75.

Mettlin, C. (1984). Epidemiologic studies on vitamin A and cancer. *Adv in Nutrition Res* 6, 47–65.

Mettlin, C, Graham S, Swanson M. (1979). Vitamin A and lung cancer. *J Nat Cancer Instit.* 62, 1435–1438.

Moertel, C. G., Fleming, T. R., Creagan, E. T., *et al.* (1985). High dose vitamin C versus placebo in treatment of patients with advanced cancer who have had no prior chemotherapy A randomized double blind comparison. *New England Journal of Medicine*, **312**, 137–41.

Moss, R. W., Wiewel, F. D., Bedell, B., *et al.* (1996). Pharmacological and biological treatments. In *Alternative medicine. Expanding medical horizons.* A report to the NIH on alternative Medical systems and practices in the United States (ed. B. M. Berman and D. B. Larson), pp. 159–82.

Olson, J. A. (1983). Adverse effects of large doses of vitamin A and retinoids. *Seminars in Oncology*, 10, 290–3.

Pendergrass, T. W. and Davis, S. (1981). Knowledge and use of alternative cancer therapies in children. *Am J Pediatr Hematol Oncol*, 3, 339–45.

Pressman, A. H. (1999). Herbs. In *Idiots guide to alternative medicine.* p 201. Simon & Shuster Macmillan, New York.

Reed, A., James, N., Sikora, K. (1990). Mexico, juices, coffee enemas and cancer. *Lancet*, **336**, 676–7.

Robison, L. (1997). General principles of the epidemiology of childhood cancer. In *Principles and practice of paediatric oncology, 3rd edn* (eds. P. A. Pizzo and D. G. Poplack), pp. 1–10. Lippincott–Raven, Philadelphia.

Rosenfeld, I. (1996*a*). In *Dr Rosenfeld's guide to alternative medicine*, pp. 10–18, Ballantine's books.

Rosenfeld, I. (1996*b*). In *Dr Rosenfeld's guide to alternative medicine*, pp.19–28, Ballantine's books

Sawyer, M. F., Gannoni, A. F., Toogood, I. R., *et al.* (1994). The use of alternative therapies in children with cancer. *Medical Journal of Australia*, **160**, 320–2.

Schink, M. (1997). Mistletoe therapy for human cancer, the role of the natural killer cells. *Anticancer Drugs*, 8, Suppl 1:S 47–51.

Spiegel, D., Bloom, J. R., Kraemer, H. C., Gottheil, E. (1989). Effect of psychosocial treatment on survival of patients with metastatic breast cancer. *Lancet*, 2, 888–91.

Weinhouse, S., Bal, D. G., Adamson, R., *et al.* (1991). American Cancer Society guidelines on diet, nutrition and cancer. *CA–A Cancer Journal for Clinicians*, **41**, 334–8.

Zambelli, G. C., Clark, E. J., and Heegard, M. (1989). Art therapy for bereaved children. In *Advances in art therapy* (ed. H. Wadeson, J. Durkin, and D. Perach), pp. 60–80. Wiley and Sons, New York.

Chapter 23

Providing complementary therapies in a cancer hospital

Judy Young and Nest Howells

Judy Young qualified as a radiotherapy radiographer in 1967 and continued to treat cancer patients until 1989 when she undertook a further training in psychotherapy and counselling. In 1993 she was involved in setting up the Lynda Jackson Macmillan Centre for Cancer Support and Information at Mount Vernon Hospital where she now works as Director of Services and head of the counselling team.

Nest Howells qualified as a nurse in 1974 and worked in oncology for 15 years before training in holistic massage, aromatherapy, reflexology, and Reiki healing. In 1993 she was appointed as Complementary Therapy Co-ordinator at the Lynda Jackson Macmillan Centre at Mount Vernon Hospital where she worked for four years before returning to Wales.

In the past decade, complementary therapies have become increasingly used by people with cancer (Downer *et al.* 1994) and are gradually changing the face of cancer patient care. In some hospitals they are now available within cancer treatment centres as part of the package of supportive care, although universal acceptance, particularly by the medical establishment, is still a long way off.

The growth of complementary therapies within healthcare has generally been fragmented, and uncoordinated. Wood (1994) found that of sixty-six cancer centres audited within the United Kingdom, only 63% had a recognized structure of patient support (including complementary therapies) with funding being an important determining factor. The range of therapies was limited, with half the centres offering one or two types of therapy, the most popular being aromatherapy and relaxation, followed by reflexology.

The models for therapy provision ranged from a well established support service with several multi-skilled therapists, to individual therapists working in isolation, often part-time and sometimes in a voluntary capacity. Availability tended to be determined by local interest, motivation, and resources.

Funding limitations suggest that the situation may not improve dramatically except where major charities or fund-raising is involved, although Lewith (1996) insists that complementary therapies in cancer hospitals are here to stay. Furthermore, one of the most important reasons for the provision of complementary therapies is that they are high on the list of patient priorities, particularly as a source of emotional and physical support (Maher *et al.*1994). Indeed Brigden (1995) reports that more than half of all cancer patients use some form of complementary therapy during the course of their illness.

Traditionally complementary therapies were only available to patients with advanced cancer and were offered as part of the palliative care package. The use of complementary therapies has now expanded to encompass patients at all stages of disease and in many centres forms part of an integrated programme of psychosocial care and support. However because of the wide-ranging needs of cancer patients and carers it is important that the complementary and orthodox approaches to cancer care and treatment are fully integrated, and that a whole range of supportive interventions (including complementary therapy) is available for patients.

This chapter will explore the cancer journey and look at some of the philosophical and practical issues of providing complementary therapies within a cancer hospital.

The cancer journey

The journey undertaken by cancer patients generally begins with an awareness of an abnormality, either on the part of the patient or discovered at routine screening, and for the unfortunate, may end in death from the disease.

At every stage of the cancer journey the patient and relatives experience a number of difficulties and a range of emotions, requiring various levels of information and support. It is difficult to provide a standard package of psychosocial care for each patient as there are no standard patients. However it is possible to provide a range of supportive care, including complementary therapies, at each stage of the cancer journey, and to educate professionals to obtain help from a number of sources as and when required by the individual patient.

The experience of diagnosis

There are few individuals in life who have the courage or indeed desire to face their own mortality, until confronted with a situation which has the potential to force the issue into the foreground of consciousness. As a result of a diagnosis of cancer, many patients experience an existential crisis which for some can have a paralysing effect until some sort of understanding is reached about the meaning of such shocking news to the individual. The shock, fear, and anger of diagnosis for many patients often changes into anticipatory anxiety about treatments and technology, and concern that despite the long treatment path ahead there are no guarantees of cure.

Negotiating the stages of the journey through the hospital system can generate both fear and frustration, leading to an increase in anxiety, making the more unpleasant side-effects of treatment feel even less bearable. Even when treatment ends, the threat of recurrence looms overhead like a sword of Damocles, and maintaining a constant vigil over the intent of this sword for many proves exhausting. Fallowfield (1990) suggests that this psychological impact is likely to be a serious long term complication of cancer treatment.

Loss and change after treatment

The psychosocial and physical impact of a cancer diagnosis and treatment can be traumatic and far reaching (Massie and Holland 1990) causing more chaos and panic than is usual in other serious illnesses (Slevin 1992). Treatment may include one or more modalities, such as surgery, chemotherapy, or radiotherapy, and may be given over several months. It might be presumed that the end of treatment would be a time of relief, even celebration. Unfortunately, evidence suggests otherwise. Survival may extract a considerable physical, social, psychological, and financial price (Zampini and Orstroff 1993).

Increased survival, even with disease present, has led to the redefinition of cancer as a chronic illness and resulting concern over the many issues of survivorship. Studies suggest that the years following cancer treatment can be fraught with difficulties and that physical and psychological well-being may actually deteriorate (Wyatt and Friedman 1996). Furthermore, psychological burnout may result where physical symptoms persist (Rapoport *et al.* 1993).

The end of treatment then is a time of transition, from being an ill person having cancer, to one regarded as well and 'normal' again. A study of patients completing treatment found that this stage was like reaching the end of a long road, facing the unknown, and without sign-posts (Howells 1997). There was loss of direction, isolation, and confusion.

> There's a sense of anticlimax, you've been looking forward for so long, but you think, what do I do now?

> There's no agenda, nothing planned.

Physical energy in this study group diminished towards the end of treatment, along with stoicism and the motivation for it, there being nothing left to fight against, to put up with, or to be brave about.

One patient described this ambivalent state:

> Much as I hated the chemotherapy and dreaded it, when I came to the last one, I didn't want it, I really didn't want it, because after that, I would be on my own.

Some patients felt abandoned, especially when care was shared between hospitals, leaving them unsure of who had primary responsibility and to whom they should turn if help was needed. Confidence was lost in the self, the body, health, the future, and the doctor's ability to detect recurrence. There was wariness of rebuilding confidence in case it was destroyed again.

Many losses were described by this group of patients, including personal, social and professional, finances and freedom of choice in many aspects of life. Temporary losses of hair, energy, and libido, could be replaced by permanent scarring, impaired function, changed appearance, compromised fertility, and chronic fatigue. Loss of control over physical health, concentration and thoughts were described, and emotional 'flashbacks' to the time of diagnosis seemed to threaten sanity.

Psychological and emotional responses varied and fluctuated in intensity but were persistent, causing surprise and dismay as, even when they faded, they were easily resurrected by events such as media items, out-patient appointments, or hearing of friends or relatives being diagnosed or dying from the disease.

Physical problems interact with psychological state and are influenced by cancer site and treatment. Fatigue, debility, and recovery can be unexpectedly prolonged (Forsberg and Cedermark 1996). Patients with some types of cancers, such as head and neck, may find physical problems more significant with the relief of cure soon overtaken by psychological distress (Rapoport *et al.* 1993). Permanent after-effects such as dry mouth, taste changes, swallowing difficulties, and changed physical appearance have been described as so bad that patients regretted having the treatment in the first place (Howells 1997).

Thus the whole experience of cancer, both diagnosis and after, has long-term physical and emotional side-effects which sadly for many cannot be left at the exit from the cancer centre.

The cancer hospital and treatments

In 1995 the Calman Hine report was published regarding the reorganization of cancer services in the UK into primary, secondary, and tertiary levels of care.

The Cancer Centre or Cancer Hospital would represent the hub of a network of cancer services, with community services being the primary level of care, through the District General Hospitals as the secondary level to the cancer centre itself as the tertiary level. Patients would visit community primary care services via the general practitioner (GP), be referred for investigations and diagnosis at the secondary level, and be referred for specialist treatment to the cancer centre. Patients would negotiate the system through channels which for them were unseen, before finally arriving for their first appointment for radiotherapy or chemotherapy at the cancer centre, which for many may be a journey of up to thirty or forty miles.

This hub and spoke model has largely been implemented throughout the UK, and although structurally this may prove to be a sound model, for the individual with cancer having to travel to a specialist centre at some distance from home can prove to be an extremely frightening and traumatic experience. In addition, the myths, fears, and apprehensions which surround cancer treatment can compound these negative experiences.

Most cancer centres include radiotherapy departments, chemotherapy suites, and two or three dedicated cancer wards. In addition, some offer certain specialist treatments such as bone marrow transplants and have specific areas which house the relevant staff and technology. By their very nature cancer centres contain 'hi-tech' rapid throughput equipment which can provoke fear and anxiety in many patients.

Patients arrive at the cancer centre often in a state of anxiety which may have been generated by a lack of information and communication. They are now not only in a state of shock over the diagnosis, but are also fearful of the treatments and the anticipated horrific side-effects.

The first appointment may be in a clinic, at the radiotherapy simulator, or in the chemotherapy suite. Each of these areas has the potential to generate further anxiety, particularly as patients often have to wait for hours to be seen. Furthermore, patients with particular difficulties such as needle phobia, dislike of being enclosed in small rooms, or a general fear of hospitals may suffer acute anxiety attacks which may be so severe as to require anxiolytic medication.

Daily visits for radiotherapy can result in tiredness, depression, and in some cases nausea and vomiting. Weekly or monthly chemotherapy treatment either as an in-patient or out-patient can result in the numerous side-effects associated with combinations of chemotherapy drugs. Tiredness, inability to sleep, hair-loss, nausea, and vomiting are amongst the more common side-effects experienced by cancer patients.

Patients who are admitted into the wards for some or all of their treatment can quickly become isolated from friends and families, becoming dependent on the medical and nursing staff.

Feelings of frustration and disappointment may arise in patients whose blood count falls too low for treatment, which ultimately may prolong the overall length of treatment causing further depression and feelings of loss of control.

Some of the drugs given to patients to offset side-effects, or enhance the body's response to treatments, are not without their own side-effects. The prescribing of steroids as an adjunct to many of the chemotherapy combinations may enhance the effect of treatment, but in addition may cause sleep disturbance, agitation, and psychosis in a small percentage of patients. Many adjuvant treatments can cause side-effects (such as menopausal symptoms from Tamoxifen) which are an additional burden for the cancer patient.

Overall the experience of cancer treatments for many patients can be one of anxiety, fatigue, stress, tension, and depression, and the provision of complementary therapies as an integral part of cancer treatment can help to improve the way in which many patients cope with this.

Some patients cope with treatments better than others, often by developing a fighting spirit and determination to do well. Patients such as these may also seek out complementary and alternative therapies to help cope with the rigours of orthodox medicine and to feel that they are contributing in some way to their own healing process. There are many patients who do **not** overtly display symptoms of anxiety, stress, or depression either during or after their treatment, and who appear to deal with the whole issue of cancer effectively without the need for additional support.

The experience of the Lynda Jackson Macmillan Centre at Mount Vernon Hospital

Setting the Scene

Mount Vernon Centre for Cancer Treatment is the centre of a network of 14 District General Hospitals in a catchment population of two million people, from which approximately 5000 cancer patients per year are referred for specialist treatment to the hospital's cancer centre.

The Lynda Jackson Macmillan Centre (LJMC) at Mount Vernon Hospital was opened in 1993 to provide support and information for people affected by cancer from within the catchment area of the cancer centre. It is an integral part of the main cancer centre service, but is housed in an adjacent purpose built building, designed and furnished to look and feel as unlike the hospital as possible.

The aims of the LJMC are to provide the cancer centre with a comprehensive back up service, supporting the staff of the cancer centre to treat and in turn support their patients. To fulfil its objectives the LJMC therefore has a number of functions all of which are interlinked with each other and with the cancer centre itself.

Functions

The LJMC acts as a drop-in centre with telephone helpline, as well as offering individual appointments for counselling and complementary therapies. Information on cancer, its treatments and side-effects, together with information on community resources, local and national support groups and other organizations is available. Psychological interventions are provided: psychiatric assessment, interventional counselling, cognitive behaviour therapy, relaxation, and visualization are offered to patients assessed as in need of these services.

A range of complementary therapies including aromatherapy, reflexology, Alexander technique, Shiatsu, and relaxation classes is offered to both in-patients and out-patients. In addition, a comprehensive network of therapists throughout the entire catchment area of the hospital has been developed for patients to access after treatment has finished.

Support groups are organized through the centre, some of which may offer a relaxation session as a component part. Because the centre acts as a safety net for patients and carers, a range of interventions is required to cover the wide-ranging needs of all those affected by cancer.

The role of complementary therapies

Most of the patients attending the LJMC are currently undergoing cancer treatment (either chemotherapy or radiotherapy), and are experiencing many of the side-effects associated with these treatments. A minority of patients attending the centre for its range of interventions have finished active treatment and are struggling to adjust to issues of survivorship. Others are experiencing a gradual deterioration in their physical condition and are feeling unwell.

The complementary therapies provided are aimed at improving the emotional well-being of the individual with cancer as well as helping to relieve some of the distress, anxiety, and pain sometimes associated with both the diagnosis and treatment.

Alexander technique, Shiatsu, reflexology, and aromatherapy are provided on an out-patient basis, and staff of the cancer centre either refer patients for therapies, or suggest that the patients drop in themselves to discuss appropriate interventions with the support staff.

Because of the popularity of these therapies and the limitation of resources, it is sometimes necessary to implement a short waiting list for individual appointments, and thus the three-times weekly relaxation classes can be used as a holding net to sustain the patient until an individual appointment slot becomes available.

However, many of these therapies are not necessarily interchangeable with each other, some being more appropriate than others for individual patients at different stages of the cancer journey. Assessment of the individual's needs and concerns therefore becomes of paramount importance before any form of complementary therapy is offered.

As part of a multicentre randomized study of complementary therapies, the psychosocial research team at the LJMC ran focus groups (1999) to investigate users' experiences of aromatherapy and relaxation classes. The key themes which emerged were that:

- relaxation was active, portable, and long-term;
- aromatherapy was more passive, non-transferable, and short-term, but gave immediate relaxation and stress relief;

- individual appointments were more motivating when lack of confidence prevented attendance at the group;
- therapies were not interchangeable, but appropriate for different people at different times.

Patients said that when they were undergoing aromatherapy they were suffering from low energy levels and needed the short term benefit of this therapy to get over the crisis, where-as the relaxation patients had slightly higher energy levels and were looking for longer term benefit for maximum impact.

Staffing

The core staff of the LJMC are oncology trained health professionals with additional qualifications in one of the complementary therapies or counselling.

The complementary therapy service was originally started by an experienced oncology nurse trained in holistic massage and reflexology, someone well-regarded by the medical staff of the cancer centre. This allowed a smoother path to the introduction of the complementary therapy service because of the implicit level of credibility and respect gained from working with cancer patients.

The development of the service has continued with a mixture of health professionals and experienced complementary therapists. The complementary therapy network has been used to increase the range of therapies provided by making use of volunteer therapists to offer *ad hoc* therapy sessions to in-patients on the cancer wards. Thus a 'rapid response team' has developed which responds to immediate requests from ward or chemotherapy staff to see patients in acute states of anxiety or pain.

Introducing a complementary therapy service

Breaking down barriers

In recent years complementary therapies have become more acceptable to the orthodox medical fraternity (BMA 1993), although there still remain many barriers to analyse and address. When starting up a complementary therapy service, any promotional or publicity material must state clearly that the aim of such therapies is to support patients through diagnosis and treatment, and that they make no attempts or claims to cure their cancer.

The practice of evidence-based medicine has developed into a sophisticated science, giving little credence to anecdotal evidence based on small numbers without any form of rigorous investigation. Unfortunately, the unsubstantiated claims of 'curing' by a minority of **alternative** practitioners, have undermined the whole of the complementary therapy movement, making it unacceptable to those with a more rigorous scientific mind. If complementary therapies are to be fully accepted and integrated into routine cancer treatment then it is important that from the outset the intended outcomes for patients are clearly and sensibly presented. Complementary therapy should be used to complement rather than replace conventional medicine (Lis-Balchin 1997).

When starting a service it can be helpful to offer therapeutic sessions to the medical staff so that they can experience first hand some of the benefits of complementary therapy. In this way some of the myths and fantasies regarding these therapies can be debunked by offering what for many is a relaxing and pleasurable experience.

Introducing therapies to the treating team

The introduction of a new service or change to existing services requires careful planning and preparation as existing personnel can feel threatened, deskilled, or suspicious of change. Furthermore, the complementary therapies should be seen as a **complement**, not an **alternative**, and in marketing the service this should be clearly understood. It can be helpful when introducing a new service to set up a project advisory team or co-ordinating committee, and to invite representation from key stakeholders. In addition to a skilled and highly experienced complementary therapist, the composition of such a team should represent the range of healthcare professionals working within a cancer centre, and thus may include an oncologist, nurse, therapy radiographer, physiotherapist, and others deemed relevant locally. The breaking down of inter-professional barriers is made easier by the multidisciplinary nature of such a project team.

User representation on such a committee is highly desirable, so to invite a patient with interest in complementary therapies to join and advise will ensure a patient-focused service. Many patients attending local support groups are familiar with the use and benefits of complementary therapies, and some support group leaders can be very helpful in advising a project team on introducing these therapies.

The functions and purpose of this committee are both to debate the needs for such a service and to define the requirements within it. The team will need to decide on a strategy for introducing complementary therapies and as such will need to clarify and define the following:

1. The aims and objectives;
2. An operational policy;
3. A referral policy;
4. A marketing and publicity strategy.

The appointment of a skilled project team leader with a knowledge of complementary therapies, an understanding of the NHS and local politics, and the communication skills to negotiate is of paramount importance if this is to be a successful venture. It is also important at the outset to determine whether the therapists should be oncology trained with additional qualifications in one of the therapies, or whether a background in oncology is desirable but not essential. Regardless of this, the person managing the service should ideally have a good working knowledge of cancer and its treatments, and understand the relevance of the provision of complementary therapies to patients at various stages of the cancer journey.

When starting a complementary therapy service a lone therapist can feel very isolated and unsupported without access to support and supervision by peers and managers with a knowledge and understanding of the subject. The establishment of a network of local therapists is helpful in providing a forum for the discussion of relevant issues.

Which therapies?

An ever-increasing range of available therapies creates difficulty in deciding which should be offered, when they should be offered and which would confer most benefit on the patient. This is made more difficult by the reduction in anxiety levels experienced by patients with most of the therapies, anxiety which is present at diagnosis, during treatment and at all stages of the disease. In addition, resource limitation may considerably restrict the availability of a range of therapies and decisions regarding service provision may sadly be determined by economics. Setting criteria to be met will facilitate the decision, and it may help to consider that all therapies should:

1. Aim to reduce anxiety and stress;
2. Aim to enhance coping;
3. Be acceptable to the patients;
4. Be acceptable to the medical establishment;
5. Not be contraindicated for use with mainstream cancer medicine;
6. Be as cost-effective as possible, for example aiming at best results with the maximum number of patients and the minimum resource implications.

Examples of therapies which may fulfil some of these criteria are: aromatherapy, reflexology, acupuncture, relaxation and visualization, and the Alexander technique. It is more cost-effective to offer group therapies rather than individual therapies, and relaxation and Alexander technique lend themselves to this approach more than the others. However the need for greater self-confidence to enter a group must be considered when planning the service.

Individual therapies can benefit patients because of the personal attention which they receive, although relaxation tapes which patients may purchase or borrow are a useful adjunct to any service, and can help to reinforce both the individual and group sessions.

Many cancer patients seek other complementary and alternative therapies as a means of taking control over their lives, and sometimes as a desperate attempt to find the ultimate cure. It can be very difficult to achieve a balance between helping to empower the patient, and tempering the situation with reality and risk destroying hope. Patients may seek extreme diets, shark's cartilage treatment, crystal therapy, or other less well-known adjuncts to help them in their struggle. Although some of these may do no harm, and indeed in some instances may help through the placebo effect, some therapies may be perceived as extreme and if the patient's condition is poor may result in physical deterioration.

If patients are to receive complementary therapies which are integrated with mainstream cancer treatments, then these therapies need to be transferable and portable to include in-patients (reflexology, aromatherapy, massage), patients waiting for chemotherapy (hand massage, Indian head massage, and personal relaxation tapes), and other out-patient sessions. The playing of relaxation tapes and relaxing music in radiotherapy treatment rooms can help to reduce levels of anxiety, and they can also be beneficial during long chemotherapy infusions. The burning of aromatherapy oils in special burners can also help in clinical areas, but care needs to be taken not to offend sensitive nostrils.

Many health professionals are now taking additional training in complementary therapies, and it is possible for some component parts of these therapies to be provided during routine cancer treatment. Simple strategies such as breathing techniques to relieve tension may often be thought appropriate, and the health professional may consider that such therapeutic skills enhance care and can be used in a clinical setting. Being distanced from the patient by high-technology and sophisticated treatments is often quoted as a reason for this interest (Stevenson 1992); Corner (1997) argues that cancer nurses should be developing the therapeutic nursing role and this could equally be applied to various professionals in the context of the supportive and therapeutic strategies considered here. Some recent innovations are team based, with some pain and symptom relief clinics using a range of therapies, whilst nurse-led clinics for patients with breathlessness are incorporating relaxation techniques (Bailey 1995).

An interdisciplinary and multiprofessional approach must be one of the main ways to progress in the future, although this may not be without problems and frustrations such as attempted medicalization and reductionism (Donnelly 1995).

The therapists

There is much debate regarding the necessity for complementary therapists working within a cancer hospital to have an oncology background, in addition to their complementary therapy training and experience. It is helpful for the co-ordinator of complementary therapies to have trained in one of the oncology disciplines as not only will they then understand the disease process and the treatments fully, but will also be able to communicate with the medical establishment in appropriate terminology. This will promote the credibility of the service.

In the focus group study at the LJMC (1999) patients felt much more confident being taught relaxation by a therapist with a wide knowledge of cancer, and felt that links with the oncology team in the cancer centre offered considerable benefit. In the study by Howells (1997) it was strongly felt that the therapist needed knowledge about cancer patients and their specific problems to work effectively and empathically with people who might be distressed, had lost hair or a part of their body, looked or felt ill, or had a potentially embarassing symptom.

All therapists must be accredited with their professional bodies, maintain a high standard of professionalism and follow the guidelines for practice developed by the co-ordinator of the service.In addition they should be able to form good relationships with patients, particularly vital with such a vulnerable client group. Much of the success of these therapies depends on the quality of the therapeutic relationship as well as the actual therapy itself. There is currently a movement towards the accreditation of all therapists with recognized professional bodies which will result in a standardization of all training and supervision.

All complementary therapists employed within the NHS should be subject to the same selection and employment criteria as any other health worker. Many complementary therapists offer their time on a voluntary basis, and although this allows a much wider provision of services, it could be argued that it will prevent the recognition of the value of these therapies if they are always assigned to the voluntary sector.

Regardless of the funding issues, any therapists paid or unpaid should be given a contract of employment by the NHS Trust, which will provide them with indemnity insurance against patient injury. The following criteria will help to ensure that the therapists are sufficiently well-qualified:

1. Qualifications recognized by the relevant governing bodies;
2. Registration with the relevant professional body;
3. Professional insurance cover;
4. Knowledge of cancer and its treatments;
5. Knowledge of the issues of people with cancer;
6. Regular updates on new developments.

Criteria for referral

Cancer centres or cancer hospitals probably treat between 3000–5000 new cases of cancer per year. If it is accepted that most cancer patients experience some degree of psychological morbidity during their cancer journey, and that anxiety related to the diagnosis and treatment is felt by a large proportion of patients attending the cancer centre, then the potential numbers of patients who might benefit from complementary interventions could be quite overwhelming. In addition, many individuals receiving complementary therapies express enjoyment and pleasure in having them, and in the experience of the author, many patients request complementary therapies because they want them, rather than fulfilling the criteria for referral. It is therefore important to develop strict referral criteria for patients who may receive these therapies, and to educate the treating staff into recognizing appropriate and inappropriate referrals.

One of the ethical dilemmas experienced by oncology professionals is how to restrict a complementary therapy service to those who might really benefit from it, when the evidence for specific conditions is still unclear. Few people will derive no benefit from complementary therapies, and each therapy has its own recognized set of contraindications. The following symptoms generally respond, and so might be considered for inclusion in the referral criteria:

1. Depression;
2. Acute/chronic anxiety and panic attacks;
3. Poor body image;
4. Loss of confidence/control;
5. General anxiety and apprehension during treatment;
6. Patients with advanced disease;
7. Nausea and vomiting, pain, loss of energy, insomnia;
8. Other physical symptoms caused by disease or treatment.

Alternatively, it is possible to set up a funded clinical trial to evaluate the benefits of some therapies, and in this case the criteria for referral will be set within the trial conditions.

Where should therapies be offered?

If a complementary therapy service has the philosophy of providing a patient-centred service, then the therapies should be offered where they will most benefit the patients. The aim of the therapies should be to support patients through treatment, and this means that some therapies may need to be offered directly where treatments are being given (e.g. relaxation therapy during infusion of chemotherapy) whereas others may need to be given away from the treatment areas altogether. Many in-patients are unable to move far from the bedside and thus appropriate therapies should be provided there. However a busy cancer ward is far from the tranquil oasis of a specially dedicated and furnished therapy room, and it is preferable to provide additional facilities away from the general hubbub of everyday hospital life.

The range of therapies provided will both determine and be determined by the facilities in which they are provided. Ideally, a dedicated suite of rooms or separate therapy centre should be available, furnished in soft, tranquil colours and materials to promote peace and relaxation. Institutionalized decor should be avoided as the ambience of the therapy room contributes to the beneficial effects of the therapy. Where space is limited it may be necessary to use clinic space for therapy, which is less than ideal, but with the addition of soft music and other portable artefacts the clinic room can quickly be transformed into a slightly 'softer' environment. Equipment such as reflexology chairs, massage couches, and oils will require storage space.

Many patients find that experiencing these therapies in the same place as their medical treatment can be counter-therapeutic. In the study at the LJMC, some patients who were offered complementary therapies in a purpose-built building in close proximity to the chemotherapy suite found it difficult not to recall their unpleasant experiences of chemotherapy, and it often brought back the feelings of nausea which they had hoped to conquer. If group therapeutic activities are to be introduced, then a room of sufficient size to house a class of 10–12 people will need to be identified, which needs to be furnished softly and be away from the noise of the main hospital.

Getting the balance between offering therapies as an integrated part of the cancer centre, but creating the right environment for maximum therapeutic gain is difficult, and requires careful planning.

Funding

The funding of complementary therapies in cancer care has traditionally been the domain of the voluntary and charitable sectors, with little money being made available from the statutory provision of mainstream cancer services. Unfortunately, the paucity of research evidence to establish identifiable benefits has made health providers reluctant to allocate over-stretched resources to such a service. Until more cost-benefit studies are undertaken, and complementary therapy gains greater status as a support for patients through treatment, then the funding of these services may largely be supported by charitable donations. The development of the complementary therapy service will depend largely on funds available, and will require careful consideration.

The set-up costs will include the purchase of equipment and the building or refurbishment of appropriate rooms. In some cancer centres, trust funds may be available to support start-up costs, with additional monies being raised by local fund-raising events and Leagues of Friends. Local fundraisers are often keen to support such ventures as they are directly patient-centred, and capital outlay may be small, particularly if refurbishment rather than rebuilding is required. However such fundraisers may wish to purchase something specific rather than simply support service provision, and selling a service to fundraisers by breaking it down into 'bite sized chunks' can help. For instance stating that £x will provide a course of complementary therapy for y patients becomes a marketable commodity and those offering charitable donations are often willing to support such packages of service provision.

Staff costs become an ongoing problem, and whereas some charities may be willing to support staff salaries, they are unwilling to provide the funding for selection and recruitment. This should be clarified from the outset as advertising can prove expensive and may exceed any planned budget allocation.

The employment of volunteer therapists has been mentioned above. However, if funding is an issue and there are sufficient therapists willing to offer their services on a voluntary basis, then providing they are managed effectively this is one solution to the lack of available resources. It could be argued that patients should be charged a nominal amount for their therapy, which would cover the cost of the therapist's time. However, many individuals with cancer are unable to afford to contribute financially in this way, and if such a policy were implemented it could pave the way for an elitist service, available only for the better off.

Many patients suffer from loss of self-worth and self-esteem as a result of developing the disease, and such a policy in this instance could reinforce these negative feelings and would therefore be counter-therapeutic.

In the experience of the author, many patients who can afford to do so make donations to the complementary therapy service, which contribute considerably to the running costs.

Networking

Most cancer centres now are based on the hub-and-spoke model described in the Calman Hine report, and are the centre of a network of a number of referring District General Hospitals in their catchment area. Patients attending the cancer centre may do so for a relatively short period of time in comparison with the amount of time they are cared for back in their own communities. In addition patients may travel long distances for cancer treatment, and thus when the treatment is finished they are happy never to set foot in the cancer hospital again! However, during their treatment they may have experienced complementary therapies which they found helpful in coping with the side-effects of the treatment as well as the impact of the diagnosis. Many patients wish to continue receiving complementary therapies for some time after their medical treatment has finished, but find difficulty in accessing suitably qualified and experienced therapists near to home. If time and staffing allows, it can therefore be very helpful to patients to develop a networking strategy throughout the catchment area of the cancer centre, aimed at identifying suitably qualified complementary therapists in the vicinity of the referring District General Hospitals. These therapists can be accessed through the relevant complementary therapy registers, and can be offered training on the specific issues of working with cancer patients. They can then be placed on a networking list which can be given to patients when leaving the cancer centre, thus allowing them to access suitably qualified and experienced therapists close to home.

Developing these networks can provide a rich source of ideas and voluntary help for the cancer centre, as well as providing patients with the wherewithal to continue therapy should they wish to do so. In addition, the local District General Hospitals can be given local contacts for complementary therapy for their own patients, thus increasing the network and offering patients further sources of support.

Conclusion

This chapter has outlined both the emotional experience for patients attending a cancer centre, as well as offering practical advice (based on the authors' experience) on the introduction of complementary therapies into this environment. There is unquestionably much further work required in this area if these therapies are to be accepted into routine cancer practice. The breaking down of some of the barriers to integration has begun, but attempting to adhere a holistic approach on to a medical model will always prove challenging.

References

Bailey, C. (1995). Nursing as therapy in the management of breathlessness in lung cancer. *European Journal of Cancer Care*, **4**, 184–90.

Brigden, M. L. (1995). Unproven cancer therapies. *Western Journal of Medicine*, **163**, 463–9.

British Medical Association (1993). *Complementary medicine: new approaches to good practice*. Oxford University Press.

Calman, K., Hine, D. (1995). A policy framework for commissioning cancer services: a report by the Expert Advisory Group on Cancer to the Chief Medical Officers of England and Wales. Department of Health, London.

Corner, J. (1997). Beyond survival rates and side-effects: cancer nursing as therapy. *Cancer Nursing*, **20**, 3–11.

Donnelly, D. (1995). Integrating complementary medicine within the NHS: a therapist's view of the Liverpool Centre for Health. *Complementary Therapies in Medicine*, **3**, 84–7.

Downer, S. M., Cody, M. M., McCluskey, P., *et al.* (1994). Pursuit and practice of complementary therapies by cancer patients receiving conventional treatment. *British Medical Journal*, **309**, 86–9.

Fallowfield, L. J. (1990). *Quality of Life: the missing measurement in health care*. Souvenir Press, London.

Forsberg, C. and Cedermark, B. (1996). Well-being, general health and coping ability; 1 year follow-up of patients treated for colo-rectal and gastric cancer. *European Journal of Cancer Care*, **5**, 209–16.

Howells, N. (1997). *Bridging the gap in cancer patient care*. MSc in Complementary Therapy Studies. University of Westminster.

Lewith, G. (1996). Cancer. *Complementary Therapies in Medicine*, **4**, 242–6.

Lis-Balchin, M. (1997). Essential oils and aromatherapy: their modern role in healing. *Journal of Royal Society of Health*, **117**, 324–9.

LJMC, Walker, G., and Adewuyi-Dalton, R. (1999). A qualitative evaluation of users' experiences of group relaxation classes and aromatherapy massage in a cancer support and information centre. Focus group study (unpublished report for the Cancer Research Campaign).

Maher, E. J., Young, T., Feigel, I. (1994). Complementary therapies used by patients with cancer. Letter *British Medical Journal*, **309**, 671–2.

Massie, M. J. and Holland, J. C. (1990). Overview of normal reactions and prevalence of psychiatric disorders. In *Handbook of psycho-oncology* (ed. J. C. Holland and J. H. Rowland). Oxford University Press.

Rapoport, Y., Kreitler, S., Chaitchik, S., *et al.* (1993). Psychosocial problems in head and neck cancer patients and their change with time since diagnosis. *Annals of Oncology*, **4**, 69–73.

Slevin, M. L. (1992). Quality of life, philosophical question or clinical reality? *British Medical Journal*, **305**, 466–9.

Stevensen, C. (1992). The psycho-physiological effects of aromatherapy massage following cardiac surgery. *Nursing Times*, **82**, 47–50.

Wood, J. (1994). Support and information for cancer patients in the UK today. *Radiography Today*. August, 16–18.

Wyatt, G. and Friedman L. L. (1996). Long-term female cancer survivors: quality of life issues and clinical implications. *Cancer Nursing*, **19**, 1–7.

Zampini, K. and Orstroff J. S. (1993). The post treatment resource program: portrait of a program for cancer survivors. *Psycho-Oncology*, **2**, 1–9.

Chapter 24

The patient's path to integration

Beata Bishop

Beata Bishop is a psychotherapist working along Jungian and transpersonal lines. Her interests include the mind-body connection in sickness and health, and its therapeutic use in working with cancer patients.

What I have to offer is based on two kinds of life experience. One is personal, for I am a former cancer patient myself, having recovered from metastasized malignant melanoma in 1983; the other is professional, gleaned from working with cancer patients as a psychotherapist ever since. My personal experience is a valuable asset in my professional work. It enables me to establish instant rapport with cancer sufferers, since they know that I know what they are going through, having travelled along that path myself. They need not be coy about the subject, use euphemisms or present a brave front. Cancer has a sinister aura of its own. The best way to dispel that is to handle the subject openly, calmly, and without fear, pointing out that cancer need not equal a death sentence. As a long-term survivor, I am in a good position to do that.

Over the years I have explored many complementary therapies, both through personal use and through my patients' experiences, although my perspective, which is also that of this paper, has remained psychotherapeutic. What I have learned is that complementary therapies can significantly improve the patients' chances of recovery, or at least their quality of life. They inject hope, comfort, and physical and spiritual healing into the most dismal situations. Beyond immediate benefits they also have a deeper purpose; by involving the patient in therapeutic activities they awaken what Albert Schweitzer called the wise healer dwelling in us all.

It is precisely the individual's self-healing ability and inner being that is ignored in a medical setting where the Cartesian principle of body-mind split still rules, and attention is focused on the body alone. This neglect means wasting a potentially powerful healing aid that costs nothing, has no harmful side-effects and can work amazingly well. Besides, evoking that inner ability is not hare-brained novelty: 'Let no-one persuade you to cure the body until he has first given you his soul to be cured', wrote Plato some 2500 years ago. Only by healing the Cartesian split can we catch up with that advice.

What follows is a loosely structured account of the methods and approaches which I have found successful in my work. It is neither complete nor definitive in any way. I may be the therapist, but the patients are my teachers, and I shall always have something to learn from them.

Emotional first aid

I may be accused of professional bias for claiming that psychotherapy, combined with training in relaxation and visualization, should have precedence over all other complementary approaches. But I do so, because having cancer is a deeply traumatic experience, a descent into fear, despair, and powerlessness; in brief, into a state of emotional turmoil which health professionals, who need to protect themselves from personal involvement in their work, can hardly imagine — and which most sufferers dare not discuss. This trauma and turmoil must be dealt with before all else. Psychotherapy has the fastest, most direct access to the patient's inner self, and the best tools to deal with its distress. And this has to be done urgently, not only out of ordinary human compassion, but also for sound medical reasons.

Psychoneuroimmunology has demonstrated the direct link between emotional state and immune competence, producing scientific proof of what psychotherapists, healers and observant physicians have long maintained, namely that a positive, hopeful, optimistic attitude boosts the immune system, while a negative, pessimistic, despairing one undermines it. One can assume that cancer patients' immune competence is below par, so they should receive swift, effective help before despair takes a hold, weakening their resistance even further. And they should receive it at the very start, when a cancer diagnosis is announced. As a rule this is done badly. The patient is faced not only with a life-threatening disease but also with a doctor who doesn't know how to break the bad news, how to communicate with the scared stranger across the desk. The resulting exchange, as reported by patients, ranges from 'Brief, correct, and ice-cold' and 'Tried to sound hopeful, but I knew he didn't mean it', to 'Couldn't wait to get me out of the room'.

As for being given the bad news, I remember my own feelings which have been echoed by many patients over the years: a sharp animal fear in the pit of the stomach, heart stopping, then speeding up with a downward lurch, a great need for air, clammy hands, paper-dry mouth. Then numbness, the world switching to slow motion, followed by a blast of icy loneliness, the sense of being cut off from the cancer-free part of humanity, like a medieval leper banished from the community. And underneath it all, profound dread.

It is at such moments that the patient would need help. What comes instead normally is a cheery remark from a nurse, an appointment card, and a sense of being sucked into a vast, impersonal system that has taken over one's destiny, stripped away one's adult autonomy, and provided no-one to lighten one's distress. In official terms the patient's psychosocial needs are not being met. In human terms the patient is in hell.

I know of cases when the numbness became so overwhelming that the patient sank into apathy, didn't keep appointments, didn't tell anybody what was going on. Precious weeks, sometimes months were wasted like that, making the outlook even bleaker. And all because communication, human touch and support are not part of the medical programme. Introducing them would be the first step towards integration.

The dread inspired by cancer has much to do with the lay person's perception of the disease, which bears no resemblance to reality, but has a powerful effect. Being invaded is what patients experience. The imagery they use has a touch of Star Wars about it, for they see the tumour as a hostile alien intruder, an enemy from some outer space, determined to destroy its host. (Significantly, heart disease, which in this country kills more people than cancer, does not excite the same dread, presumably because it is one's own familiar organ that is causing trouble, not some alien thing.)

Working through his shocked feelings, a client of mine recalled a recurring dream which conveys vividly the theme of invasion. During the year preceding his diagnosis he repeatedly dreamt that he was fleeing from an unknown enemy, running towards his fortress home, and just managing to shut the heavy gate and pull up the drawbridge in the nick of time. Safe at last — but as he looked around, he noticed a breach in the outer wall and woke up in terror as a dark presence loomed up in the undefended gap. Now, he said, he knew what the dream meant (and was never haunted by it again).

Not being heard, not being listened to is what patients find most hurtful. It makes their loneliness worse. The doctor won't listen — it's not his job. The nurse-counsellor, if there is one, only gives practical advice — there is no time for anything else. Family members must be spared — they would worry themselves sick. 'I can only cry at night when they can't hear me', a very sick girl once told me.

That leaves the therapist to act as bridge and buffer between the patient's raw emotions and the outside world. The task is to provide a safe space, total listening and open communication with no holds barred; or to sit silently, in a cocoon of acceptance and containment, until the patient is able to release the fear, shock, rage, despair, or whatever else needs to find expression. It takes skill and experience to let that happen without rushing in with premature comfort or soothing words which might help the therapist but would block the patient. (Only those who have clarified their own feelings about disease, suffering and death should undertake this work.)

The next task is to dispel the sense of powerlessness and apprehension that most hospitals evoke. The more up-to-date the hi-tech equipment is, the more it dwarfs and alienates the vulnerable outsider with its hard, cold perfection and incomprehensible workings. 'Are they more interested in their machines than in the patient?' one client mused after some tests. I recall having similar thoughts during my first CAT scan. Did the medical staff handling the machinery have any idea of what it was like to lie inside that cruel plastic pod and think that it was worse than a coffin which would at least have a lining? There was nothing to ease the loneliness and the lack of human touch. No doubt unfairly I fantasized that if I called for help, I would be answered by a computer, offering a drop-down menu of assistance options.

Consolidation

So much for the early, damage-limiting phase of psychological support. The real work comes later, and is made easier by the fact that people who contact a complementary therapist are pre-selected, having realized the need for something extra beyond medical treatment. Some patients come only once or twice, in the first post-diagnosis confusion. They pick up new ideas and guidelines and don't return. Others engage in long-term therapy. Under the impact of serious illness they choose to come to grips with some non-physical factor which they suspect has contributed to their ill-health.

It may be unfinished business from the past which has lost all relevance long ago, yet has left behind pain, guilt or repressed anger. Others may realize that they have fallen into a life trap, that is into a situation that seems both unbearable and unalterable, with serious illness or even death as the only honourable way out. A miserable marriage that can't be ended because of the children, a soul-destroying job that must be endured because past the age of forty jobs are hard to come by — these tough no-win situations are described in tones of quiet, civilized despair, heavy with resignation.

Life traps are carcinogenic. Not for nothing has cancer been called a socially acceptable form of suicide.

As a rule, life trap situations come to a head between one year and eighteen months before cancer is diagnosed. Without exception — not excepting myself, either — all patients who reviewed their immediate past in search of clues could remember a moment when they genuinely didn't care whether they lived or died. The stories were different, the outcome identical: the homesick Continental woman who loved her English husband but couldn't bear living in the North-East; the ageing unmarried daughter, trapped by duty to care for an insanely demanding, half-senile mother; the gentle young man desperate to leave his bullying, hysterical wife, but equally desperate not to lose his adored baby daughter, and so on. In such cases the psychosomatic trigger is unmistakable. Urgent mental reorientation is needed, for somatizing emotional pain into a tumour is easier than reversing the process.

Patients must be shown that serious illness or death is never the only escape from a life trap. Even if the alternative seems destructive, it's bound to be less destructive than dying.

Breaking the pattern

By now it should be clear why it is important to explore the patient's background in which the disease developed and to identify the necessary life changes. Here, again, we cannot expect much help from the medical side. Doctors and nurses tend to value patient compliance over all else and resent self-help initiatives from lay people. My own infinitely caring and dedicated consultant way back in 1979 also preferred patient passivity. He assured me that there was nothing I could or should do to speed up my recovery after major surgery, except to take it easy and leave the rest to him. Later, as I was leaving hospital, he urged me to resume the life I had lived before my illness and get on with it, as if nothing had happened.

He meant well, and he was wrong, for I followed his advice — and had a recurrence one year later. Sending patients back into the same circumstances in which they became ill, without showing any interest in those circumstances, makes little sense either medically or psychologically.

What I have learned over the years is that the indispensable first step towards healing is to make a major change in some area of life. Something must have been wrong in one's existence to allow serious disease to strike. Something, or rather some things, ranging from lifestyle, diet, self-destructive habits, and persistent stress, to pollution, poor relationships, and ordinary unhappiness — in one of many possible combinations. In this area there is no room for 'either/or', only for 'and/also'. It is almost immaterial which of the available changes the patient starts with — although obviously aiding the sick body should come first — as long as a start is made by a no longer helpless active player.

For example, a young woman I worked with started by adopting a fairly strict dietary regime, designed to cleanse her system and build up her resistance. After a lifetime of junk foods and self-neglect this was a drastic change which inevitably led to others, for she also had to stop smoking, cut out alcohol and recreational drugs, and accept a disciplined existence. The new physical routine began to change her inner state, too. After a while she felt the need to learn to relax and meditate, turn inwards and take stock of her life, which in turn led to an honest revision of her energy-sapping relationships. And so the transformation went on, followed by physical improvement.

'Remove the obstacle and the result will appear', says an ancient yoga teaching. In a health crisis the main obstacle often is a loss of purpose and meaning, or a sense of inner paralysis, but, ironically enough, the crisis itself may be the necessary goad to move us on.

Discovering imagery

Visualization is a powerful way to harness the imagination and turn it into an instrument of healing. It yields a clear, unretouched picture of the patient's true feelings, beliefs, unspoken wishes and expectations. The images that emerge by-pass the censorship of the brain. I take them seriously, even if — or especially if — they contradict the patient's statements, like in the case of a breast cancer patient who assured me that she very much wanted to live, but in a freestyle visualization chose to witness her very splendid funeral attended by countless mourners.

Beside its diagnostic value visualization is also an excellent tool for inner reprogramming and goal-setting. The images arise from the same unconscious layer as dreams, but as the subject is awake and follows some kind of softly spoken guidance, the imagery can be easily recalled and interpreted. Some clients try to reject displeasing images, but this is a mistake. Whatever crops up must be accepted. I liken the process to sitting in a darkened cinema, watching the film: one doesn't rewrite the script, change the cast around or object to the special effects, one simply sits still and pays attention. When the inner film is over, the patient draws the images, for analysis and future reference. Over time pictures and symbols change, often accurately mirroring physical processes.

My favourite types of visualization are spot imaging, and the longer guided fantasy. Spot imaging is quick and effective when words fail. If, for instance, a patient struggled to describe her feeling of stuckness, I would ask, 'What would it look like if you wanted to paint or draw it?' 'Like an endless concrete corridor, between tall grey walls, no windows … and I'm walking along it,' came the answer after a moment's pause. 'See if there is a door somewhere.' Yes, there was one, narrow and concealed, on the left, and yes, she was able to open it — and saw a beautiful wildflower meadow in full sunshine, with children playing. But no, she couldn't go through the door and even had to shut it quickly. Back in the endless grey corridor. But now she knew about the door and the meadow. Next time round she might be able to step over the threshold.

I also use the Simonton technique, the best-known visualization method for cancer work, which has been around since 1978, adapting it to suit individual needs. It is a kind of self-hypnosis which, practised twice a day over a period of time, can have some effect through subtle mind-body connections. The patient gets images for the tumour, the treatment, and the body's immune defences; what these elements look like and how they interact suggests the current state of affairs. I know that the method works. At one stage during my illness I experimented with it, concentrating on the secondary tumour in my groin for 10 minutes at a time, twice a day. After 3 days this produced a healthy inflammation around the groin that spread down my thigh right down to the knee, a convincing red-hot proof of the power of self-hypnosis that vanished when I discontinued the exercise. Who knows what it would have done to the tumour, had I persisted.

To conclude the Simonton visualization the patient is asked to see him or herself as being healthy, fit, active, enjoying life, able to give and receive love. Patients in a bad state bristle against that: the contrast between how they feel and what they should imagine is too sharp. Yet that is not the point. The purpose of the exercise is not to play make-believe games, but to set goals and focus on a desired outcome.

Everybody can visualize, except those who decide in advance that they can't. Men find it more difficult than women, but then in general they don't take easily to complementary therapies which they say aren't scientific enough. One man I worked with attempted imaging twice. The first time he promptly fell asleep. The second time he saw a chalet in his much-loved Alps, but couldn't find the entrance (a message in itself, which he chose to ignore). Another man, asked to attempt an overview of his chaotic problems, found himself on a hilltop overlooking a pine forest. In front of him there were several boxes containing his problems and their solutions, but he panicked and refused to open them. Instead, he asked for advice from a venerable Japanese sage who had suddenly appeared, but the sage only smiled, as if saying, 'You know the answers'. This scared him again and he refused to do further image work.

Sometimes during image work or meditation a symbol emerges that clearly points towards the spiritual dimension of life. As I work along Jungian and transpersonal lines, I consider that dimension all-important, particularly in life-or-death situations when the normal criteria of ordinary existence lose their validity, and something else, something greater and more meaningful is needed to hold on to. It is as if the strict limitations set up by physical illness demanded a non-physical antidote, something that transcends material conditions by unveiling another kind of reality.

How patients fulfil this need is purely individual. Some rediscover the faith they were brought up in and find warmth and security in it. For others the answer is not religious in nature but more akin to what is known as a peak experience in transpersonal psychology: a sudden brief glimpse of a higher dimension beyond normal ego consciousness, an understanding of the unity of all life, and the realization that everything is exactly as it should be, however unjustified this may seem through the lens of everyday consciousness. Peak experiences can transform patients' perception of their disease, not by denying reality but by seeing it from a different perspective where despite everything it makes sense, and may even be seen as a tremendous learning experience.

Peak experiences fade. It is their nature. But they leave behind a certain flavour, a whiff of another kind of knowing. Those who have had the experience, with or without physical illness, know its power. Those who have not, and find the concept alien, should give it the benefit of the doubt: it may hit them, too, when least expected. I have experienced and witnessed in others its transformative power.

'I cannot tell you what God is,' Carl Jung wrote to a British friend towards the end of his long life, 'but experience has shown me that the pattern of God is present in every human psyche.'

Whatever we call it, spiritual dimension or divine principle, it is a pattern of great healing potential, even when a cure seems unlikely. Once we have tuned in to the inner processes of patients, that statement no longer sounds contradictory.

Making peace with the body

Many cancer patients I worked with had a bad relationship with their body; bad or non-existent, insofar as they ignored it until it developed a serious illness and could no longer be used as a kind of flesh-and-blood taxi, a disregarded utilitarian vehicle of little importance.

Having neglected its needs and dismissed its messages, they blamed it bitterly when it ultimately broke down. They felt betrayed by their body and took a while to accept that they themselves had betrayed it through inner–outer disharmony and a lifestyle it had not been designed for.

Cancer can inflict cruel changes on the body which are hard to come to terms with, especially for women who tend to identify with their looks and physical integrity. Often the result is self-disgust, and a rejection of the mutilated, debilitated physical self. Doctors may find it difficult to strike the right balance in this sensitive area. On the one hand they sympathize with the distress of women who grieve for a lost breast or a disfigured face; on the other, they need to remain sufficiently objective and detached to value the patients' hoped-for recovery above all else. To send out the right message under the circumstances would demand communication skills which most doctors lack. The result is often harrowing for patients who don't feel that survival can be traded in for ruined looks and a wounded sense of identity. I still remember with sorrow how admiringly my consultant used to gaze at my horribly mutilated leg which I could hardly bear to look at, calling the skin graft a lovely job, as if it had been my most important part, with the rest of me attached to it as an unoptional extra. It was a chilling example of unholistic attitudes, but it taught me to relate very sensitively to similarly afflicted patients whom I met later through my work.

One of these was a formerly athletic breast cancer sufferer who had grown to hate her body which no longer allowed her to run, play tennis, and swim in the sea. Another patient, a plain woman, expressed her self-loathing in vivid, horrible dreams in which large pieces of her flesh fell away and could not be restored. By way of contrast, a male client suffering from bowel cancer and increasing weakness expressed his self-disgust by forcing himself to exercise hard, wanting to show his body who was boss. Sadly, his sick body had the last word.

Self-hatred must be dispelled. An organism that keeps getting messages of loathing and rejection is unlikely to heal well. The simplest way is to shift the patient's focus of identity away from the body, not denying its reality, only its apparent all-importance. I often use a disidentification exercise devised by Roberto Assagioli, founder of psychosynthesis and pioneer of transpersonal psychology. This is a guided meditation in which the patient is made to contemplate his or her body, mind, emotions, and desires, acknowledging and honouring them all, but not identifying with any of them. What remains is the essence of all human beings, a centre of pure consciousness and self-realization, the permanent factor in the constant ebb and flow of daily existence. What has begun with shifting the emphasis away from the body ends with a direct experience of the spiritual dimension, which allows a new approach to the physical problem.

It doesn't solve it, though. Other complementary therapies are needed for that. I find that many patients at war with their bodies did not get enough touching, holding and cuddling in early childhood. They grew up in austere, rigidly non-physical families where tenderness was unknown. So they never developed a tender relationship to themselves, either, and find the body an embarrassing nuisance.

What they need now is to experience pleasant physical sensations, the non-verbal communication of caring through touch, our first and last way to contact another human being. Chief among the available options are the gentlest kind of massage which is barely stronger than a caress; cranial osteopathy which despite its butterfly-wing touch can release long-repressed emotions; acupuncture to rebalance energies, aromatherapy to lull anxiety and give comfort and pleasure. Being cherished, pampered, held and reassured by touch dissolves the old, hostile barriers between the body and its owner, and makes patients realize that the body is not an enemy but an ally in trouble whose chief goal, just like theirs, is to survive.

The need for relaxation is too well known to need discussing here, except to say that I teach simple 10-minute exercises to all patients who are not familiar with the technique before introducing visualization or any other inner work. I also observe how patients breathe, watching for signs of hyperventilation which is easily brought on by anxiety and tension. In turn, fast, shallow, rhythmic breathing increases stress and fear, and can even bring on panic attacks. The ancient yogis of India knew and taught what Western medicine still has to explore. 'He who controls breath controls life itself,' was their way of putting it. In modern terms hyperventilation deprives the blood of the necessary amount of carbon dioxide which acts as a chemical regulator for the organism. Without it the haemoglobin does not release enough oxygen, the subject breathes more and more rapidly, which increases stress and feelings of panic, and the vicious circle grows harder to break.

It doesn't take long to re-educate hyperventilators, but the benefits can be permanent: greater calm, better groundedness, a sense of being at home in the body, and fully at peace with it.

In conclusion

Towards integration — yes, if it means that medicine accepts the validity and otherness of complementary therapies and tries to understand but not swallow them up, for as separate and independent disciplines they have much to offer that modern hi-tech medicine lacks. Let each side do what it can do best, and communicate across the necessary gap that separates them.

Orthodox attitudes are changing. Only a few years ago today's complementary therapies were contemptuously lumped together under the label of fringe medicine. The next move forward will come when doctors agree not to focus exclusively on large-scale double-blind randomized trials but also pay attention to unusual recoveries and successful unorthodox procedures which cannot be tested in the same way as new drugs, instead of dismissing them as anecdotal evidence. The insistence on statistically significant data prevents the discovery of new ways of healing, while lack of funding stops the complementary camp from engaging in large-scale research.

A kind of one-sided integration has already been going on for a while at grassroot levels, carried out by cancer patients themselves who track down and use complementary therapies alongside their medical treatment which leaves too many of their needs unmet. Typically, many keep their extra-curricular activities to themselves, for fear that their doctors might disapprove. Some doctors, I gather, tend to disapprove rather vigorously, so they never hear about the scope and potential of complementary approaches, and the chance of a constructive dialogue is lost.

But this, too, is bound to change. If I were asked to find an image for integration, I would choose the archetypal one of Asclepios, the ancient Greek god of medicine, with his two daughters: Hygeia, goddess of health and prevention, and Panacea, all-healing goddess of natural remedies. Traditionally they are represented as a closely knit group. Asclepios with his staff and sacred serpent in the middle, flanked by his two daughters. All that remains of that venerable image is the serpent gazing into a chalice, which is still the symbol of Western medicine. Now is the time to bring back to life the rest of that fully integrated group.

Recommended reading

Achterberg, J. (1985). *Imagery in healing — Shamanism and modern medicine*. New Science Library, Shambhala, Boston.

Assagioli, R. (1965). *Psychosynthesis — A collection of basic writings*. Turnstone Books, London.

Benson, H. (1976). *The relaxation response*. William Collins Sons & Co. London.

Connell, C. (1998). *Something understood — Art therapy in cancer care*. Wrexham Publications, London.

Cousins, N. (1979). *Anatomy of an illness as perceived by the patient*. Bantam Books, Toronto.

Cousins, N. (1989). *Head first — The biology of hope*. E. P. Dutton, New York.

Dossey, L. (1984). *Beyond illness — Discovering the experience of health*. New Science Library, Shambhala, Boston.

Dossey, L. (1991). *Healing breakthroughs — How your attitudes and beliefs can affect your health*. Piatkus, London.

LeShan, L. (1984). *You can fight for your life — Emotional factors in the treatment of cancer*. Thorsons Publishers Limited, Wellingborough.

LeShan, L. (1989). *Cancer as a turning point — A handbook for people with cancer, their families and health professionals*. Gateway Books, Bath.

Pert, C. B. (1997). *Molecules of emotion — Why you feel the way you feel*. Simon & Schuster Ltd, London.

Siegel, B. S. (1986). *Love, medicine and miracles*. Arrow Books Limited, London.

Siegel, B. S. (1990). *Peace, love and healing — The path to self-healing*. Arrow Books Limited, London.

Chapter 25

Guiding patients through the maze

Catherine Zollman

Catherine Zollman graduated in 1989 from Oxford University and the Royal Free Hospital School of Medicine, London, where she developed an interest in holistic medicine by becoming a member, and then a trustee, of the British Holistic Medical Association. During her training in medical oncology, palliative care, and then general practice, she worked at the Bristol Cancer Help Centre and the Hammersmith Hospital Oncology Department, and was on the executive committee of the British Psycho-Oncology Society. Between 1996 and 1999 she was part-time director of medical education with the Research Council for Complementary Medicine, where she was involved in educating conventional healthcare professionals about complementary medicine and was co-author of an ABC of Complementary Medicine, published in journal (1999) and book (2000) form by the British Medical Journal.

'Everything was turned upside down. Nothing felt the same as it had been a moment before. I felt there was nothing I could rely on, nothing in my life I could trust to carry on and be just as it had always been. All my plans about the future, all my dreams, all my purpose and direction were taken away in an instant. I felt as if I had been left on my own at the start of a mystery journey with several sets of incomplete instructions all contradicting one another. I didn't know what to take with me. I wasn't sure which direction to go in, or what to expect along the way. Even worse, I had no idea of where I was eventually going to end up or how long it was all going to take.'

For many people, being diagnosed with cancer is a bewildering and overwhelming experience, often the biggest crisis they have ever faced in their lives. Initially there may be waves of strong emotion — anger, fear, or sadness — but it seems that, of all the problems involved in coming to terms with a diagnosis of cancer, uncertainty is often one of the most difficult to bear.

At first sight, this seems surprising. Cancer is not a new illness. People have probably been living and dying with cancer for thousands of years. Surely some of the questions should have been answered, even if we haven't yet found a cure? But there is no doubt that cancer isn't regarded in the same way as other well researched, but still largely incurable, diseases of our time like rheumatoid arthritis, heart failure, and dementia. What makes it different? Why do so many people embarking on that 'cancer journey' described above feel that they are negotiating a maze full of difficult decisions with no clear guidance? This chapter will examine the reasons why decision-making in cancer may be so difficult and why the dominant healthcare system often makes the situation worse, not better. It will then go on to describe ways in which guidance from a skilled third party may make the process easier, and look at ways in which this role could be incorporated into standard practice. It is based on personal observations and reflections from several years of working with people with cancer in various medical settings—medical oncology, palliative care, a complementary cancer centre, and now general practice.

Why is there a maze?

One of the most obvious reasons for uncertainty about cancer is the huge individual variation in people's response to cancer treatments and in the natural course of cancers in different people. Nowhere is Pasteur's recognition of both the 'soil' (the patient) and the 'seed' (the disease) in illness more true. Had he lived today, he might have added the 'herbicide' (the treatment) too, although, with a few notable exceptions, the herbicide's role is generally still less important than that of the soil and the seed. Even in the case of one specific type of cancer in one specific gender and age group, the best doctors in the world can only calculate average life expectancy, or talk in terms of percentages of people who are alive at certain time-points after their diagnosis. Being told that a certain percentage of people with a given condition will be alive 10 years after diagnosis, but that actual life expectancy could be anything from under 2 years to over 30 years, is of little practical help for anyone attempting to plan their own, individual future. A number of retrospective studies of 'remarkable recoveries' from cancer and 'exceptional cancer patients' have been done but results are preliminary and are still a long way from being developed into reliable tools for predicting precise individual prognoses prospectively and reliably. To give a concrete example, a patient with advanced breast cancer who is offered chemotherapy will be faced with the knowledge that some people never survive to the end of treatment but others have several years remission. How is she supposed to estimate her own risk and, once she has decided whether to accept the treatment or not, what can she rely on to reassure her that she has made the right choice? Decisions are made more difficult because of the significant 'costs' associated with many of the options. The side-effects of conventional (and some complementary) cancer treatments are often more predictable than the outcome and have to be weighed against the realistic chances of benefit.

Misunderstanding and frustration are also caused by different responses to the fact that cancer today is often an incurable disease. The dominant rational-scientific model of western medicine regards this as a challenge that will soon yield to the 'truth' of bioscientific enquiry, when the scourge of cancer, like so many other illnesses in the past, will be tamed by a scientific breakthrough.

For a patient who is diagnosed with a mysterious and potentially incurable condition, promises of cures in the future are not necessarily enough. Help in finding a way to die, or to live with a greatly heightened awareness of mortality — something which may require acceptance of states beyond the physical — may be a much more pressing need, and one which is often difficult to meet within the philosophical framework of an acute oncology unit.

Because cancer generally progresses, there are often feelings of 'I'll only get one chance at this decision, so I've got to make the right choice now' and 'If I make the wrong decision now, there's no turning the clock back. I will have blown my chances for ever.' The fear of wrong turnings or blind alleys with no way back adds extra pressure and urgency to decision-making and can make the process much more painful and difficult.

It is often said in medicine, that when there is a wide range of treatments on offer for any condition, it usually means that none of them are really much good. This may certainly be the case for some cancers but may also reflect important inequalities in care. For example, if a particular treatment, which is widely used in the USA, is not available in the UK, this may mean that there is still insufficient research evidence to establish whether it offers any significant benefit over standard treatment. On the other hand, it may mean that the UK has been slow to take up, or cannot afford, some real therapeutic advance. Likewise, if a particular complementary regime is available somewhere else, there is always the suspicion that it may prove to be the 'magic bullet' that everyone has been waiting for. Delays in information flow about best-demonstrated practice and inequalities in health service provision always fuel uncertainty.

When two treatment approaches have philosophical or paradigmatic differences, choices can become polarized and seem more drastic. Many complementary approaches to cancer regard 'detoxifying' the body and 'boosting the immune system' to mobilize the body's own defences against cancer as the best way of achieving long term benefit. In contrast, most conventional treatments are toxic to body cells and depress the immune system, because this approach considers killing cancer cells to be the best way of achieving long term benefit. It is obvious that, in the eyes of those taking the former approach, choosing conventional treatment might actually make the situation worse, and vice versa. Fifteen to twenty years ago this inevitably meant that the two styles of treatment were regarded as incompatible alternatives, rather than as approaches which could be used together to complement one another. Recently, there have been significant moves to reconcile some of these differences and to bring the best of each of these two approaches together to provide more integrated cancer care. These developments have been mirrored by the contemporaneous shift in nomenclature from 'alternative' to 'complementary' medicine, but the philosophical contradictions remain and can induce guilt and self-blame if decisions which have been made do not lead to positive outcomes.

The current health system is very hierarchical and advice from doctors is still usually given more weight than advice from other professionals, regardless of how congruent it is with a person's own feelings and beliefs. People often choose to defer decisions to their doctors, believing that 'they know best' and 'they wouldn't offer it to me if it wasn't going to do me some good'. Others may feel pushed into making decisions which go against their own inclinations, by the fear that their doctors will reject or abandon them if they do not follow their advice. It can be very difficult to resist the pressure and go against the flow. Doctors, particularly hospital doctors, are becoming more and more specialized as technical experts within ever-narrower disciplines. Their increasing tendency to focus on the part, rather than the whole, can result in an understanding of the patient that is often far removed from the patient's own view of themselves, and recommendations that may not always be appropriate. This throws into question whether doctors, as they are currently trained, are the best-qualified people to hold this position of central influence.

Is there a role for a guide?

Does the maze of someone's personal cancer journey need to be so difficult, or is there anything anyone can do to make things easier? To some extent, people do have to make their own decisions and live by the consequences, tough though this may be. But many people want some guidance, ideally from an informed, but neutral, third party who can help put things in perspective, act as an advocate and be a source of further information, and who can also draw out and support their own feelings about how they want to proceed. In reality, many people seek out such 'guides' informally, turning, for example, to wise friends or relatives, cancer support groups, compassionate doctors, nurses or complementary therapists, counsellors or psychotherapists, and sometimes a combination of these. Unfortunately many others feel lonely and confused, without support or non-partisan guidance. It is these people who might benefit most if the health service could recognize their needs and make some more systematic provision to meet them.

But before we embark on a 'mission to guide all cancer patients', it is important to realize that not everyone needs a professional guide. There are some people who find it relatively easy to make complex choices about their cancer journey. Sometimes this is because they have a form of cancer, for example acute leukaemia or testicular cancer, for which there is a very high chance of cure with conventional treatment and therefore much less of a dilemma about choice of treatment. But others, who face more difficult decisions, may have strong principles or have had powerful experiences, which give them clear internal guidance as to the correct path to take. For example one person might have nursed a relative with cancer and have formed firm views on the type of treatment that he or she would want, should the situation arise. Another may have strong faith and may receive guidance in prayer. Another may have read about or know someone who has recovered from cancer and feel inspired to seek out whatever treatment they used. Another may meet an inspirational health practitioner (either conventional or complementary) in whose hands they feel safe and in whose treatment they can trust. These people often successfully manage to put doubts aside and move forward without regret. They probably only need a guide to question, and possibly challenge, their convictions if they appear to be putting themselves or their families at risk. Such a situation might arise, for example, if potentially life-saving treatment is being missed, if family relationships are being damaged, or when it has become obvious that someone is wasting precious time or money chasing an unattainable cure when they could be preparing for a conscious and graceful death. In general, people's autonomy should be respected and they should be supported in the choices they have made, even if they are not decisions which the guide would have taken himself or herself. Suggestions or advice to the contrary may, at best, be ignored and, at worst, induce those same negative feelings of guilt, inadequacy, and insecurity which the guide should be trying to reduce.

Other people may not find such strong conviction at the time when they face their important decisions. For them a guide may have several important functions. Firstly he or she can help by preventing information overload by helping to assess and think through the consequences of the various options available. This can make the difference between people feeling completely overwhelmed by too many contradictory choices and feeling they are capable of making informed decisions. It may involve helping people consider the quality of evidence regarding various different approaches, the likelihood of benefit and the possible downside of treatments (cost, side-effects, etc.). It may also involve helping patients translate the statistical evidence into more human terms and trying to help them understand the likely implications in their particular case. But people also need permission to be more subjective and should be encouraged to take a personal view on the positive and negative features of each approach. For example, if someone hates staying in hospital, participation in a clinical trial involving intensive in-patient monitoring of people taking a new chemotherapy drug may not be appropriate. Likewise, someone who does not like raw vegetables will find life very difficult on a metabolic dietary regime such as the Gerson diet. People need help to build up the confidence to trust their own feelings and inclinations. Sometimes it will be the right decision to choose an approach for which there is very little supporting evidence, if the pros and cons appear *to the individual concerned* to be in favour of going ahead. They need to be reassured that there is no 'one right way to tackle cancer' that applies to everyone, and encouraged to find the way that feels most congruent and constructive in their particular situation.

A guide can also be there as a source of experience and additional information. He or she may be able to direct someone towards a potentially meaningful book, a useful and well-informed website, a meeting with someone else going through similar experiences, or a new type of approach that might enhance care. Importantly, even if the guide does not know about something himself or herself, he or she may well know someone else who does have specific knowledge in that area. A guide may be able to recognize whether, and when, a person with cancer might benefit from a more creative and exploratory approach to their disease and to their life. At this point, they may be able to help that person articulate their own wishes and vision as to how this transformative work may best be done. A skilful guide will aim to sow the right seed-idea at the right time, when the person is receptive and ready for change. He or she will try to help people able to see beyond their own viewpoint and consider other ways of looking at the same situation.

A guide should also be on the lookout for times of more negative emotions and will intervene early to help people challenge self-blame and guilt. These feelings are often the 'flip side' of the positive messages of empowerment that can help people feel more in control of their cancer. If things are going well and the cancer is in remission, the belief that one's attitude and behaviour is partly responsible can be very affirming. If disease is progressing, it can be very difficult not to slide into feelings of 'I didn't try hard enough' or 'I haven't been positive enough', or even 'I'm not a good enough person, I don't deserve to get well'. Guides can help to balance both extremes of attitude. They will know when to be positive and encouraging, and when to allow people to express their frustration, anger, or despair. A guide can encourage people to voice their disappointment, without turning it in on themselves, and then help them to move on to find new and sustaining sources of hope and fulfilment.

It is also important to have knowledge of their patient's personal and social situation and to be able to apply this knowledge to help people be realistic about the constraints they are under and what can be achieved. Circumstances such as the continuing need to earn money or look after children, can profoundly influence the amount of freedom people feel they have to explore, take time out to re-evaluate their lives, and experiment with various forms of complementary or creative therapies. What their peer group believes and does will have a bearing on what they will accept as 'the norm', what they will seek out, and what they are prepared to try. Their financial situation will obviously determine the amount of non-statutory help they can access.

However, though actual constraints may be a significant 'barrier to entry' for some forms or complementary and creative therapies, perceived constraints may play an even greater role. Thus two people in identical circumstances may make radically different responses to a cancer diagnosis according to the way they feel about their obligations to themselves and to others. A guide who is sensitive to what their patient is bringing to his or her cancer journey will be able to help ensure that any intervention is at the appropriate level for the patient and their family.

Where will these guides come from?

Obviously the 'job description' for a guide or facilitator outlined above has been idealized. Very few people need someone to fulfil all these roles. Many will have their needs met by a variety of people in a variety of ways. Others, who are not so lucky, may have many unmet needs.

One model by which a guiding role could be provided more equitably is through a 'key worker', adequately supervised and supported, who would be allocated to each person diagnosed with cancer. Specialist breast care nurses who work with breast cancer patients from the moment of diagnosis onwards, are probably the closest example of this type of worker, although in practice, time constraints often limit their role. GPs also often take on aspects of the guiding role. Some centres use a well-supervised network of volunteer patients and ex-patients. Possibly the notion of a dedicated guide who could fulfil all the roles described above, for all patients in his or her caseload, is unrealistic. Much will depend on the individual nature of the relationships between the guide and each cancer patient he or she comes into contact with. Furthermore, if there are only a few professionals who are delegated to take the holistic view (especially if that professional is not a doctor) within a healthcare system that is otherwise dominated by a reductionist, materialist attitude towards cancer, there is the potential for even more confusion and chaos.

Perhaps the most sustainable way forward is through a change in the education of conventional healthcare workers, managers, and politicians to consider a more holistic, less mechanistic view of health and disease. Moves in this direction are already well established, with documents such as the General Medical Council's *Tomorrow's Doctors* showing that the very core of the medical establishment recognizes the need for change. Renewed appreciation of the power of the therapeutic relationship and the need to come alongside patients, rather than simply provide them with medical treatment, will radically alter the way healthcare is delivered. But all this will take time, probably at least a generation. In the meantime, perhaps the best we can hope for is to make health professionals aware of the maze that confronts cancer patients today, and show them how their attitudes and actions can help or hinder their patients in finding a way through.

What makes a 'good guide'?

Whoever undertakes this role, and wherever they fit in the healthcare system, certain attitudes seem to be key in achieving a good guiding relationship.

A good guide needs to be able to empathize well and see things from their patient's perspective. This may involve having prior knowledge of how that person has dealt with challenges or difficulties in the past (something which may be relatively easy for a GP), or developing open and easy communication so that the guide understands how things are for the patient and why. A guide needs enough time and space to make patients feel they are available, as moments of crisis do not always come when expected. A good guide needs to be skilled at putting his or her own preferences and beliefs aside and at really hearing what the patient is communicating. It is important that the guide doesn't have a product to 'sell' or a personal axe to grind.

Ultimately what seems essential is a holistic vision, which embraces people's living and dying, and an appreciation and a celebration of the uniqueness of each individual. A guide should recognize that the person in front of them is not an 'average patient', but is someone whose emotional and spiritual motivation may be as, if not more, important than their mental or physical functioning. A guide should know, and explicitly acknowledge, that the decisions that any human makes about themselves, particularly when knowledge is incomplete, cannot be, should not be and will not be completely logical. A guide who understands and values the fact that every patient is a 'remarkable patient' will undoubtedly, just by that very attitude, help and support people with cancer in finding their own 'right way' through the maze.

Index